CHOLERA

Edited by **Sivakumar Joghi Thatha Gowder**

Cholera
Edited by Sivakumar Joghi Thatha Gowder

Published by InTech
Janeza Trdine 9, 51000 Rijeka, Croatia

Publishing Process Manager Sandra Bakic

Technical Editor Teodora Smiljanic

Cover Designer InTech Design Team

Additional hard copies can be obtained from orders@intechopen.com

Cholera, Edited by Sivakumar Joghi Thatha Gowder
p. cm.
ISBN 978-953-51-0415-5

For EU product safety concerns:
IN TECH d.o.o., Prolaz Marije Krucifikse Kozulić 3, 51000 Rijeka, Croatia,
info@intechopen.com or visit our website at intechopen.com.

Meet the editor

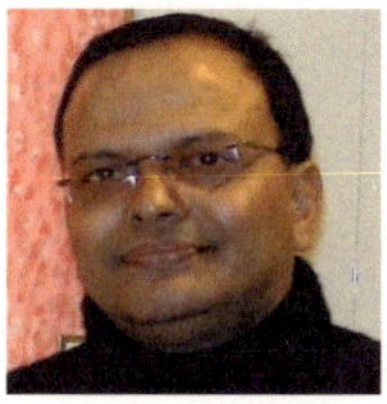

Dr Sivakumar Joghi Thatha Gowder got his academic training and carried out his research in institutions of high academic ranking in India and US. He earned his PhD from the University of Madras, India and continued his research at AIIMS, India. He then moved to US to continue his research at the UT Southwestern Medical Center, LSU Medical Center, and University of Pittsburgh School of Medicine. Currently, he is working as an Associate Professor of Pharmacology and Biochemistry at the Qassim University, KSA. Sivakumar received several prizes / awards during his academic career. He developed his own methods / techniques relevant to his research projects. Currently, he serves as an author / editor for books; an editorial member; and a reviewer for international journals and is a fellow of various international organizations. Sivakumar has also served as an invited speaker and a chairperson for international conferences.

Contents

Preface

On 21 October, 2010 Haitian public health authorities confirmed an outbreak of cholera. Ten months later the toll of this outbreak tallied 386,429 cases, including 5,885 deaths, with the outbreak spreading to the neighboring Dominican Republic and Florida, United States. Cholera is a world problem. One of the most basic lessons, which was so elegantly restated in an editorial in the New England Journal of Medicine, is that no one should lack access to clean water and sanitation. If we are to control and ultimately eradicate the deadly threat of cholera, the approach must include healthcare workers, scientists, and general public. The book Cholera focuses on various aspects of this disease with information significant for all people, from scientist and educators to general public.

This book is comprised of four parts: Epidemiology, Biology of Vibrio cholerae, Cholera Toxin, and Antagonists and Treatment. First two parts describe the history of cholera, its geographical distribution, mode of transmission, and structural and functional activities of V. cholerae. The third part deals with cholera toxin in a study of antagonist drugs used to treat cholera. The author's detailed discussion of the structural and functional aspects of cholera toxin paves the way for future drug discovery to both prevent and cure cholera. In addition to W.H.O. and other regulatory treatment regimens, the fourth part adds to an overall understanding of current methods and potential areas for enhancement of outcomes for the welfare of individuals and society. Some key points of interest in Cholera include: the emergence of an epidemiologically dominant new strain of V. cholerae, the importance of the bacterial flagellum, biotechnological utilities of cholera toxin and methods to design cholera drugs, and the spatial epidemiologic tools applied in cholera studies. This book is a significant resource not only for cholera researchers but also for scientists, physicians, healthcare professionals, faculty and students, local administrators, and general public and it is my privilege to present this book.

I extend my gratitude to my mother, my late father and my brothers for introducing me to higher education. My thanks to higher authorities, and colleagues of Qassim University for their motivation to carry out this project. I am indebted to my wife Anitha for her encouragement and technical support for this project. I also acknowledge the interest and commitment from the Publishing Process Manager at InTech, Ms. Irena Voric, whose patience and focus were an immense support in this project. Finally, I express deep and sincere gratitude to all the authors for their valuable contributions and scholarly cooperation for timely completion of this book.

Dr. Sivakumar Joghi Thatha Gowder
Department of Pharmacology & Biochemistry,
Al-Qassim University,
College of Pharmacy, Buraidah,
Saudi Arabia

Part 1

Epidemiology

1

Cholera and Spatial Epidemiology

Frank B Osei[1], Alfred A Duker[2] and Alfred Stein[3]
[1]*Faculty of Public Health and Allied Sciences, Catholic University College of Ghana, Sunyani*
[2]*Department of Geomatic Engineering, Kwame Nkrumah University of Science and Technology, Kumasi,*
[3]*Faculty of Geo-Information Science and Earth Observation (ITC), Twente University,*
[1, 2]*Ghana*
[3]*Netherlands*

1. Introduction

Cholera is an acute intestinal infection caused by the water borne bacteria *Vibrio cholerae* O1 or O139 (*V. cholerae*). Infection is mainly through ingestion of contaminated water or food (Kelly, 2001). Approximately 10^2-10^3 cells are required to cause severe diarrhea and dehydration (Sack et al., 1998; Hornich et al., 1971). Ingested cholera *vibrios* from contaminated water or food must pass through the acid stomach before they are able to colonize the upper part of the small intestine. After penetrating the mucus layer, *V. cholerae* colonizes the epithelial lining of the gut, secreting cholera toxin which affects the small intestine.

Clinically, the majority of cholera episodes are characterized by a sudden onset of massive diarrhea and vomiting. This is accompanied by the loss of profuse amounts of protein-free fluid along with electrolytes, bicarbonates and ions. The resulting dehydration produces tachycardia, hypotension, and vascular collapse, which can lead to sudden death. The diagnosis of cholera is commonly established by isolating the causative organism from the stools of infected individuals. The main mode of treatment is the replacement of electrolyte loss through the intake of a rehydration fluid, i.e. Oral Rehydration Salts (ORS) (Sack et al., 2004). Without prompt treatment, fatality rate can be as high as 50% (WHO, 1993; Sack et al., 2004). With adequate treatment, i.e. intravenous and oral rehydration therapy, supplemented with appropriate antibiotics, the fatality rate can drop to approximately 1.0% (Carpenter et al., 1966; Mahalanabis et al., 1992).

In its extreme manifestation, cholera is one of the most rapidly fatal infectious illnesses known. Within 3–4 hours of onset of symptoms, a previously healthy person may become severely dehydrated and if not treated may die within 24 hours (WHO, 2010). The disease is one of the most researched in the world today; nevertheless, it is still an important public health problem despite more than a century of study, especially in developing tropical countries. Cholera is currently listed as one of three internationally quarantinable diseases by the World Health Organization (WHO), along with plague and yellow fever (WHO, 2000a). The growing number and frequency of major cholera outbreaks, especially in countries on the African continent, have heightened concerns of focusing epidemiological research on the underlying risk factors and the identification of high risk areas.

Using simple geographical mapping, John Snow (1855) first associated cholera with contaminated drinking water in the 1850s even before any bacterium was known to exist. After Snow's seminal work, most epidemiological studies of cholera have focused on the pathogenesis and biological characteristics of *V. cholerae* (Yamai et al., 1977; Faruque et al., 1998; Ramamurthy et al., 1993; Felsenfeld, 1966; Singleton et al., 1982a, 1982b; Colwell et al., 1977; Barua and Paguio, 1977; Glass et al., 1985). However useful these studies are, they usually cannot establish accurate individual exposure levels for the critical risk factors of the disease (Haining, 1998). Spatial epidemiological tools applied in cholera studies can facilitate the identification of high risk areas and the formulation of hypotheses about the causal factors responsible for such variations, as well as the optimal allocation of health facilities to improve health care provision. The objective of this study is to present from published literature the general epidemiology of cholera, its spatial epidemiology as well as important spatial epidemiologic tools utilized in cholera studies.

2. Biology and ecology of *V. cholerae*

The biology and ecology of *V. cholerae* has been described by many authors (Yamai et al., 1977; Faruque et al., 1998; Ramamurthy et al., 1993; Felsenfeld, 1966; Singleton et al., 1982a, 1982b; Colwell et al., 1977; Barua and Paguio, 1977; Glass et al., 1985). *V. cholerae* is an aerobic, motile, Gram-negative rod that is shaped like a comma (Hamer and Cash, 1999). When ingested in the body, *V. cholerae* produces an exotoxin that either stimulates the mucosal cells to secrete large quantities of isotonic fluid, or increases the permeability of the vascular endothelium, thus allowing isotonic fluid to pass through in abnormal amount, resulting in watery diarrhea.

V. cholerae is differentiated serologically by the O antigen of its lipopolysaccharide. Over 200 serogroups of *V. cholerae* have been documented (Yamai et al., 1997). The toxigenic *V. cholerae* serogroups, which cause epidemic cholera, are the O1 and O139 (Faruque et al., 1998). Until 1992 when a newly serogroup designated O139 was identified after unusual outbreaks in India and Bangladesh (Ramamurthy et al., 1993), only the O1 serogroup was known to cause epidemic. The two major biotypes of the *V. cholerae* O1 serogroup are the classical and the El Tor (named after the El Tor quarantine camp on the Sinai peninsula where it was first isolated in 1905 from the intestines of pilgrims returning from Mecca) (Hamer and Cash, 1999). Admirably, *V. cholerae* O1 infection induces adaptive immune responses that are protective against subsequent infection. Volunteer studies in non-endemic regions have demonstrated that infection with classical biotype of *V. cholerae* O1 provides 100% protection for 3 years from subsequent challenge with a classical biotype strain, while infection with the El Tor biotype of *V. cholerae* O1 provides 90% protection for 3 years from subsequent challenge with an El Tor strain (Levine et al., 1981). In an endemic region, an initial episode of El Tor cholera reduces the risk of a second clinically apparent infection by 90% over the next several years (Glass et al., 1982).

The general assumption by most workers, until the mid 1960's, was that *V. cholerae* was an organism whose normal habitat was the human gut and/or intestine, and incapable of surviving for more than a few days outside the gut (Falsenfeld, 1966). *V. cholerae* is now known to be a water-borne bacterium that is natural inhabitant of brackish aquatic environments, which survives and multiplies in association with zooplankton and phytoplankton, quite independently of infected human beings (Colwell and Spira, 1993; Colwell and Huq, 1994; Islam et al; 1994; Nair et al., 1988; Huq et al., 1983; Islam et al., 1990). Colwell et al. (1977) first proposed that *V. cholerae* is ecologically autochthonous in estuarine and coastal waters. Colwell et al. (1977, 1980) isolated *V. cholerae* from plankton samples from Bangladesh waters and Chesapeake Bay (United States) and suggested that an association between *V. cholerae* and chitinous plankton may exist. Survival of *V. cholerae* in the aquatic environment, abundance and expression of virulence factors including cholera toxin (CT), and colonization factors such as the toxin-coregulated pilus (TCP), are strongly influenced by both biotic and abiotic factors. Abiotic factors such as sunlight, pH, temperature, salinity and nutrients enhance the growth and multiplication of aquatic lives such as phytoplankton and zooplanktons. Sequestration of CO_2 during photosynthesis of phytoplankton alter the dissolved O_2 and CO_2 contents of the surrounding which in turn leads to elevated pH in the estuarine.

3. Epidemiology

3.1 Global distribution

The Ganges Delta region (India) is believed to be the traditional home of cholera from the time of recorded history (Harmer and Cash, 1999). From this region, cholera has spread throughout the world, causing six major pandemics between 1817 and 1961 (Faruque et al., 1998). It is believed that the European invasions of India and India's fostering of trade with the Dutch Indies spread the disease to other parts of the world. The seventh pandemic, which began in 1961 in Sulawesi, Indonesia, has now involved almost the whole world and is still continuing. The pandemic (i.e. the seventh) reached India in 1964, Africa in 1970 (Barua, 1972; Cvjetanovic and Barua, 1972; Goodgame and Greenough, 1975; Küstner et al., 1981, Glass et al., 1991), southern Europe in 1970 (Editorial, 1971), and South America in 1991 (Swerdlow et al., 1992; Weil and Berche, 1992). The seventh pandemic was confined in Asia for nearly 10 years which later reached the west coast of Africa, the south coast of Europe, and the western Pacific islands in 1970. The seventh pandemic reached the Americas in 1991, starting from the Peruvian coast (Blake, 1994). The fifth and the sixth pandemics epidemiologically incriminated the classical biotype as the causative agent. The earlier pandemics are also believed to have been caused by the classical biotype as well, although there is no hard evidence. The seventh pandemic this time caused by the El Tor biotype has subsequently spread worldwide and largely replaced the classical biotype.

The burden of cholera is characterized by both endemic disease and epidemics. Globally, cholera cases and deaths have increased steadily since the beginning of the 21st century. From 2004 to 2008, a total of 838,315 cases were notified to WHO, compared with 676,651 cases between 2000 and 2004, representing a 24% increase in the number of cases (WHO, 2009). The burden of the disease is currently enormous on developing countries and catastrophically on the African continent. The seventh pandemic is the first to have established persistent residence on the African continent. Africa alone has recorded over 2.4 million cases and 120,000 deaths from 1970 to 2005. This accounts for over 90% of both worldwide cases and deaths (WHO, 2000b, 2001, 2002, 20003, 2004, 2005, 2006). The burden of the disease on the African continent, however, is possibly worse than officially reported owing to underreporting, limitations in the surveillance and reporting system, as well as fear of unjustified restrictions on travel and trade (WHO, 2000a).

3.2 Transmission hypothesis

Two routes of cholera transmission have been described, primary and secondary transmission. Primary transmission occurs through exposure to an environmental reservoir of *V. cholerae* (Hartley et al., 2006) or contaminated water sources regardless of previously infected persons, and thus responsible for the beginning of initial outbreaks. Primary transmission is enabled by both micro-and macro-level environmental and climatic factors that affect the seasonal patterns of infection (Islam et al., 1994; Alam et al., 2006; Lipp et al., 2002; Sack et al., 2003; Colwell, 1996; Huq and Colwell, 1996; Islam et al, 1989, 1990a, 1990b, 1999). In locations like Africa and South America where one yearly peak of cholera is often observed, the beginning of the epidemics has been associated with environmental conditions that favor the growth and survival of the bacterium (Codeço, 2001; Glass et al., 1991; Swerdlow et al., 1992). Primary transmission appears to play a limited role in the epidemiological process since it does not fully explain the exponential growth of incidences during epidemics.

Secondary transmission or fecal-oral transmission occurs via the fecal-oral route through exposure to contaminated water sources. Fecal-oral transmission provides a mechanism for exhibiting a strong feedback between present and past levels of infection. The importance of fecal-oral transmission in cholera epidemics is also supported by recent time series models fitted to the endemic dynamics of cholera in Bangladesh (Koelle and Pascual, 2004; Koelle et al., 2005). In an epidemic situation, the initial reproduction rate of fecal-oral transmissions is positively affected by the degree of contamination of water supply as well as the frequency of contacts with such contaminated water supply (Codeço, 2001), which in turn is influenced by human dimensions such as local environmental factors, socioeconomic, demographic as well as sanitation conditions. Fecal-oral transmissions reflect a complicated transmission pattern since multiple factors may play a role in the spread of the disease. Although cholera control measures that target primary transmission is clearly important (from the perspective of disease persistence (Colwell et al, 2003)), the dominant role of fecal-oral transmission as observed in several studies (Ali et al., 2002a, 2002b; Mugoya et al., 2008; Borroto and Martinez-Piedra, 2000; Ackers et al., 1998; Sasaki et al., 2008; Sur et al., 2005), suggest that the containment of fecal-oral infections may be a viable and useful strategy to control epidemics.

3.3 Socioeconomic and demographic variations

Socioeconomic and demographic factors have been reported to significantly enhance the vulnerability of a population to infection and contribute to epidemic spread (Ali et al., 2002a, 2002b; Borroto and Martinez-Piedra, 2000; Ackers et al., 1998; Sasaki et al., 2008; Sur et al., 2005). Such factors also mandate the extent to which the disease will reach epidemic proportions (Miller, 1985; Emch et al., 2008) and also modulate the size of the epidemic (Pascual et al., 2002, 2006; Koelle and Pascual, 2004; Hartley et al., 2005). Known population-level (local-level) risk factors of cholera include poverty, lack of development, high population density, low education, and lack of previous exposure (Ackers et al., 1998; Ali et al., 2002). The synergy of poverty, high population density, poor sanitation, poor housing, and lack of good water supplies enhance exposure to pathogenic cholera *vibros*. In epidemic prone regions like Africa, cholera outbreaks have been linked to multiple environmental and socio-economic sources (Acosta et al., 2001; Shapiro et al., 1999). Cholera diffuses rapidly in environments that lack basic infrastructure with regard to access to safe water and proper sanitation. The cholera vibrios can survive and multiply outside the human body and can spread rapidly in environments where living conditions are overcrowded and where there is no safe disposal of solid waste, liquid waste, and human feces (Ali et al., 2002a, 2002b). Root (1997) and Siddique et al (1992) have reported that increase in population density can strain sanitation systems, thus putting people at increased risk of contracting cholera. Ali et al (2002a, 2002b) have identified high population density and low educational status as important risk factors of cholera in an endemic area of Bangladesh.

3.4 Temporal variations

Many researchers have hypothesized the temporal variation of cholera as due to environmental and climatic factors that affect the seasonal patterns of infection (Alam et al., 2006; Lipp et al., 2002; Sack et al., 2003; Colwell and Huq, 2001; Pascual and Dobson, 2005; Huq and Colwell, 1996; Huq et al., 2005; Islam, 1990; Islam et al., 1990, 1993, 1999, 2004). The temporal variation of endemic and epidemic cholera has been associated with both regional and local environmental forces such as rainfall patterns, sea surface temperature and the El Nino Southern Oscillation (Epstein, 1993; Patz et al., 1996; Colwell, 1996; Bouma and Pascual, 2001; Colwell and Huq, 2001; Pascual et al., 2002; Koelle et al., 2005, Huq et al., 2001). Outbreaks in Peru and Bangladesh have been linked to periodic climatic cycles of the El Nino Southern Oscillation (Salazar-Lindo et al., 1997; Pascual et al., 2002; Rodo et al., 2002). In Bangladesh cholera epidemics occur twice a year in the spring and fall, before and after the monsoons (Merson et al., 1980; Islam et al., 1993; Emch and Ali, 2001; Longini et al., 2002). Several studies have also described a regular seasonal cycle of outbreaks in Bangladesh, including specific studies on the different strains: classical (Samadi et al., 1984), El Tor (Khan et al., 1984) and O139 (Alam et al., 2006). Temporal variation of cholera has also been related to variations in physical and nutritional aquatic parameters, including conditions in both coastal and estuarine environments (Faruque et al., 2005). Studies in Bangladesh have also shown environmental associations with *V. cholerae*, including water temperature and depth, rainfall, and copepod counts (Huq et al., 2005). These factors may contribute to the seasonality and secular trends seen in cholera outbreaks. In Dhaka Lobitz et al (2000) were the first to observe that both sea surface temperature and sea surface height are correlated with temporal fluctuations of cholera. In Ghana, de Magny et al (2007) observed a coherence between cholera outbreak resurgences and climatic/environmental parameters such as rainfall, Southern Oscillation Index and Land Surface Temperature.

4. Spatial epidemiology and cholera

The analysis of the spatial distribution of disease incidence and its relationship to potential risk factors (referred to in general in this paper as *spatial epidemiology*) has an important role to play in various kinds of public health and epidemiological studies. Recent advancements in technology and the increasingly powerful and versatile spatial statistical tools developed in this application area are capable of addressing more complex health issues than was hitherto the case. The field of spatial statistics involves the statistical analysis of observations with associated geographical location. Often these observations are not Gaussian distribution and are not independent (two main-stays in the development of statistical methods). Fortunately, a wide variety of statistical techniques for spatial epidemiologic inference have developed in recent years, coalescing into a collection of approaches which address specific questions. Consequently, the field of spatial epidemiology has been a subject of several lengthy texts (Elliott et al., 2000, Lawson, 2001, Waller and Gotway, 2004). Yet, few authors have addressed the spatial epidemiology of cholera (Ali et al, 2002a, 2002b; Ali et al., 2006; Borroto and Martinez-Piedra, 2000). Following Elliot et al (2000) and Lawson (2001), spatial epidemiology generically comprises at least three types of study focus: These are (1) *disease mapping*, (2) *disease clustering* and (3) *ecological analysis* (geographical correlation analysis). In this regard, we discuss methodological significance of *disease mapping, disease clustering* and *ecological analysis* with special emphasis on their applications in cholera studies.

4.1 Disease mapping and cholera

Disease maps have played a key descriptive role in spatial epidemiology. Disease maps are useful in suggesting hypotheses for further investigation or as part of general health surveillance and the monitoring of health problems. A famous historical example is the classical epidemiological work of John Snow. Mapping the locations of cholera victims, Snow was able to trace the cause of the disease to a contaminated water source. Surprisingly, this was done 20 years before Koch and Pasteur established the beginnings of microbiology (Koch, 1884). Disease mapping has long been in the form of plotting the observed disease cases or prevalence. Borroto and Martinez-Piedra (2000) used Geographic Information System (GIS) to map cumulative incidence rates of cholera in 32 Mexican states. Chevallier et al (2004) used cartographic representation of cholera incidence rates to study the spatial distribution of cholera in Ecuador. Raw disease rates yield less precise estimates for small populations and vice versa; hence, mapping the raw estimates of disease occurrence can lead to spurious spatial features. Thus, maps of raw disease incidences are not suitable for appropriate epidemiologic inferences. Bithel (2000), Diggle (2000), Lawson (2001), and Lawson and Clark (2002) provide recent reviews of current appropriate disease mapping methods. Several statistical smoothing techniques have been proposed to filter out the noise (rate variations) caused by population variability (e.g. *median-based head-banging* (Hansen, 1991), *spatial filtering* (Bithel, 1990; Rushton and Lolonis, 1996), *empirical Bayes smoothing* (Clayton and Kaldor, 1987), *full Bayesian smoothing* (Besag et al., 1991, 1995), and *geostatisticsal methods* (Oliver et al., 1998; Webster et al., 1994; Carrat and Valleron, 1992; Goovaerts, 2005; Goovaerts and Jacquez, 2004; Berke, 2004)). However, few have been applied in cholera studies. Kuo and Fukui (2007) have used the inverse distance weighted (IDW) interpolation technique to map the temporal features of cholera in the Fukushima prefecture Japan. Ali et al (2002) used kriging to interpolate and map the spatial risk of cholera in Bangladesh at regularly space interval. Ali et al (2006) presented the first application of Poisson kriging to the spatial interpolation of local cholera rates, resulting in continuous maps of cholera rate estimates and associated prediction variance.

4.2 Disease clustering and cholera

Fundamental to the spatial epidemiologist is the investigation of possible disease clusters. Cluster analysis provides opportunities for the epidemiologist to understand possible associations between demographic and environmental exposures and the spatial distribution of diseases (Besag and Newell, 1991; Kulldorff and Nagarwalla, 1995; Kulldorff et al., 1997). There are numerous methods for testing global clustering, including those methods proposed by Alt and Vach (1991), Besag and Newell (1991), Cuzick and Edwards (1990), Diggle and Chetwynd (1991), Grimson (1991), Moran (1950), Tango (1995, 1999, 2000), Walter (1992a, 1992b, 1993) and Whittemore et al (1987). Siddiqui et al (2006) applied Cuzick-Edward's k-Nearest Neighbors test (Cuzick and Edwards, 1990) to evaluate clustering of cholera cases in Pakistan. Using the Moran's Index, Borroto and Martinez-Piedra (2000) have described the spatial distribution of cholera in Mexican states as clustered. This clustering reflects a north-south gradient and spatial clustering of southern states with higher incidence and spatial clustering of northern states with low incidence. Likewise, the Moran's Index has been used to evaluate the clustering of cholera in the Lusaka area of Zambia (Sasaki et al., 2008) and in Madras (India) (Ruiz-Moreno et al., 2007). Osei et al (2008) have also used the Moran's Index to evaluate global clustering of cholera in the Ashanti Region of Ghana. However, global cluster analysis ran the risk of obscuring local effects since the assumption of stationarity is rarely met. Locating and/or defining the characteristics of disease clusters, i.e. local cluster analysis, can inform hypothesis of population or environmental drivers of ill-health, as well as direct the prevention or treatment efforts of health care workers. Using the popular spatial statistics approach, i.e. Ripley's K index, Ruiz-Moreno et al (2007) observed that clustering of cholera in Bangladesh occur at different spatial scales. Local clustering methods such as the Circular Scan Statistic (Kulldorff, 1997) and the Flexible Scan Statistic (Tango and Takahashi, 2005) have been used to detect and map the clustering of cholera in the city of Kumasi-Ghana (Osei et al., 2010; 2011). They emphasize that the Circular Scan Statistic can underestimate the relative risk of cholera clusters compared with the Flexible Scan Statistic. Emch and Ali (2003) have also used the spatial scan statistic to evaluate clustering of cholera.

4.3 Ecological analysis and cholera

A significant interest in spatial epidemiology also lies in identifying associated risk factors which enhance the risk of infection, the so called *ecological analysis* (Lawson et al., 1999a, 1999b; Lawson, 2001) or *geographic correlations studies* (Elliott et al., 2000). Understanding the spatial relationship between cholera and ecological risk factors has always been a challenge. Most authors ignore the geographical structure (spatial autocorrelation) of the data in the statistical analysis. For instance, Ali et al (2001, 2002a, 2002b) have utilized logistic regression, simple and multiple regression models to study the spatial epidemiology of cholera in an endemic area of Bangladesh. In their study, spatial filtering methods (Talbot et al., 2000), typically spatial moving average (Kafadar, 1996), and traditional geostatistics were only used to remove noise and transform cholera and environmental data into a spatially continuous form. This notwithstanding, the effect of spatial proximity or geographical structure of the data was not incorporated in the statistical model. Sasaki et al (2008) investigated risk factors of cholera with a GIS and matched case-case control in a peri-urban area of Luzaka, Zambia. Although a spatial autocorrelation analysis using Moran's Index was found to be statistically significant, this was never incorporated in the logistic and multiple regression models. Other authors have also used classical statistical methods to analyze the risk factors of cholera. Sasaki et al (2008) applied logistic and multiple regression models to examine risk factors of cholera in a peri-urban area of Luzaka, Zambia. Mugoya et al (2005) used logistic regression analysis to investigate the spread of cholera in Kenya. Ackers et al (1998) used Pearson correlation coefficient to determine the correlation between cholera incidence rates and socioeconomic and environmental risk factors in Latin America. Kuo and Fukui (2007) used a logarithmic regression to model the diffusion of cholera in Japan. De Magny et al (2008) used a Poisson regression to model environmental variables associated with cholera in Bangladesh.

Geographical data are correlated in space; therefore, data in close geographical proximity is more likely to be influenced by similar ecological factors and therefore affected in a similar way, i.e. spatial autocorrelation. Consequently, when these standard statistical methods are used to analyze geographically correlated data, the standard error of the covariate parameters is underestimated and thus the statistical significance is overestimated (Cressie, 1993). Yet, few studies have incorporated the effect of geographical proximity in cholera studies (Ali et al., 2002a, 2002b, 2006; Borroto and Martinez-Piedra, 2000). Spatial statistical methods, such as spatial regression models, incorporate spatial autocorrelation according to the way geographical neighbors are defined. Osei and Duker (2008) have used spatial regression models (both spatial lag and spatial error models) to explore the spatial dependency of cholera prevalence on an important local environmental factor (open-space refuse dumps) in Kumasi, Ghana. Inhabitants with high density of refuse dumps were observed to have higher cholera prevalence than those with lower density of refuse dumps (Osei and Duker, 2008). Moreover, inhabitants close to refuse dumps were observed to have higher cholera prevalence than those farther. Similarly, Osei et al (2010) have used spatial regression models to explore the spatial dependency of cholera on potential contaminated water bodies.

5. Conclusion

Cholera has been a public health burden for ages. Unlike the biological characteristics, relatively little effort has been made to understand the spatial epidemiology. Understanding the spatial patterns is useful for effective health planning and resource allocation. This review emphasized on the generic and spatial epidemiology of cholera. Important spatial epidemiologic tools applied in cholera studies have also been discussed in this review. However, not all the knowledge of cholera epidemiology has been captured in this review. Further studies are required to fully explain the spatial epidemiology of cholera.

6. References

Ackers, M-L.; Quick, R.E.; Drasbek, C.J; Hutwagner, L. & Tauxe, R.V. (1998). Are there national risk factors for epidemic cholera? The correlation between socioeconomic and demographic indices and cholera incidence in Latin America. *Int. J. Epidemiol.* 27(2):330-334

Acosta, J.C; Galindo, C.M; Kimario, J; Senkoro, K; Urassa, H.; Casals, C.; Corachán, M.; Eseko, N.; Tanner, M.; Mshinda, H.; Lwilla, F.; Vila, J. & Alonso, P.L (2001). Cholera outbreak in southern Tanzania: risk factors and patterns of transmission. *Emerg. Infect. Dis.* 7(3):583-587

Alam, M.; Hasan, N.A.; Sadique, A.; Bhuiyan, N.A.; Ahmed, K.U.; Nusrin, S.; Nair, G.B.; Siddique, A.K.; Sack, R.B.; Sack, D.A.; et al. (2006). Seasonal cholera caused by Vibrio cholerae serogroups O1 and O139 in the coastal aquatic environment of Bangladesh. *Appl Environ Microbiol* 72(6):4096-4104.

Ali, M.; Emch, M.; Donnay, J.P.; Yunus, M. & Sack, R.B. (2002b): The spatial epidemiology of cholera in an endemic area of Bangladesh. *Soc. Sci. & Med.* 55(6):1015-1024

Ali, M.; Emch, M.; Donnay, J.P; Yunus, M. & Sack R.B. (2002a). Identifying environmental risk factors of endemic cholera: a raster GIS approach. *Health & Place* 8 (3): 201-210

Ali, M.; Emch, M.; Yunus, M. & Sack, R.B. (2001). Are the environmental niches of vibrio cholerae 0139 different from those of vibrio cholerae 01 El Tor? *Int. J. Infect. Dis.* 5(4):214-219

Ali, M.; Goovaerts, P.; Nazia, N.; Haq, M. Z.; Yunus, M. & Emch, M. (2006). Application of Poisson kriging to the mapping of cholera and dysentery incidence in an endemic area of Bangladesh. *Int. J. Health Geogr.* 5:45

Alt, K.W. & Vach, W. (1991). The reconstruction of "genetic kinship" in prehistoric burial complexes: Problems and statistics. In: *Classification, Data Analysis; and Knowledge Organization: Models and Methods with Applications.* Bock, H.H. & Ihm, P. (Eds.). Springer, Berlin pp 299-310

Barua, D. & Paguio, A.S. (1977). ABO blood groups and cholera. *Ann. Hum. Biol.* 4:489-92

Barua, D. (1972). The global epidemiology of cholera in recent years. *Proc. R. Soc. Med.* 65:423-28

Berke, O. (2004): Exploratory disease mapping: kriging the spatial risk function from regional count data. *Int. J. Health. Geogr.*3:18

Besag, J. & Newell, J. (1991). The detection of clusters in rare disease. *J. R. Stat. Soc. A* 154(1): 143-155

Besag, J.; Green, P.; Higdon, D.; & Mengersen, K. (1995). Bayesian computation and stochastic systems. *Stat. Sci.* 10:3–66.

Besag, J.; York, J.; & Molli´e, A. (1991). Bayesian image restoration with two applications in spatial statistics. *Ann. Inst. Stat. Math.* 43:1–59.

Bithell, J.F. (1990). An application of density estimation to geographical epidemiology. *Stat. Med.* 9:691–701

Bithell, J.F. (2000). A classification of disease mapping methods. *Stat. Med.* 19(17–18): 2203-2215.

Blake, P.A. (1993). Epidemiology of cholera in the Americas. *Gastroenterol. Clin. North Am.* 22(3):639-660

Borroto, R.J & Martinez-Piedra, R. (2000). Geographical patterns of cholera in Mexico; 1991-1996. *Int. J. Epidemiol.* 29(4):764-772

Bouma, M.J. & Pascual, M. (2001). Seasonal and interannual cycles of endemic cholera in Bengal 1891-1940 in relation to climate and geography. *Hydrobioogia* 460:147-156

Carpenter, C.; Barua, D. & Sack, R. (1966). Clinical studies in asiatic cholera. IV. Antibiotic therapy in cholera. *Bull. Johns. Hopkins Hosp.* 118:230-242

Carrat, F. & Valleron, A.J. (1992). Epidemiologic mapping using the "kriging" method: application to an influenza-like illness epidemic in France. *Am. J. Epidemiol.* 135:1293–1300.

Chevallier, E.; Grand, A. & Azais, J-M. (2004). Spatial and temporal distribution of cholera in Ecuador between 1991 and 1996. *Eur. J. Public Health* 14(3):274-279

Clayton, D. & Kaldor, J. (1987). Empirical Bayes estimates of age standardized relative risks for use in disease mapping. *Biometrics*, 43:671–681

Codeço, C.T. (2001). Endemic and epidemic dynamics of cholera: the role of the aquatic reservoir. *BMC Infect. Dis.* 1:1

Colwell, R.R. & Huq, A. (2001). Marine ecosystems and cholera. *Hydrobiologia* 460:141-145

Colwell, R.R. (1996). Global climate and infectious disease: the cholera paradigm. *Science* 274(5295):2025-2031

Colwell, R.R.; Huq, A, (1994). Vibrios in the environment: viable but nonculturable vibrio cholerae. In: *Vibrio Cholerae and Cholera: Molecular to Global Perspectives.* Wachsmoth, I.; Blaker, P.; Olsvik O. (Eds.), pp 117-134, American Society of Microbiology, Washington DC

Colwell, R.R.; Huq, A.; Islam, M.S.; Aziz, K.M.A.; Yunus, M.; Kahn, N.H.; Mahmud, A.; Sack, R.B.; Nair, G.B.; Chakraborty, J.; Sack, D.A. & Russek-Cohen, E. (2003). Reduction of cholera in Bangladeshi villages by simple filtration. *Proc. Natl. Acad. Sci.* 100(3):1051-1055

Colwell, R.R.; Kaper, J. & Joseph, S.W. (1977). Vibrio cholerae; Vibrio parahaemolyticus; and other vibrios: occurrence and distribution in Chesapeake Bay. *Science* 198(4315):394-396

Cressie, N. (1993). Statistics for Spatial Data. John Wiley & Sons, New York

Cuzick, J.C. & Edwards, R. (1990). Spatial clustering for inhomogeneous populations. *J. R. Stat. Soc. B* 52:73-104

Cvjetanovic, B. & Barua, D. (1972). The seventh pandemic of cholera. *Nature* 239:137-38

De Magny, G.C.; Cazelles, B. & Guegan, J.F. (2007). Cholera threats to humans in Ghana as influenced by both global and regional climatic variability. *EcoHealth* 3(4):223-231

Diggle, P. & Chetwynd, A. (1991). Second order analysis of spatial clustering for inhomogeneous populations. *Biometrics* 47:1155-1163

Diggle, P. (2000). Overview of statistical methods for disease mapping and its relationship to cluster detection. In: *Spatial Epidemiology: Methods and Applications.* Elliot, P.; Wakefield, J.C.; Best, N.G.; Briggs, D.J. Oxford University Press, Oxford

Editorial, (1971): Cholera in Spain. *Br. Med. J.* 3: 266

Elliot, P.; Wakefield, J.C.; Best, N.G. & Briggs, D.J. (2000). *Spatial Epidemiology: Methods and Applications*. Oxford University Press, Oxford

Emch, M. & Ali, M. (2001). Spatial and temporal patterns of diarrheal disease in Matlab, Bangladesh. *Environ Plan A* 33: 339–350.

Emch, M. & Ali, M. (2003). Spatial cluster analysis for etiological research and identification of socio-environmental risk factors. In: *Geographic Information Systems and Health Applications*. Khan, O.A.; Skinner, R. (Eds.). Idea Group Publications, Hershey, PA, pp. 172–187.

Emch, M.; Feldacker, C.; Yunus, M.; Streatfield, P.K.; DinhThiem, V.; Canh, D.G. & Ali, M. (2008). Local Environmental Predictors of Cholera in Bangladesh and Vietnam. *Am. J. Trop. Med. Hyg.* 78(5):823-832

Epstein, P.R. (1993). Algal blooms in the spread and persistence of cholera. *Biosystems* 31:209–221

Falsenfeld, O. (1966). A review of recent trends in cholera research and control. *Bull. World Health Organ.* 34(2): 161-195

Faruque, S.M.; Albert, M.J. & Mekalanos, J.J. (1998). Epidemiology; genetics and ecology of toxigenic Vibrio cholerae. *Microbiol. Mol. Biol. Rev.* 62(4):1301-1314

Faruque, S.M.; Naser, I.B.; Islam, M.J.; Faruque, A.S.G.; Ghosh, A.N.; Nair, G.B.; Sack, D.A. & Mekalanos, J.J. (2005). Seasonal epidemics of cholera inversely correlate with the prevalence of environmental cholera phages. *Proc. Natl. Acad. Sci.* USA 102: 1702-1707

Fotedar, R.; Banerjee, U.; Singh, S.; Shriniwas & Verma, A.K. (1992b). The housefly (*Musca domestica*) as a carrier of pathogenic microorganisms in a hospital environment. *J. Hosp. Infect.* 20(3):209-215

Glass, R.; Claeson, M.; Blake, P.; Waldman, R. & Pierce, N. (1991). Cholera in Africa: Lessons on transmission and control for Latin America. *Lancet* 338(8770):791-795

Glass, R.I.; Holmgren, J.; Haley, C.E.; Khan, M.R.; Svennerholm, A.; Stoll, B.J.; Hossain, K.M.B.; Black, R.E.; Yunus, M. & Barua, D. (1985). Predisposition for cholera of individuals with O blood group: possible evolutionary significance. *Am. J. Epidemiol.* 121(6):791-796

Goodgame, R.W. & Greenough, B. (1975). Cholera in Africa: a message for the West. *Ann. Intern. Med.* 82(1):101-06

Goovaerts, P. & Jacquez, G.M. (2004). Accounting for regional background and population size in the detection of spatial clusters and outliers using geostatistical filtering and spatial neutral models: the case of lung cancer in Long Island; New York. *Int. J. Health. Geogr.* 3:14.

Goovaerts, P. (2005). Geostatistical analysis of disease data: estimation of cancer mortality risk from empirical frequencies using Poisson kriging. *Int. J. Health. Geogr.* 4:31

Greenberg, B. (1973). *Flies & Disease. II. Biology and Disease Transmission.* Princeton University Press; Princeton; pp 15

Grimson, R.C.; Wang, K.C. & Johnson, P.W.C. (1981). Searching for hierarchical clusters of disease: spatial patterns of sudden infant death syndrome. *Soc. Sci. Med. D* 15(2):287-293

Haining, R. (1998). Spatial statistics and the analysis of health data. In. *GIS and health,* A.C. Gatrell, & M. Loytonen (Eds.); GISDATA Series 6, Taylor & Francis, London

Hansen, K.M. (1991). Head-banging: Robust smoothing in the plane. IEEE Transactions on Geoscience and Remote Sensing, 29:369–378

Harmer, D.H. & Cash, R.A. (1999). Secretory Diarrheas: Cholera and Enterotoxigenic Escherichia Coli. In: *Infectious Diseases,* Donald, A. & Cohen, J. (Eds.), Harcourt Publishers Ltd, Mosby

Hartley, D.M.; Morris, M. & Smith, D.L. (2005). Hyperinfectivity: A Critical Element in the Ability of V. Cholerae to Cause Epidemics? *PLoS Med.* 3(1): e7

Hornick, R.B.; Music, S.I.; Wensel, R.; Cash, R.; Libonati, J.P.; Snyder, M.J. & Woodward, T.E. (1971). The Broad Street pump revisited; response of volunteers to ingested cholera *vibrios. Bull. NY Acad. Med.* 47(10):1181-1191

Huq, A. & Colwell, R.R. (1996). Environmental factors associated with emergence of disease with special reference to cholera. *Eastern Mediterraneal Health Journal* 2:37-45.

Huq, A.; Sack, R.B. & Colwell, R.R. (2001). *Cholera and global ecosystems. Ecosystem change and public health: A global perspective.* The Johns Hopkins University PressAron JL; Patz JA. 327-352.

Huq, A.; Sack, R.B.; Nizam, A.; Longini, I.M.; Nair, G.B.; Ali, A.; Morris, J.G.; Khan, M.N.H.; Siddique, A.K.; Yunus, M.; Albert, M.J.; Sack, D.A. & Colwell, R.R. (2005). Critical factors influencing the occurrence of vibrio cholerae in an environment of Bangladesh. *Appl. Environ. Microbiol.* 71(8):4645-4654

Huq, A.; Small, E.B.; West, P.A.; Huq, M.I.; Rahman, R. & Colwell, R.R. (1983). Ecologic relationships between *Vibrio cholerae* and Planktonic crustacean copepods. *Appl. Environ. Microbiol.* 45(1):275-283

Islam, M.S. (1990). Effect of various biophysicochemical conditions on toxigenicity of Vibrio cholerae 01 during survival with a green alga; Rhizoclonium fontanum; in an artificial aquatic environment. *Can. J. Microbiol.* 36(7):464-468.

Islam, M.S.; Drasar, B.S. & Bradley, D.J. (1990). Survival of toxigenic Vibrio cholerae O1 with a common duckweed; Lemna minor; in artificial aquatic ecosystems. *Trans. R. Soc. Trop. Med. Hyg.* 84(3):422-424.

Islam, M.S.; Drasar, B.S. & Sack, R.B. (1993). The aquatic environment as a reservoir of Vibrio cholerae: a review. *J. Diarrhoeal. Dis. Res.* 11(4):197-206.

Islam, M.S.; Drasar, B.S. & Sack, R.B. (1994). Probable Role of Blue-Green-Algae in Maintaining Endemicity and Seasonality of Cholera in Bangladesh-a Hypothesis. *J. Diarrhoeal Dis. Res.* 12(4):245-256

Islam, M.S.; Draser, B.S. & Bradley, D.J. (1989). Attachment of toxigenic *Vibrio cholerae* O1 to various freshwater plants and survival with filamentous green algae *Rhizoclonium fontanum*. *J. Trop. Med. Hyg.* 92(6):396-401

Islam, M.S.; Rahim, Z.; Alam, M.J.; Begum, S.; Moniruzzaman, S.M.; Umeda, A.; Amako, K.; Albert, M.J.; Sack, R.B.; Huq, A.; et al. (1999). Association of Vibrio cholerae O1 with the cyanobacterium; Anabaena sp.; elucidated by polymerase chain reaction and transmission electron microscopy. *Trans. R. Soc. Trop. Med. Hyg.* 93(1):36-40.

Islam, M.S.; Talukder, K.A.; Khan, N.H.; Mahmud, Z.H.; Rahman, M.Z.; Nair, G.B.; Siddique, A.K.; Yunus, M.; Sack, D.A.; Sack, R.B.; et al. (2004). Variation of toxigenic Vibrio cholerae O1 in the aquatic environment of Bangladesh and its correlation with the clinical strains. *Microbiol. Immunol.* 48(10):773-777.

Kafadar, K. (1996). Smoothing geographical data; particularly rates of disease. *Stat. Med.* 15(23):2539-2560

Kelly, L. (2001). The global dimension of cholera. *Glob. Chang. Hum. Health* 2(1):6-17

Khan, M.U.; Samadi, A.R.; Huq, M.I.; Yunus, M.; Eusof, A. (1984): Simultaneous classical and El Tor cholera in Bangladesh. *J. Diarrhoeal. Dis. Res.* 2(1):13-18.

Kobayashi, M.; Sasaki, T.; Saito, N.; Tamura, K.; Suzuki, K.; Watanabe, H. & Agui, N. (1999). Houseflies: not simple mechanical vectors of enterohemorrhagic Escherichia coli 0157:H7. *Am. J. Trop. Med. Hyg.* 61(4):625-629

Koch, R. (1884). An address on cholera and its bacillus. *Br. Med. J.* 2(1235):453-59

Koelle, K. & Pascual, M. (2004). Disentangling extrinsic from intrinsic factors in disease dynamics: A nonlinear time series approach with an application to cholera. *The Am. Nat.* 163(6):901-913

Koelle, K.; Rodo, X.; Pascual, M.; Yunus, M. & Mostafa, G. (2005). Refractory periods to climate forcing in cholera dynamics. *Nature* 436:696-700

Kulldorff, M. & Nagarwalla, N. (1995). Spatial disease clusters: detection and inference. *Stat. Med.* 14(8):799-810

Kulldorff, M.; Feuer, E.J.; Miller, B.A. & Freedman, L.S. (1997). Breast Cancer clustering in the northeast United State; a geographic approach. *Am. J. Epidemiol.* 146(2):161-170

Kulldroff, M. (1997). A spatial scan statistics. *Communications in Statistics*: Theory and Methods 1997; 26:1481-1496.

Kuo, C-L. & Fukui, H. (2007). Geographical structures and the cholera epidemic in modern Japan: Fukushima prefecture in 1882 and 1895. *Int. J. Health Geogr.* 6:25

Küstner, H.G.V.; Gibson, I.H.N; Carmichael, T.R.; Van Zyl, L.; Chouler, C.A.; Hyde, J.P. & du Plessis, J.N. (1981). The spread of cholera in South Africa. *S. Afr. Med. J.* 60(3):87-90

Lawson, A.B. & Clark, A. (2002). Spatial mixture relative risk models applied to disease mapping. *Stat. Med.* 21(3):359-70.

Lawson, A.B. (2001). Disease map reconstruction. *Stat. Med.* 20(14):2183-204.

Lawson, A.B. (2001). Tutorial in biostatistics: disease map reconstruction. *Stat. Med.* 20:2183-2203.

Lawson, A.B.; Biggeri, A. & Dreassi, E. (1999a). Edge effects in disease mapping. In: *Disease Mapping and Risk Assessment for Public Health*, Lawson, A.; Biggeri, A.; Bohning, L.E.; Viel, J-F.; Bertollini, R. (Eds). pp 85-98. John Wiley & Sons, Chichester

Lawson, A.B.; Biggeri, A.; Bohning, L.E.; Viel, J-F. & Bertollini, R. (1999b). Introduction to spatial models in ecological analysis Disease. In: *Disease Mapping and Risk Assessment for Public Health*, Lawson, A.B.; Biggeri, A.; Bohning, L.E.; Viel J-F.; Bertollini, R. (Eds). pp 181-191. John Wiley & Sons, Chichester

Levine, M.M.; Black, R.E.; Clements, M.L.; Cisneros, L.; Nalin, D.R. & Young, C.R. (1981). Duration of infection-derived immunity to cholera. *J. Infect. Dis.* 143(6): 818-820

Lipp, E.K.; Huq, A. & Colwell, R.R. (2002). Effects of global climate on infectious disease: the cholera model. *Clin. Micro. Rev.* 15(4):757

Lobitz, B.; Beck, L.; Huq, A.; Wood, B.; Fuchs, G.; Faruque, A.S.G. & Colwell, R.R. (2000). Climate and infectious disease: Use of remote sensing for detection of Vibrio cholerae by indirect measurement. *Proc. Natl. Aced. Sci. USA* 97(4):1438-1443

Longini, I.M. Jr.; Yunus, M.; Zaman, K.; Siddique, A.K.; Sack, R.B. & Nizam, A. (2002). Epidemic and endemic cholera trends over a 33-year period in Bangladesh. *J. Infect. Dis.* 186: 246–251.

Mahalanabis, D.; Molla, A. & Sack, D. (1992). Clinical Management of Cholera. In *Cholera*, D. Barua, & W. Greenough III (Eds.). Plenum Medical Book Company, New York, pp 253-283

Margaret, C.; Emch, M.; Streatfield, P. & Yunus, M. (2009): Spatio-temporal clustering of cholera: The impact of flood control in Matlab, Bangladesh, 1983–2003. *Health & Place* 15:771–782

Merson, M.H.; Black, R.E.; Khan, M.U. & Huq, I. (1980). Enterotoxigenic Escherichia coli diarrhea: acquired immunity and transmission in an endemic area. Cholera and Related Diarrheas: Molecular Basis of a Global Health Problem. 43rd Nobel Symposium. Basel; Switzerland: S. Karger; 34–45.

Miller, C.J.; Feachem, R.G. & Drasar, B.S. (1985). Cholera epidemiology in developed and developing countries: new thoughts on transmission; seasonality; and control. *Lancet* 1(8423):261-263

Moran, P.A.P. (1950). Notes on continuous stochastic phenomena. *Biometrika* 37(1-2):17-23

Mugoya, I.; Kariuki, S.; Galgalo, T.; Njuguna, C.; Omollo, J.; Njoroge, J.; Kalani, R.; Nzioka, C.; Tetteh, C.; Bedno, S.; Breiman, R.F. & Feikin, D.R. (2008). Rapid Spread of *Vibrio cholerae* O1 Throughout Kenya, 2005. *Am. J. Trop. Med. Hyg.* 78(3):527-533

Nair, G.B.; Oku, Y.; Takeda, Y.; Ghosh, A.; Ghosh, R.K.; Chattopadhyay, S.; Pal, S.C.; Kaper, J.B. & Takeda, T. (1988). Toxin profiles of Vibrio cholerae non-O1 from environmental sources in Calcutta; India. *Appl. Environ. Microbiol.* 54(12):3180-3182

Oliver, M.A.; Webster, R.; Lajuanie, C.; Muir, K.R.; Parkes, S.E.; Cameron, A.H.; Stevens, M.C.G. & Mann, J.R. (1998). Binomial cokriging for estimating and mapping the risk of childhood cancer. *Math. Med. Biol.* 15 (3):279-297

Osei, F.B. & Duker, A.A. (2008b). Spatial dependency of V. cholerae prevalence on open space refuse dumps in Kumasi; Ghana: a spatial statistical modeling. *Int. J. Health Geogr.* 7:62

Osei, F.B.; Duker, A.A.; Augustijn, E-W. & Stein, A. (2010). Spatial dependency of cholera prevalence on potential cholera reservoirs in an urban area; Kumasi; Ghana. *Int. J. Appl. Earth Obs. Geoinf.* 12(5):331-339

Pascual, M. & Dobson, A. (2005). Seasonal patterns of infectious diseases. *Plos Med.* 2(1):18-20.

Pascual, M.; Bouma, M.J. & Dobson, A.P. (2002). Cholera and climate: revisiting the quantitative evidence. *Microbes. Infect.* 4(2):237-45

Pascual, M.; Bouma, M.J. & Dobson, A.P. (2002). Cholera and climate: revisiting the quantitative evidence. *Microbes. Infect.* 4(2):237-45

Pascual, M.; Koelle, K. & Dobson, A.P. (2006). Hyperinfectivity in Cholera: A New Mechanism for an Old Epidemiological Model? *PLoS Med.* 3(6): e280

Ramamurthy, T.; Garg, S.; Sharma, R.; Bhattacharya, S.K.; Nair, G.B.; Shimada, T.; Takeda, T.; Karasawa, T.; Kurazano, H.; Pal, A. & Takeda, Y. (1993). Emergence of novel strain of *Vibrio cholerae* with epidemic potential in southern and eastern India. *Lancet* 341(8846):703-04

Rodo, X.; Pascual, M.; Fuchs, G. & Faruque, A.S. (2002). ENSO and cholera: a nonstationary link related to climate change? *Proceedings Proc. Natl. Aced. Sci. USA* 99:12901–12906

Root, G. (1997). Population density and spatial differentials in child mortality in Zimbabwe. *Soc. Sci. Med.* 44 (3):413-421

Rosenberg, M.S.; Sokal, R.R.; Oden, N.L. & DiGiovann, D. (1999). Spatial autocorrelation of cancer in Western Europe. *Eur. J. Epidemiol.* 15(1):15-22

Ruiz-Moreno, D.; Pascual, M.; Bouma, M.; Dobson, A. & Cash, B. (2007). Cholera Seasonality in Madras (1901-1940): Dual Role for Rainfall in Endemic and Epidemic Regions. *EcoHealth* 4(1):52-62

Rushton, G. & Lolonis, P. (1996). Exploratory spatial analysis of birth defect rates in an urban population. *Stat. Med.* 15:717–726

Sack, D.A.; Sack, R.B.; Nair, G.B. & Siddique, A.K. (2004). Cholera. *Lancet* 363(9404):223-233

Sack, D.A.; Tacket, C.O.; Cohen, M.B.; Sack, R.B.; Losonsky, G.A.; Shimko, J.; Nataro, J.P.; Edelman, R.; Levine, M.M.; Giannella, R.A.; Schiff, G. & Lang, D. (1998): Validation of a volunteer model of cholera with frozen bacteria as the challenge. *Infect. Immun.* 66(5):1968-1972

Sack, R.B.; Siddique, A.K.; Longini, I.M.; Nizam, A.; Yunus, M.; Islam, M.S.; Morris, J.G.; Ali, A.; Huq, A.; Nair, G.B.; et al. (2003). A 4-year study of the epidemiology of Vibrio cholerae in four rural areas of Bangladesh. *J. Inf. Dis.* 187(1):96-101.

Salazar-Lindo, E.; Pinell-Salles, P.; Maruy, A. & Chea-Woo, E. (1997). El Nino and diarrhoea and dehydration in Lima; Peru. *Lancet* 350:1597–1598

Samadi, A.R.; Chowdhury, M.K.; Huq, M.I. & Khan, M.U. (1983). Seasonality of classical and El Tor cholera in Dhaka; Bangladesh: 17-year trends. *Trans. R. Soc. Trop. Med. Hyg.* 77(6):853-856

Sasaki, S.; Suzuki, H.; Igarashi, K.; Tambatamba, B. & Mulenga, P. (2008). Spatial Analysis of Risk Factor of Cholera Outbreak for 2003-2004 in a Peri-urban Area of Lusaka, Zambia. *Am. J. Trop. Med. Hyg.* 79(3):414-421

Shapiro, R.L.; Muga, R.O.; Adcock, P.M.; Phillips-Howard, P.A.; Hawley, W.A.; Waiyaki, P.; Nahlen, B.L. & Slutsker, L. (1999). Transmission of epidemic Vibrio cholerae O1 in rural western Kenya associated with drinking water from Lake Victoria: an environmental reservoir for cholera? *Am. J. Trop. Med. Hyg.* 60(2):271-276

Siddique, A.K.; Zaman, K.; Baqui, A.H.; Akram, K.A.; Mutsuddy, P.; Eusof, A.; Haider, K.; Islam, S. & Sack, R.B. (1992). Cholera epidemics in Bangladesh: 1985-1991. *J. Diarrhoeal Dis. Res.* 10(2):79-86

Singleton FL; Attwell RW; Jangi MS; and Colwell RR (1982a): Influence of salinity and organic nutrient concentration on survival and growth of Vibrio cholerae in aquatic microcosms. Appl. Environ. Microbiol. 43(5):1080-1085

Singleton, F.L.; Attwell, R.W.; Jangi, M.S.; & Colwell, R.R. (1982b). Effects of temperature and salinity on Vibrio cholerae growth. *Appl. Environ. Microbiol.* 44(5):1047-1058

Snow, J. (1855). *On the Mode of Communication of Cholera.* 2nd ed. John Churchill; London

Sur, D.; Deen, J.; Manna, B.; Niyogi, S.; Deb, A.; Kanungo, S.; Sarkar, B.; Kim, D.; Danovaro-Holliday, M.; Holliday, K.; Gupta, V.; Ali, M.; von Seidlein, L.; Clemens, J. & Bhattacharya, S. (2005). The burden of cholera in the slums of Kolkata, India: data from a prospective; community based study. *Arch. Dis. Child* 90(11): 1175-1181

Swerdlow, D.L.; Greene, K.D.; Tauxe, R.V.; Wells, J.G.; Bean, N.H.; Ries, A.A.; Blake, P.A.; Mintz, E.D.; Pollack, M.; Rodriguez, M.; Tejada, E.; Seminario, L.; Ocampo, C.; Vertiz, B.; Espejo, L. & Saldana, W. (1992). Waterborne transmission of epidemic cholera in Trujillo; Peru: lessons for a continent at risk. *Lancet* 340 (8810):28-32

Talbot, T.O.; Kulldroff, M.; Teven, P.F. & Haley, V.B. (2000). Evaluation of spatial filters to create smoothed maps of health data. *Sat. Med.* 18(17-18):2399-2408

Tango, T. (1995). A class of tests for detecting "general" and "focused" clustering of rare diseases. *Stat. Med.* 14(21-22):2323-2334

Tango, T. (1999). Comparison of general tests for disease clustering. In: *Disease Mapping and Risk Assessment for Public Health*, Lawson, A.B. *et al* (Eds). John Wiley & Sons, New York, pp 111-117

Tango, T. (2000). A test for spatial disease clustering adjusted for multiple testing. *Stat. Med.* 19(2):191-204

Waller, L.A. & Gotway, C.A. (2004). Applied Spatial Statistics for Public Health Data. John Wiley & Sons, New Jersey

Walter, S.D. (1992a). The analysis of regional patterns in health data: I. Distributional considerations. *Am. J. Epidemiol.* 136(6):730-741

Walter, S.D. (1992b): The analysis of regional patterns in health data: II. The power to detect environmental effects. *Am. J. Epidemiol.* 136(6):742-759

Walter, S.D. (1993): Assessing spatial patterns in disease rates. *Stat. Med.* 12(19-20):1885-1894

Watt, J. & Lindsay, D.R. (1948). Diarrheal disease control studies: effect of fly control on high morbidity area. *Public Health Rep.* 63(41):1319-1334

Webster, R; Oliver, M.A.; Munir, K.R. & Man, J.R. (1994). Kriging the local risk of rare disease from a register of diagnoses. *Geogr. Anal.* 26(2):168-185

Weil, O. & Berche, P. (1992). The cholera epidemic in Ecuador: towards an endemic in Latin America. *Rev. Epidemiol. Sante. Publique.* 40(3):145-55

Whittemore, A.S.; Friend, N.; Brown, B.W. & Holly, E.A. (1987). A test to detect clusters of disease. *Biometrika* 74(3):631-635

WHO (2000a). Report on global surveillance of epidemic prone infectious diseases. World Health Organization, Geneva.

WHO (2010). Cholera vaccines: WHO position paper. Weekly epidemiological record 85(13):117-128. http://www.who.int/wer. Last accessed 5 September 2011

WHO, (1993). Guidelines for Cholera Control. World Health Organization; Geneva. http://helid.desastres.net/en/d/Jwho90e/. Last accessed 5 September 2011

WHO (2000b). Cholera 1999. *Weekly epidemiological record* 75(31):249-256.

WHO (2001). Cholera 2000. *Weekly epidemiological record* 76(31):233-240.

WHO (2002). Cholera 2001. *Weekly epidemiological record* 77(31):257-268.

WHO (2003). Cholera 2002. *Weekly epidemiological record* 78(31):269-276.

WHO (2004). Cholera 2003. *Weekly epidemiological record* 79(31):281-288.

WHO (2005). Cholera 2004. *Weekly epidemiological record* 80(31):261-268.

WHO (2006). Cholera 2005. *Weekly epidemiological record* 81(31):297-308.

Yamai, S.; Okitsu, T.; Shimada, T. & Katsube, Y. (1997). Distribution of serogroups of *Vibrio cholerae* non-O1 non-O139 with specific reference to their ability to produce cholera toxin; and addition of novel serogroups. *Kansenshogaku Zasshi* 71(10):1037-1045

2

Evaluating Spatial and Space-Time Clustering of Cholera in Ashanti-Region-Ghana

Frank B Osei[1], Alfred A Duker[2] and Alfred Stein[3]
[1]*Faculty of Public Health and Allied Sciences, Catholic University College of Ghana, Sunyani*
[2]*Department of Geomatic Engineering, Kwame Nkrumah University of Science and Technology, Kumasi*
[3]*Faculty of Geo-Information Science and Earth Observation (ITC), Twente University*
[1,2]*Ghana*
[3]*Netherlands*

1. Introduction

Basic problems in geographical surveillance for a spatially distributed disease data are the identification of areas of exceptionally high prevalence or clusters, test of their statistical significance, and identification of the reasons behind the elevated prevalence of the disease. Knowledge of the location of high risk areas of diseases and factors leading to such elevated risk is essential to better understand human interaction with its environment, especially when the disease transmission is enhanced by environmental or demographic factors. Cluster analysis provides opportunities for environmental epidemiologist to study associations between demographic and environmental exposures and the spatial distribution of diseases (Myaux et al., 1997; Kulldorff and Nagarwalla, 1995; Besag and Newell, 1991; Kulldorff, 2001; Kulldorff et al., 1998).

Cholera is caused by specific strains of the water borne bacterial *Vibrio cholerae* O1 or O139 (*V. cholerae* here after), following ingestion of infective dose through contaminated water or food (Kelly, 2001). The disease has remained as an important cause of mortality and morbidity in the world, especially in developing tropical countries. African countries report approximately 90% of the world wide cholera cases and deaths (WHO, 2001-2006). In most African countries, the synergy of poverty, high population density, poor sanitation, poor housing, and lack of good water supplies enhance exposure to *V. cholerae*. Despite the prevalence and/or fatality and demographic overlap, little has been studied about the spatial and temporal patterns of cholera in Africa. In Ghana, the disease has been a public health problem since its introduction in the 1970s (Pobee and Grant, 1970). Cholera infection is primarily driven by environmental factors (Ali et al., 2002a, 2002b; Huq et al., 2005), and since environmental processes are spatially continuous in nature (Webster et al., 1994), high incidence rates of the disease are expected to cluster together. A previous study carried out in Ashanti Region used Moran's Index for spatial autocorrelation to explore the existence of clusters of cholera. Also in the above study, empirical Bayesians smoothed rates of cholera (i.e. visual inspection) revealed possible spatial and temporal clustering of cholera for the 5 year period, i.e. from 1997 to 2001 (Osei and Duker, 2008). However, the exact locations of these cluster, as well as the correlations with some demographic and socioeconomic factors were not systematically investigated. The purpose of this study, however, is to investigate spatial and space-time clusters of cholera in Kumasi. Correlation analysis of cholera rates with demographic factors, i.e. sanitation, drinking water and internal migration are also explored to assess the extent to which these factors might explain high rate clusters of cholera.

This study utilizes the *spatial scan statistic* (Kulldorff, 1997) to detect spatial and space-time clusters of cholera. The spatial scan statistic offers several advantages over other clustering methods: (1) it corrects for multiple comparisons, (2) adjusts for the heterogeneous population densities among the different areas in the study, (3) detects and identifies the location of the clusters without prior specification of their suspected location or size thereby overcoming pre-selection bias, (4) and the method allows for adjustment for covariates. Also Kulldorff's spatial scan statistic is both deterministic (i.e., it identifies the locations of clustering) and inferential (i.e., it allows for hypothesis testing and evaluation of significance). The spatial scan statistic has been used to detect and evaluate various disease clusters including cancer (Michelozzi et al., 2002; Viel et al., 2000; Sheehan and DeChelo, 2005; Hjalmars et al., 1996; Turnbull, 1990, Kulldorff et al., 1998), giardiasis (Odoi et al., 2004) tuberculosis (Tiwari et al., 2006), diabetes (Green et al., 2003), Creutzfeldt-Jacob disease (Cousens, 2001), granulocytic elrlichiosis (Chput et al., 2002), and sclerosis (Sabel et al., 2003). The spatial scan statistic, as implemented in SaTScan software (Kulldorff, 2005; Kulldorff, 2006) has the capabilities of detecting purely spatial clusters, temporal clusters, and space-time clusters.

2. Methods

2.1 Study area

This study was conducted in Ashanti Region, one of the ten regions in Ghana. The region lies between longitudes 0° 9'W and 2° 15'W, and latitudes 5° 30'N and 7° 27'N. The Ashanti Region is dominated by Ashantis, who constitute 14.8% of all Ghanaians by birth. The Ashantis have a great history of culture of which the influence of the Ashanti Kingdom stretches beyond the borders of Ghana. The region occupies a total land area of 24,389 square kilometers representing 10.2% of the total land area of Ghana. The region has a population density of 148.1 persons per square kilometer, which is about two times higher than the overall population density in Ghana. There are 18 administrative districts in the Ashanti region including Kumasi Metropolis of which the capital is Kumasi, and is the only district which has gained a metropolitan status. The Kumasi Metropolis is the most populous district in the region. The 2000 census recorded the region's population as 3,612,950, representing 19.1 per cent of the country's population. The urban population (51.3%) in the region exceeds that of the rural population (48.7%). In-house pit latrines and public toilets, which may be pit, Kumasi ventilated improved pit (KVIP) or bucket latrines, are the main toilet facilities used in the districts. Water closet (WC) is used by small proportions of households, ranging from 0.5 per cent in Ahafo Ano South to 27.8 per cent in the Kumasi Metropolis. The proportion of the population with access to potable (pipe-borne) water is relatively low in the districts, including the Kumasi Metropolis. A number of factors, particularly high fertility and internal migration, have accounted for the rapid population growth in the region. About two-thirds of the population in the region was born where they were enumerated; the remaining one third are in-migrants to the region. In 6 of the 18 districts, at least seven out of every ten persons were enumerated in the localities in which they were born, indicating that these districts have less in-migrant than other districts in the region (PHC, 2000).

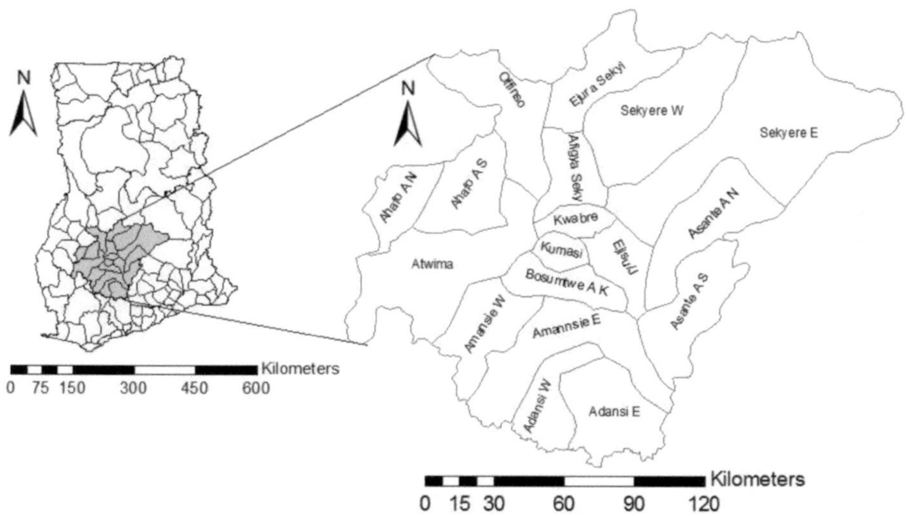

Fig. 1. A map of Ghana showing Ashanti region (in gray color). The figure also shows the spatial distribution of the various districts in Ashanti region

2.2 Data sources

The Ashanti region has a Disease Control Unit (DCU) to which all District Health Directorates (DHD) report suspected outbreaks of various infectious diseases at the end of each year. In this study, all cholera cases used were based on hospital data which were reported to the various DHD. For the detection of statistically significant clusters of cholera, the spatial scan statistic software, SaTScan, developed by Kulldorff, was used. This software requires three main data files to run:

2.2.1 Case file

Case file contains information about cholera cases for specified districts and times. Reported cases of cholera from 1997 to 2001 for each district within the region were retrieved from the DCU. Case definition of cholera was based on the WHO (1993) guidance on formulation of national policy on the control of cholera. According to this guidance, in an area where the disease is not known to be present a case of cholera should be suspected, when a patient, 5 years of age or older develops severe dehydration or dies from acute watery diarrhea, or where an epidemic is occurring, a patient, 5 years of age or older develops acute watery diarrhea, with or without vomiting.

2.2.2 Population file

The population file provides information about the background population at risk for each spatial district. The population database was obtained from the 2000 Population and Housing Census of Ghana conducted by the National Statistical Service (PHC, 2000).

2.2.3 Coordinate file

The coordinate file provides information about the spatial location of each district. In this study, the spatial scale of analysis was at the district level. The centroids of the districts were used as the coordinates of the districts.

2.3 Cluster analysis

The spatial scan statistic was used to detect the presence spatial and space-time clusters of cholera. The spatial scan statistic was developed by Kulldorff (1997, 2006) and it is been implemented in the SaTScan software. Spatial scan statistic has a disadvantage of being difficult to incorporate prior knowledge about the size and shape of an outbreak as well as its impact on disease rate (Neill et al., 2005). However, we used this as an advantage to get rid of pre-selection biases of clusters and their locations. Spatial scan statistic method is based on the principle that the number of cholera cases in a geographic area is Poisson-distributed according to a known underlying population at risk (Kulldorff, 2006). For the detection of purely spatial clusters, SaTScan imposes a circular window on the study region which is moved over the region and centered on the centroid of each district. The size of the circular window, which is also the cluster size, is expressed as a percentage of the total population at risk. This varies from 0 to a maximum (not exceeding 100), as specified by the user. The maximum window size should not exceed 50% of the total population because clusters of larger sizes would indicate areas of exceptionally low rates outside the circle rather than an area of exceptionally high rate within the circle. Possible clusters are tested within the window whenever it is centered on the centroid of each district. Whenever the window finds a new case, the software calculates a likelihood function to test for elevated risk within the window in comparison with those outside the window. The likelihood function for any given window W is proportional to:

$$L(\mathrm{W}) = \sup_{W \in \mathbf{W}} \left(\frac{Chol_{(\mathrm{C})}(W)}{Chol_{(\mathrm{E(C)})}(W)} \right)^{Chol_{(\mathrm{C})}(W)} \left(\frac{Chol_{(\mathrm{C})}(\hat{W})}{Chol_{(\mathrm{E(C)})}(\hat{W})} \right)^{Chol_{(\mathrm{C})}(\hat{W})} \times I\left(\frac{Chol_{(\mathrm{C})}(W)}{Chol_{(\mathrm{E(C)})}(W)} > \frac{Chol_{(\mathrm{C})}(\hat{W})}{Chol_{(\mathrm{E(C)})}(\hat{W})} \right) \tag{1}$$

where $\hat{W}$ indicates all the regions outside the window W, and $Chol_{(\mathrm{C})}(\ )$ and $Chol_{(\mathrm{E(C)})}(\ )$ denote the observed and expected number of cases within the specified window, respectively. The window W to be scanned by the spatial scan statistic is included in the set: $\mathbf{W} = \{W_{ik} | 1 \le i \le m, 1 \le k \le K_i\}$, where W_{ik}, $k = 1,...,K_i$, denote the window composed by the (k −1) nearest neighbors to region i. The window W^* that attains the maximum likelihood is defined as the *most likely cluster* (MLC). The indicator function

$I(\,)$ depends on the comparison between $Chol_{(E(C))}$ and $Chol_{(C)}$. $I(\,)$ is 1 when $Chol_{(C)} > Chol_{(E(C))}$, otherwise 0. The test of significance level of clusters is through the Monte Carlo hypothesis testing (Dwass, 1957). In this study, the maximum window size was set as 50% of the total population. The null hypothesis of no cluster was rejected when the simulated *p-value* was less than or equal to 0.05 for most likely clusters and 0.1 for secondary clusters since the latter have conservative *p-values* (Kulldorff, 2006).

A smaller window size (defined as ≤ 25% of the total population) was also used to investigate the possibility of smaller clusters. This varied from ≤ 25% to ≤ 50% with successive increments of 5%. This was meant to check the sensitivity of spatial scan statistic to smaller window sizes when there are larger spatial units and small number of spatial units.

For the detection of space-time clusters, SaTScan imposes a cylindrical window with a circular geographic base and with height corresponding to the time of occurrences. In this way, the base of the cylinder is centered around one of several possible centroids located throughout the study region with the radius varying continuously in size, whereas the height of the cylinder reflects any possible time interval of less than or equal to half the total study period, as well as the whole study period. The window is then moved in space and time so that for each possible geographic location and size, it also visits each possible time interval (Kulldorf et al., 1998). The likelihood ratio test statistic is constructed in the same way as for the purely spatial scan statistic. However, the computational algorithm for calculating the likelihood for each window is in three rather than two dimensions (Kulldorff, 2001). Here, we used a spatial window that could include up to 50% of population at risk and a maximum temporal window of 50%, without including purely spatial clusters. Moreover, most likely clusters for different time lengths (i.e. 1, 2, 3, or 4 year length) were scanned using a temporal cluster size of 90% of the study period and also included purely spatial clusters with temporal size of 100%. The maximum spatial cluster size was set at 50% of population at risk and included purely temporal clusters (spatial cluster size = 100%) as well.

2.4 Correlation between cholera and risk factors

Three main risk factors, i.e. sanitation, source of drinking water, and internal migration, were used to explore the extent at which these variables affect cholera prevalence within the study area. These were obtained from the 2000 Population and Housing census of Ghana (PHC, 2000). Four different types of sanitation facilities are used in the study area; WC, Pit latrine, KVIP, bucket or pan. A number of households in the districts have no access to toilet facilities. When a substantial number of households do not have toilet facilities, it is to be expected that inhabitants will defecate in the bush, drains, etc. Bucket or pan is the most unsafe sanitation method because the bucket is open and can attract filth breeding flies. Moreover, faeces have to be transferred to a different bucket when it is full; thus faeces can spread to nearby areas in the course of transfer. In this study, sanitation condition for a district is described as the percentage of the district's share of the region's population who do not have access to toilet facilities, and who use bucket or pan sanitation method. For this, larger values reflect poor or bad sanitation condition, while smaller values reflect good sanitation condition.

Since the natural reservoir of cholera is the aquatic environment, inhabitants who drink from wells, streams, rivers, ponds, dugouts and dams are assumed to be at a higher risk of cholera than those who drink from pipe borne water. Therefore, inhabitants who drink from wells, streams, rivers, ponds, dugouts and dams are classified as inhabitants who do not have access to potable water. The indicator for drinking water for each district was computed as the percentage of the district's share of the region's population who drink from wells, streams, rivers, ponds, dugouts and dams.

Internal migration is one of the important demographic characteristics that accounts for rapid population growth in a place. This variable was computed as a percentage of the district's share of the region's population in the year 2000 that were born outside the district during the time of enumeration.

Global Pearson's correlation coefficient was used to determine the correlation between cholera cumulative incidence rates from 1997 to 2001 and sanitation, drinking water, and internal migration. *P-values* were calculated to serve as a guide to access the significance of all correlation coefficients. Most health planning strategies in Ghana are based on the level of urbanization of a district. In other words, groups of districts with similar urbanization levels are planned together. With this in mind, all districts in the study region were stratified according to the level of urbanization; i.e. *low, medium and high.* Pearson's correlation analyses were repeated for each stratum of districts in order to assess the effects of the risk factors on cholera within each urbanization stratum.

3. Results and analyses

3.1 Purely spatial clusters

No cluster was detected for the years 1997 and 2000 since very few cases were reported for these years. Only most likely significant clusters were detected for the years 1998, 1999, 2001 (Table 1 and Figure 2). These clusters encompassed Kumasi, Bosumtwe AK and Kwabre in 1998 (relative risk $Chol_{(RR)} = 12.25$, $Chol_{(C)} = 733$, $Chol_{(E(C))} = 328.62$), Kumasi in 1999 ($Chol_{(RR)} = 7.42$, $Chol_{(C)} = 1033$, $Chol_{(E(C))} = 421.33$), Kumasi and Kwabre in 2001($Chol_{(RR)} = 15.60$, $Chol_{(C)} = 956$, $Chol_{(E(C))} = 383.32$), and Kumasi and Kwabre from 1998 to 2001($Chol_{(RR)} = 9.70$, $Chol_{(C)} = 2727$, $Chol_{(E(C))} = 1161.47$). No differences were observed between the results of the varying window sizes and the window size of ≤ 50% of the total population. Hence tables for these results are not shown.

3.2 Space-time clusters

While testing whether the purely spatial clusters were long term or temporary i.e. space-time analysis, a statistically significant ($p = 0.001$) most likely cluster was identified at Kumasi metropolis for the year 1998-1999. This cluster has $Chol_{(RR)} = 5.86$ with $Chol_{(C)} = 1668$ as against $Chol_{(E(C))} = 508.75$ (See Table 2). One statistically significant ($P = 0.001$) secondary cluster encompassing 3 districts (Ahafo Ano North, Ahafo Ano South, and Atwima) was detected for 1999. For this cluster $Chol_{(RR)} = 1.91$ and $Chol_{(C)} = 179$ as against $Chol_{(E(C))} = 96.34$.

Cluster Area	$Chol_{(C)}$	$Chol_{(E(C))}$	$Chol_{(RR)}$	LLR	*p-value*
Year: 1998					
Kumasi Kwabre Bosumtwe AK	733	328.62	12.253	434.73	0.001
Year: 1999					
Kumasi	1033	421.23	7.42	592.29	0.001
Year: 2001					
Kumasi Kwabre	956	383.32	15.597	673.86	0.001
Year: 1997-2001					
Kumasi Kwabre	2727	1161.47	9.699	1618.26	0.001

Table 1. Most likely purely spatial clusters of cholera in Ashanti region, Ghana, detected by retrospective spatial analysis. This Table shows the results of the purely spatial cluster analysis using a spatial window that could include up to 50% of the population at risk in Ashanti region, Ghana, during 1998-2001: LLR (Log Likelihood Ratio)

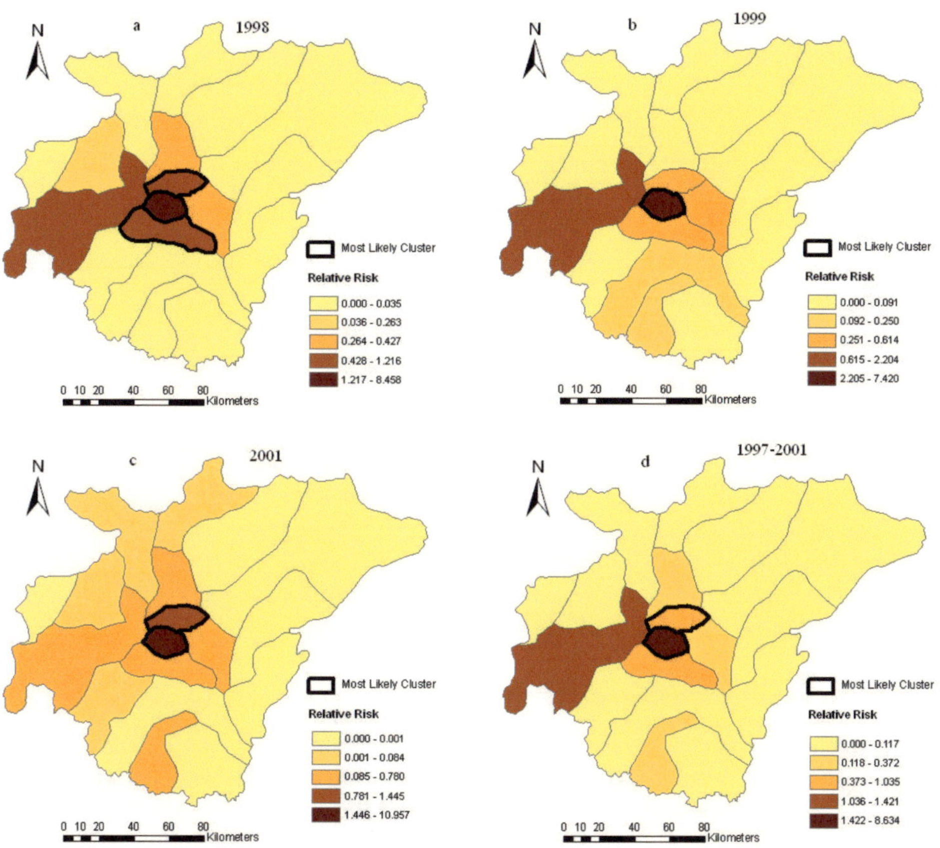

Fig. 2. Locations of the detected clusters of cholera and spatial distribution of the relative risks for 1998(2a), 1999(2b), 2001 (2c), and 1998-2001 (2c)

Cluster Area	Year	$Chol_{(C)}$	$Chol_{(E(C))}$	$Chol_{(RR)}$	LLR	*p-value*
Most Likely Cluster						
1. Kumasi Metro	1998-1999	1688	508.75	5.86	1149.02	0.001
Secondary Cluster						
2. Ahafo Ano North						
Ahafo Ano South						
Atwima	1999	179	96.34	1.908	29.34	0.001

Table 2. Significant high rate spatial clusters of cholera in Ashanti region, Ghana, detected by retrospective space-time analysis. This Table shows the results of the space-time cluster analysis using a spatial window that could include up to 50% of the population at risk and a maximum temporal window of 50% without including purely spatial clusters, in Ashanti region, Ghana, during 1998-2001: LLR (Log Likelihood Ratio).

The results of the space-time analysis when modified, i.e. when using a maximum temporal window of 90% (which included purely spatial clusters as well) and a spatial window that could include up to 50% of the population at risk (which included purely temporal clusters also) are shown in Table 3. Most likely statically significant ($p = 0.001$) cluster of high rates of cholera was again found to exist at the Kumasi Metropolis and Kwabre district for the year 1998-2001. This indicates that Kumasi Metropolis and Kwabre remained statistically significant throughout the year 1998-2001. One statistically significant ($p = 0.001$) secondary cluster encompassing Ahafo Ano South, Ahafo Ano North and Atwima for the year 1999 was also detected.

Cluster Area	Year	$Chol_{(C)}$	$Chol_{(E(C))}$	$Chol_{(RR)}$	LLR	*p-value*
Most Likely Cluster						
1. Kumasi Metro Kwabre	1998-2001	2727	1161.47	9.699	1618.26	0.001
Secondary Cluster						
2. Ahafo Ano North Ahafo Ano South Atwima	1999	179	96.34	1.91	29.33	0.001

Table 3. Significant high rate spatial clusters of cholera in Ashanti region, Ghana, detected by retrospective space-time analysis. This Table shows the results of the space-time cluster analysis when modified to find 1, 2, 3 or 4-year length clusters using a maximum temporal window of 90%, which included purely spatial clusters as well, and a spatial window of ≤50% of the population at risk, which included purely temporal clusters also, in Ashanti region, Ghana, during 1997-2001: LLR (Log Likelihood Ratio)

3.3 Correlation between cholera and risk factors

Pearson's correlation coefficients and their associated *p*-values were computed to determine the relationship between cholera cumulative incidence rate and the demographic risk factors (see Table 4). For the whole region, statistically significant relationship was observed for sanitation ($R^2 = 0.55$, $p = 0.001$), drinking water ($R^2 = 0.39$, $p = 0.001$), and internal migration ($R^2 = 0.73$, $p = 0.001$). However, when the analyses were repeated for each strata of urbanization, statistically significant correlations were observed for only the *high* urban strata (See Table 2). For instance there was a high, but non-significant correlation between cholera and drinking water within the *medium-urban* strata ($R^2 = 0.62, p = 0.12$), and no significant correlation between cholera and drinking water within the *low-urban* strata ($R^2 = 0.001, p = 0.96$). However, there was a high and significant correlation between cholera and drinking water within the *high-urban* strata ($R^2 = 0.86, p = 0.007$).

	Correlation and (*p-value*)		
	Sanitation	Drinking water	Migration
Global	[a]0.55 (0.001)	[a]0.39 (0.001)	[a]0.73 (0.001)
Low urban	[c]0.21 (0.36)	[c]0.04(0.66)	[c]0.001 (0.96)
Moderate urban	[c]0.48 (0.13)	[c]0.62 (0.12)	[c] 0.62 (0.11)
High urban	[b]0.86 (0.007)	[b]0.79 (0.018)	[b]0.89 (0.005)

Table 4. Pearson's correlation coefficients for the relationship between cholera and demographic factors. This Table depicts both the Global Pearson's correlation analyses, and Pearson's correlation analyses for each urbanization strata of districts. The associated *p-values* are shown in brackets. [a]*significant correlations at 0.1% significance level;* [b]*significant correlations at 5% significance level.* [c]*not significant.*

4. Discussion

In this study, the purely spatial and space-time scan statistic methods implemented in SaTScan software have been used to analyze cholera cases from 1998 to 2001 in Kumasi, Ghana. These methods identifies whether unusual concentration of disease cases can be explained by chance or statistically significant. The findings of this study reveal several notable points. First, there is the existence of both purely spatial and space-time clusters, not explainable by chance (See Tables 1,2, and 3). Also, the results of both the purely spatial and space-time analysis are somewhat similar. In particular, the purely spatial analysis reported an excess incidence of cholera in Kumasi during the years 1998, 1999, and 2001 (See Table 3.1 and Figure 3.2), and the space-time analysis also reported an excess incidence of cholera from 1999 to 2001 at the same area.

Second, the excess incidence of cholera mainly existed at Kumasi Metropolis throughout the period under study. Specifically, the purely spatial analysis reported excess incidence of cholera at Kumasi in 1998, 1999, and 2001. While testing whether the purely spatial clusters were long term or temporary, the space-time analysis also reported excess incidence of cholera at Kumasi Metropolis from the year 1999 to 2001. When the space-time analysis was modified to detect 1, 2, 3, 4, or 5 year length clusters, the space-time most likely cluster at Kumasi Metropolis became a purely spatial cluster (i.e. existed for 1997 to 2001, see Table 3). This indicates a sustained transmission of cholera at Kumasi Metropolis from 1997 through to 2001. Two main reasons may explain these patterns. (1) *Demographic status*: Kumasi is the most urbanized and highly commercialized district in Ashanti region, and therefore there is always a high daily influx of traders and civil workers from neighboring districts to Kumasi Metropolis. Such a high daily influx strain existing sanitation systems, thereby putting people at increased risk of cholera transmission. The rural poor also often migrate to city centers with the hope of a better life. However, due to the high cost of housing, such migrants settle at slummy and/or squatter areas where environmental sanitation is poor. This largely explains the high *northern population* (inhabitants from the northern sector of Ghana; which is the most deprived sector) within Kumasi Metropolis. (2) *Geographic location*: Kumasi Metropolis is the central nodal district of Ghana, and therefore, all road networks linking the northern sector and the southern sector of Ghana pass through Kumasi. There is the high probability of stoppage and transit by travelers, resulting in a high daily population increase and overcrowding at city centers.

Third, the findings of the space-time analysis clearly depict the statistical power of the scan statistic for detecting recently emerging clusters. The space-time analysis detected an important cluster during the year 1999 that would otherwise not be detected by a purely spatial analysis. This cluster encompassed areas surrounding Ahafo Ano North, Ahafo Ano South, and Atwima districts (See Tables 2 and 3).

Fourth, both the purely spatial and space-time cluster analysis detected no cluster during the years 1997 and 2000. This is somewhat consistent with both the overall global and national cholera trends. Although officially notified cases do not reflect the overall burden of the diseases, cholera cases reported to WHO in 1996 was 4.4 times higher than cases in 1997 (a decrease of 77% from 1996 to 1997), and cases in 1998 was 9 times higher than cases in 1997(an increase of 80.3% from 1997 to 1998). Compared to 1999, the year 2000 saw 46% global reduction in the total number of cases, and about 65% reduction in the total number of cases reported in Ghana. After a massive outbreak in Ghana from 1998 to 1999, health officials and policy makers implemented several measures to curb the menace. Notable among these measures were effective waste collection and disposal (including solid waste, sewage, industrial and clinical waste), cleansing of public areas, food hygiene, hygiene education and related programs. Consequently, the reduced number of cholera cases in the year 2000.

When the maximum window size was varied from ≤ 25% to ≤ 50% of the total population, the same results were obtained as with the window size of ≤ 50% of the total population. This clearly shows that for large geographical scales with fewer spatial units, spatial scan statistic will likely not be sensitive to varying window size. Chen et al. (2008) clearly demonstrated the sensitivity of the spatial scan statistic to the issues of varying window sizes (SaTScan scaling issues) through a geo-visual analytic technique. Their study was partly a quest to determine an optimal setting for SaTScan scaling parameters due to the confusing and even misleading results which are possible if the parameter choices are made arbitrarily. However, their data was across larger spatial geographical area with larger number of spatial units; giving SaTScan much flexibility on the varying window sizes. Contrary to our data used, there were only 18 spatial units; a number probably too small for spatial scan statistic. Therefore the interpretation of our findings should fall within the framework of the above limitation.

The findings of the correlations analysis suggest that cholera is high when majority of the people do not have access to good sanitation facilities; do not have access to potable water; and when internal migration is high. When the correlation analyses were repeated for each strata of urbanization, statistically significant correlations were observed for only the *high-urban* strata. Considering drinking water for instance, there was no significant correlation within the *low-urban* strata and the *medium-urban* strata, but a high significant correlation was observed within the *high-urban* strata (See Table 4). This implies that drinking water, sanitation and internal migration affect only *high-urban* communities in the study area. This is consistent with the findings of the cluster analysis. Both the purely spatial and space-time analysis identified Kumasi Metropolis and Kwabre district as significant high rate clusters of cholera, which are also amongst the most urbanized and overcrowded areas in Ashanti Region.

Cholera primarily attack individuals with insufficient knowledge of and inappropriate attitudes towards hygienic practices, and who live in dwellings that lack access to safe drinking water supply and to adequate facilities for sanitation, sewerage disposal and treatment (Glass and Black, 1992). Majority of the region's population who do not have access to good sanitation systems, and drink from rivers, streams and ponds are people living in most urbanized and densely populated districts. For instance, Kumasi metropolis's share of the region's population who do not have access to potable water is close to 13%, a value 2.3 times higher than the mean percentage.

Fecal contamination of rivers is a major water quality issue in many fast growing cities like the Kumasi Metropolis where population growth far exceeds the rate of development of wastewater collection and treatment. The water bodies near densely populated areas may have high fecal concentrations due to defecation and sanitation practices of the people. Ali et al. (2002a) has asserted that fecal contamination of surface water in densely populated area is higher than a sparsely populated area. Although Kumasi Metropolis and other urbanized districts are served with potable water, this water does not flow throughout the year. At certain times no water flow for a period of a week or two. Residents are therefore compelled to exploit nearby streams, rivers and ponds. If such water bodies are contaminated and is used for drinking or cooking, there is the likelihood of infection.

After several decades of research into cholera, the risk factors which contribute to its transmission have not changed. The spatial and temporal patterns that the disease displays, however, are not the same from one outbreak area to another. Although several of the findings of this research are more confirmatory, it draws the attention of health officials and policymakers about the area where there has been sustained transmission of the disease over the years. The study also provides very useful information to health officials and policymaker about the spatial and temporal patterns of cholera in Ghana. For example, this study clearly shows that there has been a sustained transmission of cholera in Kumasi during the period under study. The findings of this study will also have important implications for public health officials since control strategies would vary depending on the most important risk factors in most important districts. With the important high rate cluster locations and risk factors identified, optimal efforts can be taken at appropriate districts to prevent and control cholera. There is no doubt that the fecal oral route of cholera transmission should be of primary concern because of its importance in the development of secondary cases and in subsequent spread of the disease. It should therefore be the concern of health officials and policymakers to provide better sanitation systems to prevent fecal contamination of water bodies within *high-urban* districts. Moreover, potable (pipe-borne) water supply in urban and densely populated districts should be expanded and improved to prevent cholera outbreaks.

5. Conclusion

This study has shown the presence of both spatial and space-time hotspots of cholera in Ashanti region, suggesting that there has been sustained transmission of cholera within these hotspots. The study has also shown that drinking water, sanitation and internal migration are important risk factors of cholera in Ashanti region; however, these predictors do not have a significant impact in cholera transmission in low urban communities. This study has also demonstrated that using available health data, GIS and spatial scan statistic can provide public health officials in Ghana with new knowledge about the prevalence rate and hotspots of a disease. This new knowledge will help them to come out with optimal strategies to prevent and contain diseases outbreak. Of the three risk factors studied, the effect of internal migration on cholera is comparatively high. Measures to reduce internal migration can reduce pressure on sanitation and water supply systems. Since the studied risk factors could not explain cholera prevalence in low urban areas, a more detailed research needs to be carried out at individual levels to thoroughly understand the epidemiology of cholera in the study area.

6. Acknowledgements

We extend our sincere appreciation to the Disease Control Unit-Ashanti Region and the Ghana Statistical Service for providing all the necessary data and background information for this research.

7. References

Ali, M.; Emch, M.; Donnay, J.P.; Yunus, M. and Sack, R.B. (2002a). Identifying environmental risk factors of endemic cholera: a raster GIS approach. *Health and Place* 8: 201-210

Ali, M.; Emch, M.; Donnay, J.P.; Yunus, M. and Sack, R.B. (2002b). The spatial epidemiology of cholera in an endemic area of Bangladesh. *Soc. Sci. & Med.* 55(6):1015-1024

Besag, J. and Newell, J. (1991). The detection of clusters in rare disease. *J. R. Stat. Soc.* A 154: 143-155.

Chput, E.K.; Meek, J.I. and Heimer, R. (2002). Spatial analysis of human granulocytic ehrlichiosis near Lyme; Connecticut. *Emerg. Infect. Dis.* 8: 943-948.

Cousens, E.K.; Smith, P.G.; Ward, H.; Everington, D. and Knight, R.S.G. (2000). Geographical distribution of variant Creutzfeldt-Jakob disease in Great Britain; 1994-2000. *Lancet* 357: 1002-1007.

Dwass, M. (1957). Modified randomization tests for non-parametric hypothesis. *Ann. Math. Stat.* 28: 181-187.

Glass, R.I. and Black, R. (1992). Epidemiology of cholera. In: *Topics in infectious diseases: cholera*, Barua, D.; Greenough, W.B. pp. 129-54, Plenum Medical Company, New York

Green, C.; Hoppa, R.D.; Young, T.K. and Blanchard, J.F. (2003). Geographical analysis of diabetes prevalence in an urban area. *Soc. Sci. Med.* 57: 551-560.

Hjalmars, U.; Kullforff, M.; Gustafsson, G. and Nagarwalla, N. (1996). Childhood leukemia in Sweden: Using GIS and a spatial scan statistics for cluster detection. *Stat. Med.* 15: 707-715.

Kelly, L. (2001). The global dimension of cholera. *Glob. Chang. Hum. Health* 2(1):6-17

Kulldorff, M. (2001). Prospective time-periodic geographical disease surveillance using a scan statistic. *J. R. Stat. Soc.* A 164:61-72.

Kulldorff, M.; Athas, W.F.; Feuer, E.J.; Miller, B.A. and Key, C.R. (1998). Evaluating cluster alarms: A space-time scan statistic and brain cancer in Los Alamos, New Mexico. *Am. J. Public Health* 88: 9.

Kulldorff, M. and Nagerwalla, N. (1995). Spatial disease clusters: detection and inference. *Stat. Med.* 14:799-810.

Kulldorff, M. (1997). A spatial scan statistic. *Commun. Stat.-Theory Methods* 26:1481-1496.

Kulldorff, M. (2005): Software for the spatial space time statistics; SaTScan v6.0. Information Management Service; Inc. http:// www. Satscan.org/. Last accessed 5 September 2011

Kulldorff, M. (2006). SaTScan users guide for version 6.0. http://www.satscan.org/. Last accessed 5 September 2011

McNeill, W.H. (1976). Plagues and People. Anchor Press Doubleday, New York.

Michelozzi, P.; Capon, A.; Kirchmayer, U.; Forastiere, F.; Biggeri, A.; Barca, A. and Perucci, C.A. (2002). Adult and Childhood leukemia near a high power radio station in Rome, Italy. *Am. J. Epidemiol.* 155: 1096-1103.

Myaux, J.; Ali, M.; Chakraborty, J. and de Francisco, A. (1997). Flood control embankments contribute to the improvements of health status of children in rural Bangladesh. *Bull. WHO* 75(6): 533-539.

Osei, F.B. and Duker, A.A. (2008a). Spatial and demographic patterns of Cholera in Ashanti Region-Ghana. *Int. J. Health Geogr.* 7:44

Odoi, A.; Martin, S.W.; Michel, P.; Middleton, D.; Holt, J. and Wilson, J. (2004). Investigation of clusters of giardiasis using GIS and spatial scan statistics. *Int. J. Health Geogr.*; 3:11

PHC (2000): Population and Housing Census for 2000. Ghana statistical service

Pobee, J.O.M. and Grant, F. (1970). Case Report of Cholera. *Ghana Med. J.* 306-309

Sheehan, T.J. and DeChelo, L.M. (2005): A space-time analysis of the proportion of late stage breast cancer in Massachusetts; 1988 to 1997. *Int. J. Health Georgr.* 4:15.

Tiwari, N.; Adhikari, C.S.; Tewari, A. and Kandpal, V. (2006). Investigation of geo-spatial hotspost for the occureence of tuberculosis in Almora district; India; using GIS and spatial scan statistic. *Int J. Health Goegr.* 5:33.

Turnbull, B.W.; Iwano, E.J.; Burnett, W.S.; Howe, H.L.; and Clark, L.C. (1990). Monitoring for clusters of disease: application to leukemia incidence in upstate New York. *Am. J. Epidemiol.* 132: S136- S143.

Viel, J.F.; Arveux, P.; Baverel, J. and Cahn, J.Y. (2000). Soft-tissue sarcoma and non-Hodgkin's lymphoma clusters around a municipal solid waste incinerator with dioxin emission levels. *Am J Epidemiol.* 152: 13-19

Webster, R.; Oliver, M.A.; Munir, K.R. and Man, J.R. (1994). Kriging the local risk of rare disease from a register of diagnoses. *Geogr. Anal.* 26(2): 168-185.

WHO (2000a). Cholera, 1999. Weekly epidemiological record 75(31):249-256.

WHO (2000b). WHO report on global surveillance of epidemicprone infectious diseases. WHO/CDS/CSR/RS. Geneva 2000b:1.

WHO (2001). Cholera, 2000. *Weekly epidemiological record.* 76(31):233-240

WHO (2002). Cholera, 2001. *Weekly epidemiological record.* 77(31):257-268.

WHO (2003). Cholera, 2002. *Weekly epidemiological record.* 78(31):269-276.

WHO (2004). Cholera, 2003. *Weekly epidemiological record.* 79(31):281-288.

WHO (2005). Cholera, 2003. *Weekly epidemiological record*. 80(31):261-268.
WHO (2006). Cholera, 2004. *Weekly epidemiological record*. 81(31):297-308.

3

Cholera in Lao P. D. R.: Past and Present

Satoshi Nakamura[1,7,*,*]
[1]*Department of Tropical Medicine and Malaria,*
National Centre for Global Health and Medicine, Tokyo
[7]*Institut Pasteur du Laos, Ministry of Health, Vientiane*
[1]*Japan*
[7]*Lao People's Democratic Republic*

1. Introduction

Lao People's Democratic Republic (Lao PDR) is a mountainous country in Southeast Asia, situated along the Mekong and bordering China, Vietnam, Cambodia, Thailand, and Myanmar. Cholera epidemics are known to have occurred in Laos during the time of the French colonial era and the Kingdom of Laos period prior to the establishment of Lao PDR in 1975. There are public records of cholera epidemics in 1895 to 1902 of the French era (Monnais-Rousselot, 1999) and in the 1910s, 1953 and 1969 of the Kingdom era (Nakamura and Iwasa, 2008). However, after the establishment of Lao People's Democratic Republic (Lao PDR), it was presumed that there were no epidemics of cholera and, at the level of both rural and central government, cholera was not sufficiently recognized prior to 1993. Acquisition of pandemic information on cholera was severely restricted, due to the establishment of a socialist state system in Laos and its isolationist state from 1975 to the mid-1980s. Moreover, while diarrhea and/or fever outbreaks caused by unknown pathogens were common in remote areas of mountainous districts equipped with few health resources, case detection or confirmation was quite difficult because almost all the cases had ceased by the time the reports reached the central government. Since these areas had scant populations with a scattered distribution of small size villages, the roads to which they were connected were poor; thus, confirmed diagnoses of the diseases could not be made because the areas could not be accessed easily, and prudent control was not exercised with the

*Yutaka Midorikawa[2], Masami Nakatsu[1], Toru Watanabe[3], Rattanaphone Phethsouvanh[4], Phengta Vongphrachanh[5], Kongsap Akkhavong[6] and Paul Brey[7]
[1]*Department of Tropical Medicine and Malaria,*
National Centre for Global Health and Medicine, Tokyo
[2]*Faculty of Health Sciences, Suzuka University of Medical Sciences, Mie*
[3]*Graduate School of Agriculture, Yamagata University, Yamagata*
[4]*Laboratory of Bacteriology, National Mahosot Hospital, Ministry of Health, Vientiane*
[5]*National Centre of Laboratory and Epidemiology, Ministry of Health, Vientiane*
[6]*National Institute of Public Health, Ministry of Health, Vientiane*
[7]*Institut Pasteur du Laos, Ministry of Health, Vientiane*
[1,2,3]*Japan*
[4,5,6,7]*Lao People's Democratic Republic*
*Corresponding Author

exception of the itinerary of EPI sentinels. As a result, most of the outbreaks occurred unquestioned and health measurement in these remote areas remained limited.

We will present details of the cholera situation in Lao PDR from 1993-1996, a period during which overt epidemics were reported. Hitherto, these epidemics had been little known to other countries with the exception of some documents or reports (Anonymous, 1993; Global Task Force on Cholera Control, 2008). Hence, we would like to give details of case studies and especially to clarify some characteristics of non-O1 non-139 *Vibrio cholerae* strains which have not yet been studied as a potential causative of diarrhea in the country. These results will necessarily be limited; however, they might contribute to further epidemiological study of cholera in the Southeast Asia region.

In this chapter, we refer to non-O1 non-139 *Vibrio cholerae* simply as NAG (non-agglutinable) *V. cholerae*, a former common abbreviation.

2. Cholera epidemics in Lao PDR from 1993 to the present

In Lao PDR, a cholera outbreak began in the Napo area of Hinboun district in Khammouane Province on April 7th of 1993 and spread to Boulapa (at the end of April and in June), Gnyomalath (in July), Mahaxay (in July), Takehk (in July), other parts of Hinboun (in July), Xebanphai and Nonbok districts (in August). In the same year it spread within the entire region including Nakai district, and became an epidemic of 5276 cases (including 250 deaths; a case fatality rate of 4.8%). An outbreak even occurred in the Pin district of the neighboring province of Savannakhet on May 1st of the same year, and this spread within the four districts of Xephon (in June), Nong (in June), Vilaburi (in September), and Atsaphan (in December) with a total of 1614 cases (86; 5.3%). In 1994, cases of severe diarrhea first occurred at Ta Oy village in the Toum Laan district of Saravane Province in the south, before the epidemic spread to two further districts, Lakhopheng and Vaphi, with 1111 cases (88; 11.3%) by March. A further 53 (18; 43%) cases of cholera occurred again in two areas of Nong district in Savannakhet in April of the same year. By June, the outbreak had expanded to the nine districts of Champon, Tumphon, Khamthabuli, Phin, Thapanthong, Songkhon, Xaybuli, Sonbuli, and Atsaphan with a total of 1209 cases (126; 10.4%).The number of inpatients at the provincial hospital between May 8th and June 18th was 360; this rapidly increased to 1554 (126; 8.1%) in the following three months. In the north of the country, nine cases of severe diarrhea were reported by the provincial health office of Bokeo Province in April 1994. Cases also spread to the three provinces of Oudomxay, Xaignaburi, and Luangnamtha within the same month, and two cases of cholera were reported in Luangphabang Province in May. Severe diarrhea cases spread to Xienkhouane province in the north and to Attapeu province in the south by June but cholera bacterium was not detected in patients from Attapeu Province. The official statistic report on cases of severe diarrhea including cholera in 1994 was not very precise; however, more than 5200 cases were observed during the two months from April to May.

In the year 1995, 192 cases (36; 18.9%) of serious diarrhea occurred in Attapeu between early January and the end of February. As in the previous year, the causative bacterium was not confirmed. In June and beyond, 260 cases (25; 9.6%) of cholera broke out in the four provinces of Sekon, Xaignaburi, Luangphabang, and Khammouane. From December 11-19th, a cholera outbreak with 141 cases occurred at Ban Phailom in Xaithani district, the first of its kind in Vientiane Capital (Vientiane Municipality at the time) (Nakamura, Marui,

2000), and the epidemic had spread to the whole of the country by 1996 (Midorikawa *et al*, 1996). Table 1 shows a summary of the epidemics in Lao PDR during the above period.

Year	Province	Population*	Case	Death case	Fatality rate(%)
1993	Khammouane	275,400	5521	254	4.6
	Savannakhet	674,900	1531	84	5.5
1994	Bokeo	114,900	1077	56	5.2
	Luangnamtha	115,200	1043	81	7.8
	Oudomxai	211,300	1492	92	6.2
	Luangprabang	367,200	52	4	7.7
	Special region				
	Hongsa**	-	18	3	16.7
	Xayabury	293,300	793	66	8.3
	Khammouane	275,400	611	11	1.8
	Savannakhet	674,900	2789	151	5.4
	Saravane	258,300	1315	93	7.1
	Attapeu**	87,700	688	59	8.6
1995	Luangprabang	367,200	128	4	3.1
	Xayabury	293,300	158	3	1.9
	Vientiane Mun.	531,800	141	0	0
	Sekong	64,200	610	76	12.5
	Attapeu*	87,700	530	91	17.2
1996	Phongsaly	153,000	1	0	0
	Huaphanh	247,300	83	12	14.4
	Xayabury	293,300	78	4	5.1
	Xiengkhuang	201,200	199	14	7
	Khammuane	275,400	5	0	0
	Savannakhet	674,900	4	0	0
	Sekong	64,200	75	4	5.3

* Population census 1995

** Cholera vibrio was not confirmed

Table 1. Cholera epidemics in Lao PDR during 1993-1996.

The government of Lao PDR (GOL) responded swiftly in requesting cholera control assistance from foreign countries including NGOs through the UN Department of Humanitarian Affairs, Geneva, and received donations of 570,000 US dollars for control activities (Anonymous 1995). In addition, GOL cooperated with the WHO after 1994, a joint National Cholera Epidemic Control Committee was established in the CDD (Diarrheal Disease Control) program at the Department of Preventive Health within the Ministry of Health, GOL, and formalized control measures against cholera were advanced. Committee meetings, and training for control in the major cities took place, and more than ten examples of active surveillance were conducted up until 1996. For example, surveillance including carrier surveys was conducted in 12 districts in 4 provinces and resulted in the identification of 306 diarrheal cases and 25 confirmed death cases from May to August, 1994. The existence of NAG *V. cholerae* in the country was demonstrated for the first time prior to 1995 through this active surveillance. In the same year, the first cholera vaccination was performed, using oral killed vaccine donated by the Vietnamese government, at several villages in Xekong and Attapeu provinces (Nakamura, 2003). Moreover, the first National Conference on Diarrhea was held in Vientiane on 14-15th December, 1994.

The cholera epidemic temporarily ceased around the end of 1996. Although cholera in the country was categorized as severe diarrhea in the diseases statistic reports of GOL in 1997 and beyond, it continued sporadically. In 1998, cases of severe diarrhea rapidly increased to 6,000, and a cholera epidemic reemerged in 2000 with more than 12,000 recognized cases, although this decreased dramatically in 2002 (Figure.1). The monthly cases of severe diarrhea including cholera from 1994 to 2000 are shown in Figure 2. According to the average of the cumulated data, diarrheal cases were most frequent between April and June with a peak in May (Figure 3), results which will require further epidemiological analysis in relation to weather conditions.

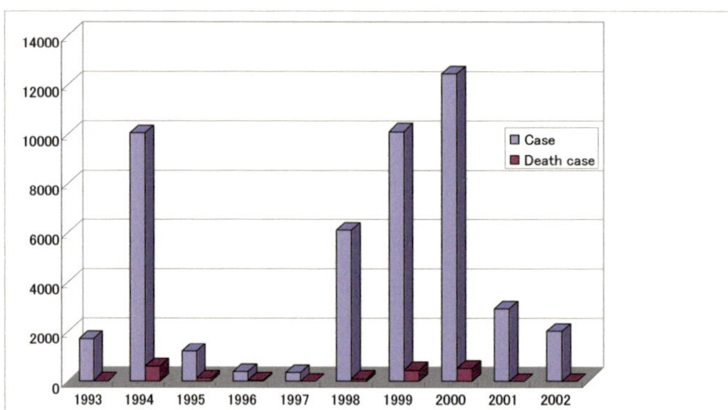

Modification of "Summarized report of surveillance on 18 symptoms/diseases classification in 2002, MOH, GOL, 2003, p.34 "

Fig. 1. Case and death case of severe diarrhea from 1993 to in Lao PDR.

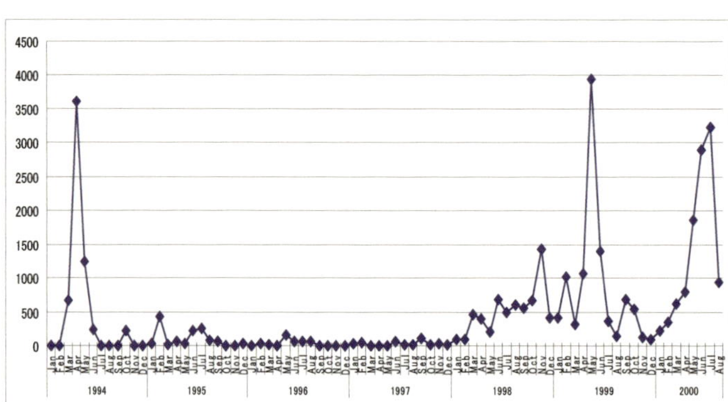

Fig. 2. Severe diarrheal cases reported by Ministry of Health, Lao PDR, Jan 1994 - Aug 2000

Although the patients' average case fatality rate exceeded 11% during the epidemic from 1993 to 1996, it henceforth fell to about 4.5% in 1998. Moreover, the rate in 2000 fell even further than previously, to 4.2%.

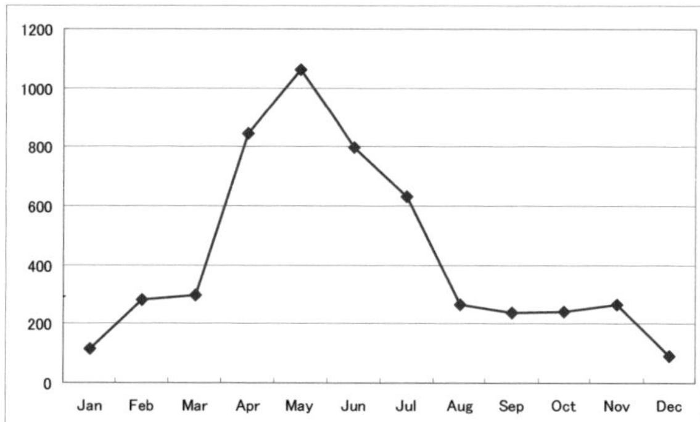

Fig. 3. Average monthly severe diarrheal cases pattern including cholera in Lao PDR from January 1994 to August 2000

In terms of epidemics in 2000-2003 and beyond, a distinct outbreak occurred in the two districts of Thateng and Lamam in Sekong Province in December 2007- January 2008 (Lenglet *et al.*, 2010).

The causative vibrios collected by the active surveillance in 1993-1995 were all identified as *Vibrio cholerae* O1 serotype Ogawa and biotype El Tor at the National Institute of Hygiene and Epidemiology (NIHE) (Nakamura *et al.* 1998), and the strains contributed for further publications (Toma *et al.*, 1997). Amongst these strains, antibiotic resistance was limited to Ampicillins. However, the characteristics of the cholera bacteria changed in the strains collected in 1996 and afterwards as reported in India, Vietnam and Thailand (Bag *et al.*, 1998; Dalsgaard *et al.*, 1999; Dalsgaard *et al.*, 2000). The genomic analyses revealed that these strains were introduced with a SXT constin gene that regulates for multidrug resistancy (Iwanaga *et al.*, 2004). We also speculate that the change was mediated by the presence of NAG vibrios in the country. Although a *V. cholerae* O139 epidemic occurred in Thailand from 1993 to1994 (Chongsa-nguan M. *et al.*, 1993; Bodhidatta L., *et al.*, 1995), we have no evidence that the strain was recovered from the country.

Even though epidemics have ceased and severe diarrheal cases have been limited to sporadic cases since 2008, it is possible that another epidemic could easily reoccur in Lao PDR because people's natural immunity to the cholera vibrios is limited to O1 serotype Ogawa, biotype El Tor and, as such, this immunity will not be very long lasting (Kabir, 2005). Moreover, in some local areas, people were indifferent about the cholera disease itself (Midorikawa *et al.*, 2010). Local people also suffer from poor food hygiene related to the common custom of eating raw materials (mixed dishes known as *laap*; fish, meat, *Tao etc.*: Nakamura *et al.*, 2008), as well as poor knowledge of water-food sanitation, which was confirmed by our experiences including active surveillance.

The following case studies focused on the characteristics of water-borne and food-borne aspects related to disease control in the northern part of Laos in 1994-1995.

3. Case studies of cholera in northern Lao PDR in the epidemic year of 1994

3.1 Cases in Luangnamtha Province

In early April of 1994, outbreaks of cholera occurred successively in northern Bokeo and Oudomxay provinces, and in Luangnamtha province.

No.	Village	Population	Case	Death case	Age distribution of death case	Date of onset
1	Pavi	152	4	0		10 May, 1994
2	Moklao	53	4	2	50y:f, 43y:m	12 April, 1994
3	Hatte	118	39	2	35y:f, 33y:m	19 April, 1994
4	Vath	205	51	4	4y:m, 3y:m, 1.6y:f 88y:f	1 May, 1994

No.	Locality	Age distribution >65	64-16	15-6	<5	Total
1	Moktou	3	31*	1	0	35
2	Hattae	0	7	0	1	8
3	Nam Heng	1	5	0	0	6
4	Phouhaun	0	1	2	2	5
5	Ponhaun	0	1	1	0	2
6	Nale	1	1	0	0	2
7	Takdeth	0	0	1	0	1
8	Vath	0	1	0	0	1
9	Vienglao	0	1	0	0	1
10	Phavy	0	0	0	1	1
11	Phattana	0	0	0	1	1
12	Unknown	0	33	7	5	45
	Total	5	81	12	10	108

Table 2. The diarrhea case detection at four onset villages in Nale district on 16th May and age distribution of recorded cases treated at Nale district hospital during April to May 1994

Based on a request by the local government of Luangnamtha province, a GOL surveillance team visited Nale district as part of a national active case finding mission on May 12th-25th, 1994. The district is 86 km in distance from the capital of Luangnamtha. There was no car-road access but the Namtha River was accessible by boat at the time. The district had a population of 20,108 consisting of 113 villages in 12 communes. A wooden-made district hospital with a director and 13 medical aids and 11 nurses was located in the capital village of Nale. The major ethnic group living in the area were *Lao Teun* (mid-mountain people). It was confirmed that 98 severe diarrhea cases including 8 death cases amongst 4 villages occurred in the district (Table 2). Also 108 cases of diarrhea inpatients were confirmed at the district hospital. Almost all the cases were of people over the age of five, as cholera epidemics are defined. The case fatality rate was confirmed as 8.2%.

Figure 4 shows that the epidemic route was from upstream to downstream along the Namtha River. The first unreported case was of a 50-year-old male who developed severe diarrhea at Moklao (or Vienglao) village on 12th April, 1994, before *Phimai Lao* (Lao New Year). The first reported case was of a 30-year-old at Hatte village, located on the opposite side of the Namtha River from Moklao, who visited relatives from Moklao and suffered from severe diarrhea for 5-6 days in the same period. Subsequently, a second case occurred in the village of a male aged over 30 who also suffered and died from diarrhea. Sixty five cases of severe diarrhea in sufferers over 10 years of age were then reported to the district health office on 19th April, 1994. Two to three days after this outbreak, an incidence of diarrhea occurred at Vath village and spread to 34 cases on 29-30th April, reported on May 1st , 1994. This village is located on the riverbank, about 3 km downstream from Hatte. A villager had returned to Vath after attending the funeral of a relative at Hatte, and subsequently contracted severe diarrhea. At the funeral, the local people had buried the body; however, the victim's clothes were washed in the Namtha River. Dwellers in the area had no toilet at the time other than excreting near the river.

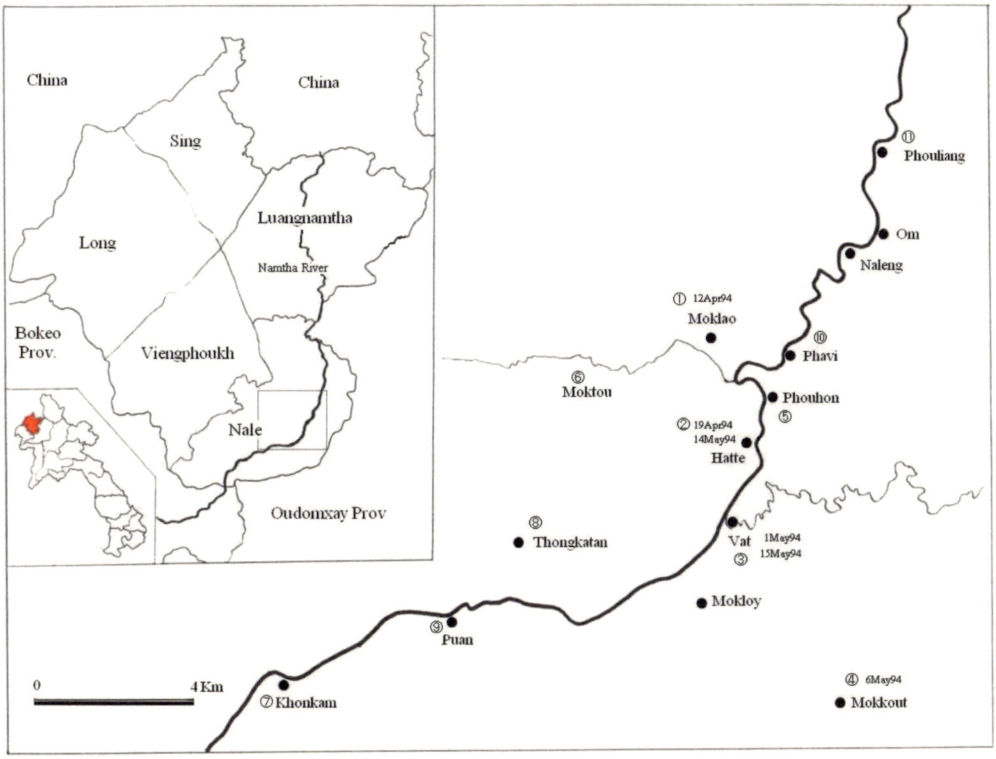

Fig. 4. Cholera transmission route in Nale district along the Nale River in Luangnamtha Province in 1994

During this mission, we also found that stools of the cholera inpatients were collected in buckets and thrown directly into the river by their family members who had stayed at the district hospital in the capital of Nale district (Picture 1). Moreover, in one case in Bokeo, the body of the deceased was also observed being thrown directly into the river by another active surveillance mission in Xaygnabouri Province in April to May 1994 (personal communication). Needless to say, cholera is a water-borne infection. It is thought that the disease was also spread through the river in a remote district of Luangnamtha Province.

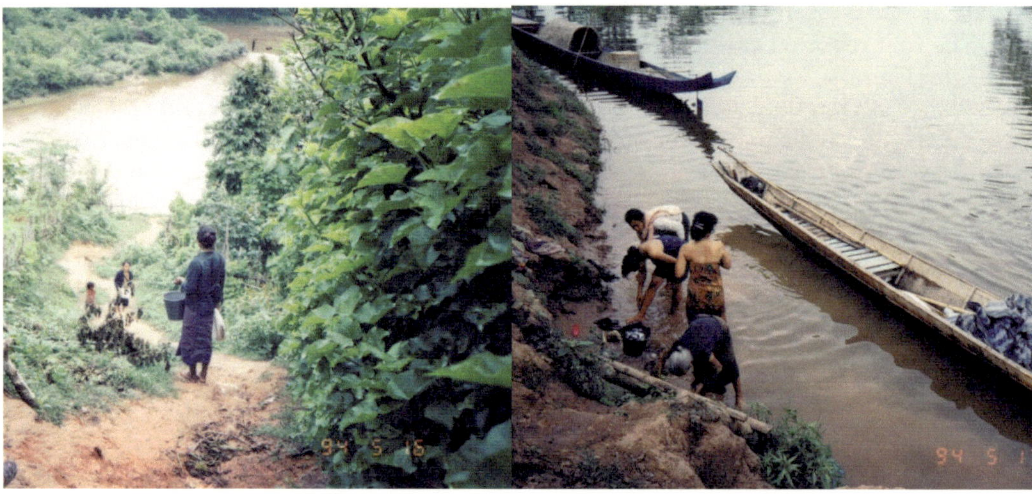

Picture 1. Namtha river (left: bringing human stools to the river; right: daily life of the riverside)

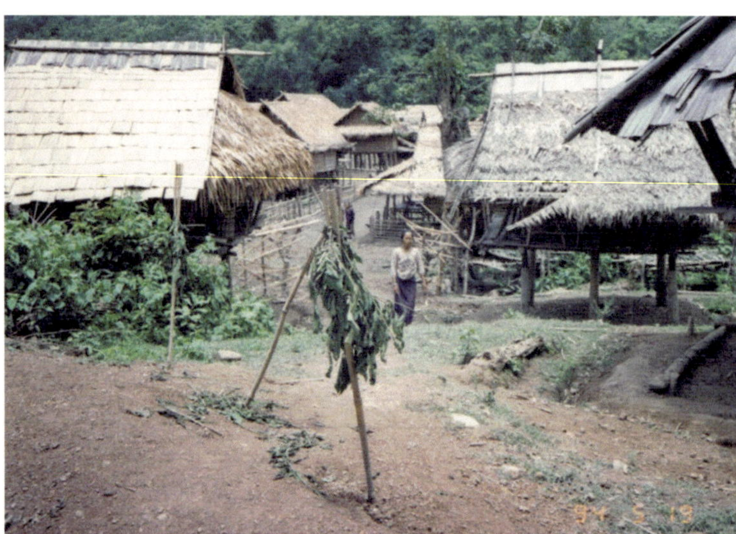

Picture 2. A "spirit gate" at the entrance of a village

Interestingly, the belief that such an epidemic had been evoked as the curse of an evil spirit (*Phi* by its Lao name; man or woman) remained strong in such remote regions of Laos

(Halpern, 1963). Throughout this survey, we witnessed many charms in front of the gates of villages and the entrances of each house of villages in the district (Picture 2). People told us that the epidemic of diseases that year was caused by a female *Phi*; therefore the target was men. It was well known that rehydration therapy, such as giving oral rehydration solution to patients, is extremely effective in diminishing the number of fatalities among cholera sufferers. However, our surveillance confirmed cases of deaths in which even water was not given to the patient for fear that it would lead to even greater possession by the *Phi*. In such situations, it was thought that a control objective should have been set to improve education regarding rehydration therapy, so that skills could be gained in order to reduce cholera deaths among the local residents, even though these beliefs still remain in the present day.

3.2 Cholera expansion due to local customs and cooking food: Cases in Oudomxay Province

We now turn to cases in Oudomxay. We conducted active surveillance in the province on 6-8th June, 1994 in response to a request by the provincial government. Through the surveillance, it was reconfirmed clearly that food played a big role in the spread of cholera because it could develop in the area as food poisoning.

			Case		Age & Sex	Death	Age &	Water	
No.	Village	Population	New	Reported*	(Reported case)	case	Sex	source**	Toilet
1	Huai Ta	209	0	0		0		Strm	-
2	Kuanoy	181	0	0		0		Strm	-
3	Lak Sip	90	1	0	2, f	0		Strm	-
4	Lak Jet	NA	0	0		0		Strm	-
5	Pang Thong	>300	0	0		0		Well	-
6	Xieng Le	>200	0	0		0		Well	-
7	Nalai	370	2	0	43, m; 24, m	0		Strm	-
8	Pong Deua	397	0	0		0		Riv	-
9	Pho Keo	519	0	0		0		Well	-
10	Kon Kham	226	1	0	12, f	0		Well	-
11	Nabone	338	4	0	48, f; 20, m; 19, m; 50, m	0		Well	-
12	Houihuk	129	4	0	40, m; 30, f; 51, m; 38, f	0		Well	-
13	Pho Kham	359	2	0	40, f; 17, f	0		Well/Riv	-
14	Sam Kang	760	2	0	22, m; 20, f	1	97,f	Well/Riv	-
15	Vang Wa	329	0	2	(31, f; 65, m)	0		Riv/Strm	-
16	Pang Som	395	1	1	50, f; (38, m)	0		Fount	-
17	Namone	170	0	0		0		Strm	-
18	Vang Tang	365	0	2	(50, m; 20, m)	0		Strm	-
19	Vang Jing	230	0	1	(30, f)	0		Strm	-
20	Nangeun	287	1	0	6, m	0		TapW	+
21	Don Kham	756	0	0		0		NA	NA
22	Nakai	157	1	2	40, f; (35, m; 50, m)	0		Riv	-
23	Nam Nhone	570	0	0		0		Riv/Strm	-
24	Done Keo	714	0	0		0		Well	+
25	Oudom	471	1	0	46, f	0		Well/Fount	-
26	Saysana	718	2	0	30, f; 50, f	0		Riv	-
27	Don Saat	300	0	0		0		TapW	-
Total			22	8		1			

* The case was already reported by the District Health Servicies
** Strm: Streamlet; Riv: River; Fount: Fountain; TapW: Tap water

Table 3. The diarrhea case detection at 27 villages along the Road No. 2 in Oudomxay province during 6-8th June 1994

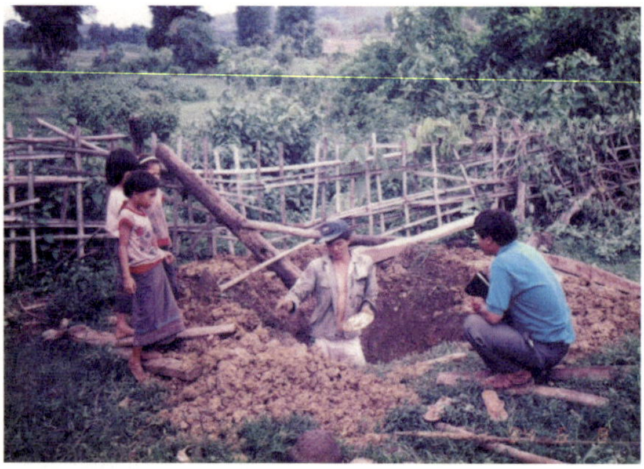

Picture 3. Making of pit for toilet

The surveillance team of GOL visited the four districts of Xai, Beng, Huon and Pak Beng in Oudomxay Province for active surveillance of cholera on June 6-8th, 1994. There were 27 villages, with a total population of 9500. There had been 1041 cholera cases in Oudomxay Province, including 44 death cases (Oudomxay Provincial Health Service, 7th June, 1994) and the epidemic was still continuing, as shown in the summary on Table 3. The surveillance was done only along the Route 2 road. There had been no reported severe diarrhea cases in Muan Namour and in Muan Xai districts. However, a total of 22 suspected cholera cases, including an infant and eight remainder cases, were confirmed in the surveillance. Most of the villagers in the areas had no toilet for disposing of or washing out the diarrheal stool. Therefore, a pit hole was made to dispose of the patient stool at each village (Pictue 3). One village, Oudom in Muan Beng district, suffered from a lack of drinking water from their fountain. Early in the dry season, this kind of water source was highly contaminated by faecal bacteria (Picture 4).

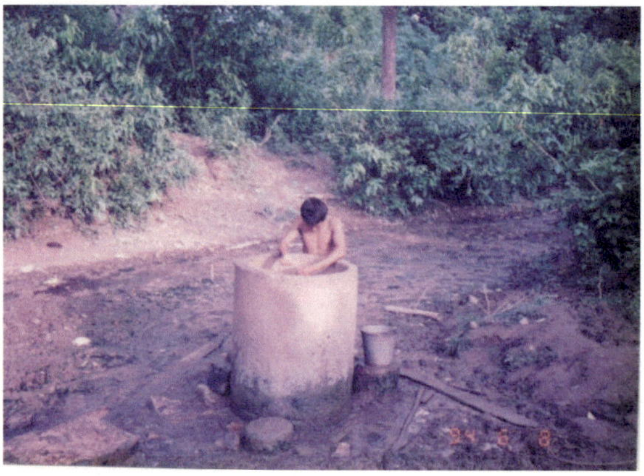

Picture 4. Well in a drying streamlet

The situation of cholera transmission in the province: Traditional customs for people preparing and taking meals together during ceremonies such as funerals was considered a factor in transmission in the province. For example, the first case found at Done Keo village in Huon district was on 16th April, 1994. This male case died with severe diarrhea on the same day as its onset, and did not come into contact with the people in epidemic areas during *Phi Mai Lao*. During his funeral ceremony, many condolence callers, including relatives in Bokeo Province, visited the village. After the ceremony, his wife and his sister got severe diarrhea within a few days. After that, the diarrhea became prevalent among the villagers. We consider this kind of transmission as similar to food poisoning and it was a factor in spreading cholera from one place to another in the province. Such cases caused by cholera-contaminated foods have been reported in Africa (Lous et al., 1990). In this surveillance, we happened to observe a funeral ceremony (Picture 5, right) at Sam Kang village in Beng district on 8th June 1994. The ceremony, which involved the sacrifice of a cow, started on 6th June and participants still cooked the cow meat to eat together in front of the house of the dead patient (Picture 5, left).

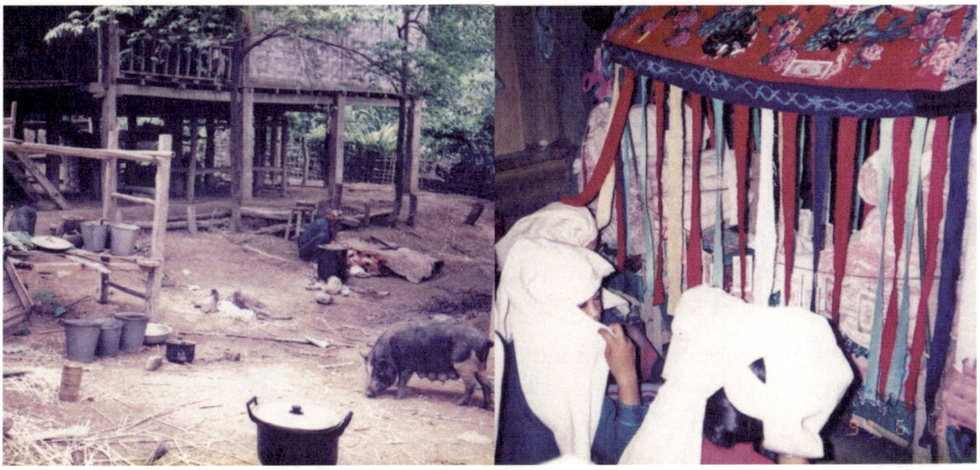

Picture 5. Meal preparation (left) and the funeral of a Thai Dam villager (right).

The people of Laos, in particular, have a custom of eating raw food materials. Our observations suggested that the transmission of cholera among people in local areas depended much on cooking meals using unsafe water and on the custom of eating them using fingers at the ceremony. It is well known that a cholera bacterium can easily be disinfected by boiling, dryness, ultraviolet rays, alcohol, acid (Mata *et al.*, 1994), and other means. Thus, clean food handling, sufficient cooking, and drying by sunlight for tableware, clothing, etc., are essential precautions against cholera. In particular, careful washing of hands with soap and clean water is essential before food handling. If no soap or clean water is available, hand-washing using the local alcohol *Lao-Lao* (ca.30%) or the juice of a local lime fruit (pH 4.2) called *maknao* (*Citrus aurantifolia*) is strongly recommended for disinfection of cholera vibrios. Although this recommendation was not introduced to the people, it seems that these methods are still useful to people in the local areas in Laos.

The actual transmission route of the cholera outbreak in northern provinces such as Bokeo is still quite obscure, but according to official provincial records, the first case might have occurred on 6th March 1994, before Phi Mai Lao. In Nale district, Luangnamtha Province, the first case was reported on 12th April, 1994, suggesting that quick diffusion and the spread of cholera was transmitted along the travel routes and waterways of rivers within the northern mountainous areas among Bokeo, Oudomxay and Luangnamtha provinces within April. Interestingly, there were nine cholera cases reported in Chiang Seng in

Thailand on 16th April, 1994 (information of the national cholera control committee meeting in 1994). The northern part of Laos is an important site of traffic with neighbouring countries of Thailand, Burma, China and Vietnam. Monitoring and comparing the molecular biological characteristics of the epidemic strains including NAG vibrios recovered from these areas will give useful information on controls beyond the border.

In the following section, the characteristics of the NAG vibrios recovered in Lao PDR is introduced.

4. Characteristics of NAG *V. cholerae* in Lao PDR

Some strains of NAG *V. cholerae* are a pathogen responsible for sporadic diarrhea in developing countries (WHO Weekly Epidemiological Record, 1993). The serogroup of O139 is the most widely known and studied since 1993 (Ramamurthy *et al.*, 1993; Albert MJ., 1993). However, another NAG *V. cholerae* has been frequently mentioned as the causative of diarrhea in the last two decades, and is now known as enteropathogenic *V. cholerae* (Sharma, C. *et al.* 1998). To date, 200 or more *V. cholerae* serogroups have been reported, and, in particular, future epidemics of CT producing O141 strains are cause for alert (Yamai S. *et al*, 1997). Taylor, D.N. *et al* mention that NAG *V. cholerae* was frequently isolated from food and drinking water among the H'mong refugees in camps in Thailand. Despite the importance of NAG *V. cholerae* as a diarrheal cause in Lao PDR, little information on the organism was available up to now.

We report here on the serogroups and tentative results of molecular patterns of the non-O1 non-O139 strains of *V. cholerae* isolated from two areas in Lao P.D.R. during two years from 1995 to 1996.

Isolation and identification: Isolation of these Vibrio strains was carried out at the NIHE, Ministry of Health in Vientiane, Lao P.D.R. These isolates were further classified serologically with monospecific sera at the Department of Bacteriology, National Institute of Infectious Disease (NIID) in Tokyo, Japan.

PFGE: For the pulsed-field gel electrophoresis (PFGE) study, 17 strains of *V. cholerae* were classified. These included reference strains of *V. cholerae* such as the O1 classical biotype (strain 569B), O37 (African strain S7: Yamamoto *et al.*, 1986) and non-typed one (strain BDD), isolated from Ban Don Daen, Khon Kaen, Thailand, respectively. *Vibrio fluvialis* O11 isolated from a diarrhea patient caused by NAG vibrio in Vientiane Capital in 1995 was also analysed as an additional reference. The genomic DNAs of the various strains were prepared in agarose plugs following the technique described by Bag P.K. *et al.* (1998). For digestion of the DNAs, 40U of *Not* I was used. PFGE of the digested plug inserts was performed by the contour-clamped homogeneous electric field method on a CHEF Mapper TM system (Bio-Rad, CA., USA) in 0.5 x TBE buffer for 40 hours 24 minutes while maintaining the temperature of the buffer at 14C. Run conditions were generated by the auto-algorithm mode of the system using a size range of 20 kb to 300 kb. A bacteriophage λ ladder (Bio-Rad) was used as the DNA molecular mass standard. The gels were stained with ethidium bromide and photographed under UV light.

PCR assay and CT production assay: A PCR-based assay was used to determine whether the *ctx*, and NAG specific heat-stable toxin (ST) were present. CT production was confirmed with RPLA commercially purchased (Denka-Seiken, Japan). The test was performed at the Department of Bacteriology, NIID, Japan.

A total of 16 strains were isolated from two areas in Laos (Table 4). Among them, three strains were isolated from 533 specimens obtained by the first national cholera carrier survey at four villages in Toum Laan district, Saravane province in the southern part of the country, where a cholera epidemic occurred in May, 1994 (Midorikawa *et al.*, 1996). The details of these specimens are: 468 human stools, 14 domestic animal stools, 50 drinking water samples, and 1 sewage sample at Hon Laon. These specimens were bacteriologically analyzed at NIHE in Vientiane. They included two strains of O68 and one strain of O14. Of the other 13 samples, 6 strains were isolated from 410 healthy persons who were examined after two months of the cholera epidemic at Ban Phailom in Xaithani district in Vientiane Capital on 12th December 1995, and 7 strains were isolated from 18 human diarrhea patients at a small village named Ban Lack Sao-et (meaning "21 Km village" in Laotian) located approximately 2 km from Ban Phailom in the same capital area of the country. There were variable serogroups among the isolates including O16, O21, O41, O43, and O68 at Ban Phailom, and 6 isolates of O169 and an O11 at Ban Lack Sao-et.

In the latter village, the health department of Vientiane Capital reported that 28 sporadic diarrhea cases found on 28th December 1995 were considered to be cholera. The diarrhea must have been caused by food poisoning, namely the consumption of a rice noodle call "*Khao Poun*", during a period from 16:00 to 21:00 on that day. Eleven severe cases were immediately referred to Sethathilath hospital in Vientiane. Among them, a strain of *V. fluvialis* O11 was isolated from a patient along with V. cholerae O169, and two strains of enteropathogenic *E coli* (EPEC) O159 were also co-isolated with *V. cholerae* O169 from each patient. Excluding three cases referred to but with unknown names, the age distribution was 2 children under 5 years of age, 8 between 6 to 15 years, 7 over 16 years and 1 of unknown age, respectively. Fortunately, no fatal cases were reported in this episode.

Organisms	O serogroup	Number	Source	Locality	Year
V. cholerae	O169	6	Diarrhoea stools	Vientiane	1995
V. cholerae	O11	1	Diarrhoea stool	Vientiane	1995
V. cholerae	O68	1	Normal stool	Vientiane	1995
V. cholerae	O43	1	Normal stool	Vientiane	1995
V. cholerae	O41	2	Normal stool	Vientiane	1995
V. cholerae	O21	1	Normal stool	Vientiane	1995
V. cholerae	O16	1	Normal stool	Vientiane	1995
V. cholerae	O68	2	Normal stools	Salavane	1996
V. cholerae	O14	1	Normal stool	Salavane	1996

Table 4. *Vibrio cholerae* non-O1 non-O139 strains isolated from humans in Lao P.D.R.

The representative patterns of *Not* I-digested PFGE of non-O1 non-139 *V. cholerae* strains isolated from Ban Lack Sao-et are shown in Figure 5. Of the O169 strains (lane no. 2 to 3, 5 to 7 and 9), their patterns were altogether identical except in one strain (lane 7). Other NAG Vibrio cholerae O11 (lane 4), and O21 (lane 10) were different from each other. The rest of the lanes 1, 8, 11 were V. cholera O37 (S'), V. fluvialis O11, and V. cholerae O1 (569B), respectively as reference strains.

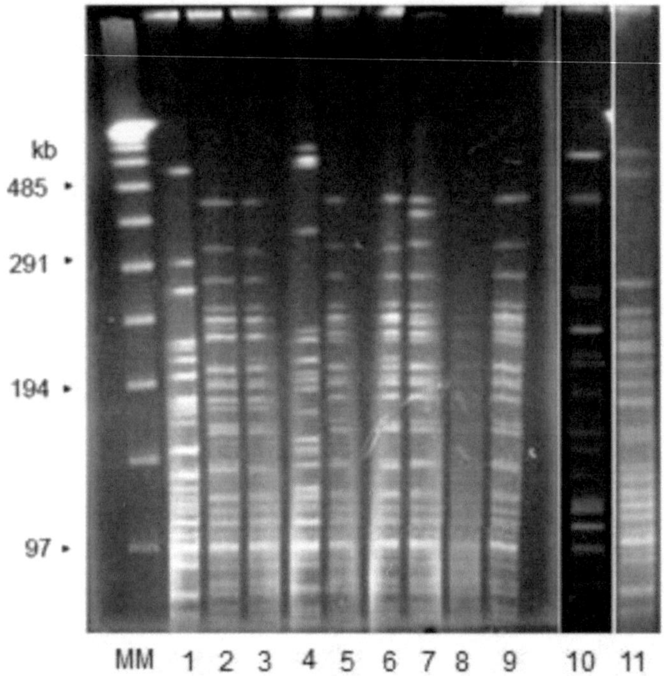

V. cholera O11:lane 4, O14:lane12, O16:lane 11, O21:lane 10, O41:lanes 13-14,O68:lanes 15-17, O169:lanes 2-3;5-7;9, *V. cholerae* BDD (Thailand):lane18, *V. cholerae* S7 (Africa):lane 1, *V.fluvialis* O11:lane 8

Fig. 5. PFGEF profiles of NAG *Vibrio cholera* strains obtained with *Not*I enzyme.

The 16 NAG *V. cholerae* strains examined had neither the cholera toxin gene nor the heat stable toxin gene. No CT producing strains were observed among them. These results may reveal that the varied strains isolated from Ban Phailom were irrelevant to the last epidemic of *V. cholera*e O1 (Nakamura S. and Marui E., 2000). However, distinct diarrhea cases were present at Ban Lack Sao-et (21 Km village) and their major isolates were *V. cholerae* O169, which had genetic homogeneity with that of the endemic strain, suggesting that the strain was a possible endemic pathogen of diarrhea in this area. Pathogen related gene (*tcp, zot, ace,* and others) and toxin assays other than CT and the ST were not yet performed. Whether some serogroups of the enteropathogenic *V. cholerae* would cause diarrhea by a mechanism quite different from that of toxin producing *V. cholerae* O1 and O139 has not been demonstrated yet (Sharma, C. *et al.* 1998). Further analyses are necessary to clarify the relationship between genomic patterns and the pathogenicity or drug susceptibility of these *V. cholerae* O169 strains as a possible enteric pathogen in this region.

Very recently, a death case caused by the serogroup of *Vibrio cholera* O21 was reported (Phethsouvanh *et al.*, 2008). This sepsis case was caused by eating a snail obtained in a swamp in the suburbs of Vientiane. For this reason, when this group was analyzed, it became clear that the serogroup has unique variation in *ompW* domain, which was named 'ompW_O21' by Nakatsu *et al.* (AB441168, GenBank, 2008). Moreover, since this strain entirely lacked the flagellum, unlike the others of O21 group included in this report, it was thought that the strain has variations in the domain of major flagellin regulation gene *fla*A (Klose KE and Mekalanos JJ, 1998). This DNA fragment related to OmpW_21 was recovered from rivers in several places in Laos, and the fragment was also reported from tap water in the United States of America (Dross, M.C. et al.; FJ462454, GenBank, 2008). Hence, it seems that the fragment might be widely distributed over environmental water, and analysis has advanced further now.

It seems that there is a strong possibility that NAG of this country will serve as a pool of the SXT constin gene of O1 O139 *V. cholerae*. Although the place where NAG and O1 O139 *V. cholerae* in epidemics meet includes the possibility of biofilm on an animal or in nature, the most probable place is the human alimentary canal. It is necessary to advance analysis further with regard to pathogenicity about the possibility that strains of specific NAG and other *Vibrionaceae* bacteria are potential reservoirs of the drug resistance gene or of the pathogenic gene cassette as transposons.

It is reported that NAG *V. cholerae* strains are frequently separated from market foods such as meat and fish, as well as environmental water in Vientiane Capital (Nakamura *et al.*, 2004, Midorikawa *et al.*, 2007). Therefore, food and water source surveillance on the vibrios and their pathogen related laboratory monitoring are indispensable to health care administration in Lao PDR, which will be shown in the next section.

5. Food market and environmental water monitoring for contaminant vibrios

5.1 Observation of contamination of food by *Vibrionaceae* bacteria in the major food markets in Vientiane Capital from 2004 to 2009

In Lao PDR, the prevalence of water-borne diseases, like diarrhea, is still very high (Midorikawa *et al.*, 1996; Rattanaphone *et al*, 1999). Recently, market food cross contamination by *Salmonella* and *Vibrio* species (vibrios) was reported (Nakamura *et al.*2004; Sano *et al*, 2004). Large cities such as Vientiane Capital and their surrounding areas, where people's life-style has changed rapidly, are facing the risk of environmental pollution, particularly with regard to drinking water and food. The aim of this research is to know the degree of contamination by vibrios on around 30 kinds of foods at the marketplace by monitoring food hygiene and to present an update of the possible diarrheal disease risk by using these results in the capital area. This small scale cross-sectional survey has been made by us from 1999 to the present. We presented a part of the study up to 2003 (Nakamura *et al.*, 2004); also, in 2008 the analysis between some *Aeromonas* species and *V. cholerae* was not performed, and therefore we report here mainly on the results of 5 years from 2004 to 2007 and 2009.

Study site and date: The food sampling survey was conducted at two major market places in the city area in Vientiane Capital, Lao PDR. The surveys were conducted once a year, in December 2004, and in September 2005, 2006, 2007, and 2009, respectively.

Sampling of food: Objective foods of various kinds were categorized as follows: domestic animal meats (beef, water buffalo, pork, chicken, duck, and domestic fowl eggs), fresh water products (fresh water fish and shellfish), marine products (marine fish and shellfish), and others (frog and/or insect), sold at the marketplaces.

Equipment for sampling: In collection of food specimens, "Fuki-Fuki test kit" (EIKEN Kagaku, Tokyo) and "Seed-swab No.1" (EIKEN Kagaku, Tokyo) of the monitoring and transport media for food-borne bacteria were used. The surfaces of food samples were wiped with this equipment.

Isolation and identification of the bacteria: The cotton part of Fuki-Fuki test kit sample and Seed-swab or Cary-Blair kit was applied to peptone water for growth culture media, and subsequently TCBS medium was employed for selective culture of vibrios at 37C for 24 hours. Colonies on the selective medium were screened with classical *InVic* system (Phetsouvanh *et al.* 1999) and the suspected bacteria were identified with commercial identification kits such as API 20e system (bioMerieux, Tokyo, Japan). Identification of the family *Vibrionaceae* was performed using the criteria of the multiply in 0% and 7% saline broths for halophilic species, string test using 0.5% solution of sodium deoxycholate in saline added (Keast & Riley, 1997), and O129 disk susceptibility for differentiate of genus *Vibrio* and *Aeromonas*. O-antigen serotype of identified *V. cholerae* strains were determined further using diagnostic anti-O1 and anti-O139 antisera (DENKA Seiken, Tokyo).

Observation of bacterial contamination in the market foods in 2004-2009: Excepting the results of the year 2008, a total of 166 food items were examined during six years from 2004 to 2009. Suspected food poisoning *Vibrionaceae* species contamination was widely confirmed on the surface of food of animal origin (Table 5). *Aeromonas* spp including *Ae. hydrophila, Ae. sobria* detected from 68 items was the most prevalent except among marine fish. NAG *V. cholerae* strains confirmed in 50 food items was the next most prevalent. Among these, 26 (52%) were confirmed in the meat of domestic animals, such as cattle and pork. Moreover, contamination by the other vibrios including *V. parahaemolyticus* was commonly detected in the same category. In particular, the recovery of *V. parahaemolyticus* and other halophile vibrios from freshwater fish is uncommon in developed countries and suggests that some cross contamination reported by us is still frequent in the markets (Nakamura *et al.*, 2004).

There are still insufficient regulations within food laws regarding food handling in the markets of Laos. It is still observed that the degree of cleanliness and the state of order change greatly according to each retailer's counter. Moreover, changes in collection time and sampling place also greatly influence these kinds of investigative results.

Food Item	Number of items examined	Number of item found of Bacteria of Vibrionaceae (%)			
		non-O1, non-O139 *V. cholerae*	*V. parahaemolyticus*	Other *Vibrio* spp.	*Aeromonas* spp.
Cattle	25	7 (28) *	2 (8) *	3 (12) *	11 (44)
Buffalo	7	2 (28.5) *	0	2 (28.5) *	1 (14.2)
Pork	33	7 (21.2) *	1 (3) *	8 (24.2) *	12 (36.3)
Chicken	23	8 (34.7) *	0	9 (39.1) *	8 (34.7) *
Duck or other poultry	9	2 (22.2)	0	2 (22.2)	3 (33.3) #
Fish	51	18 (35.2) #	2 (4) *	8 (15.6) *	26 (50.9) #
Shellfish	7	4 (57.1)	1 (14.2)	1 (14.2)	4 (57.1)
Marine fish	5	1 (20) #	0	1 (20) #	0
Marine shellfish	4	1 (25) #	2 (50)	2 (50) #	3 (75)
Others (Insect & frog)	2	0	0	2 (100)	0
Total	166	50 (30.1)	8 (4.8)	38 (22.8)	68 (40.9)

* Common contamination
# Uncommon contamination

Table 5. Number of food items found containing *Vibrionaceae* species in the major markets in Vientiane Capital during years from 2004 to 2007, and 2009

O antigen typing and analysis of diarrheagenic toxins of these NAG *V. cholerae* have not yet been performed; however, the possible risk of severe diarrheal outbreaks was evident, as mentioned in section 4 of this chapter.

The detection rate of the food items contaminated with bacteria of *Vibrionaceae* among small size sampled food items at two major markets in Vientiane Capital from 1999 to 2009 is shown in Figure 6. Due to the sample size, and variability within the sampling place, a direct comparison of each set of annual data is difficult; however, the results in 2004 and afterwards are reviewed here. The detection rate of food contaminated by NAG *V. cholerae* varied widely from 0 (December 2004) to 64% (2009). However there was a tendency of decreasing rates from 57% to 19% during the years from 2005 to 2007. According to Disease Statistics of Laos in 1999-2002, many food poisoning cases occurred from April to May, and the case occurrence was lowest in September (Anonymous: statistics, 2003). Since most of our investigations were conducted in September, it is necessary to similarly investigate in April and May when food poisoning occurs frequently, and to grasp the actual conditions of *V. cholerae* contamination among the foods. In addition, a more advanced investigation should also be performed on rats, flies, and sewage which are all regarded as reservoirs in the marketplaces.

In investigations into enteropathogenic bacteria carriers among residents in the year 2005 in the suburb of Vientiane, a carrier of *V. cholerae* (1.5%) was detected among 63 healthy volunteers. In the same investigation, Nakamura *et al.*, (2005) confirmed that some of the Salmonella recovered from humans and market foods in the capital city showed common DNA restriction patterns. It must be emphasized that the tendency towards frequent detection of NAG *V. cholerae* from livestock meats in the marketplaces of Vientiane will be a potential risk of diarrheal outbreak.

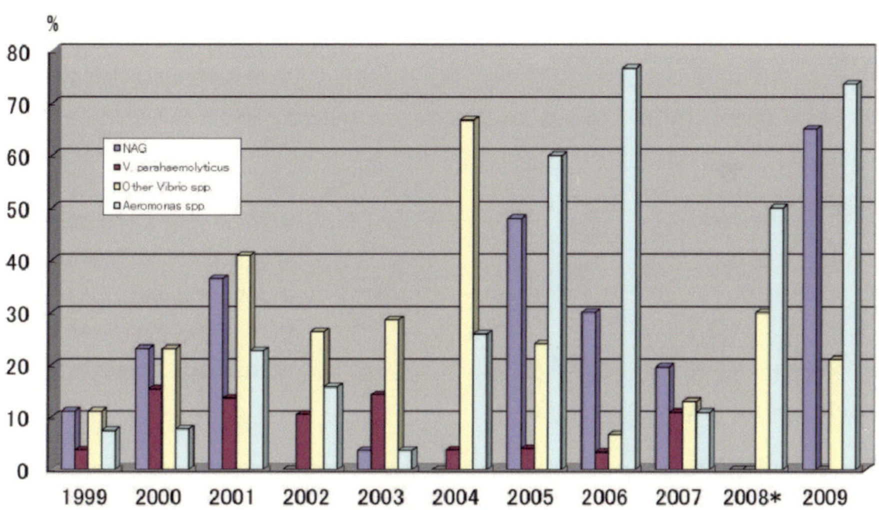

Fig. 6. Percent recovery of *Vibrionaceae* species from the foods at the two major markets in Vientiane Capital, Lao PDR. from 1999 to 2009

5.2 Environmental water monitoring on contaminant vibrios

The population density of the country is very low and it has maintained abundant water in its rivers with dense forest covering its mountainous areas. However, access to safe water is very limited among the 70% of the population living in the countryside, and risks have been pointed out about infections caused by environmental water consumption. Although the tackling of water-borne infections such as severe diarrhea among children has been an important subject for attaining MDGs of the country, there is little research in connection with actual risk, with the exception of a few study reports. In particular, research on the actual conditions of the pathogenic organisms in the country's water cannot be found. Hence, continuous monitoring research which targets vibrios and amoeba of enteropathogenic importance was conducted to clarify distribution of these pathogenic organisms in the country.

Study area, monitoring point, sampling and the detection methods during years 2006, 2009-2011: The investigation was conducted from Vientiane to Attapeu along the catchment of the Mekong (Figure 7). Collecting river water samples of the Mekong and its branches was conducted mostly at fixed locations which cross the major national road No. 16 during the year 2006 and years 2009-2010. The water sampling along the Nam Som River and from lake water was performed in Vang Vieng district, Vientiane Province and in Khammouane Province, respectively, in 2011.

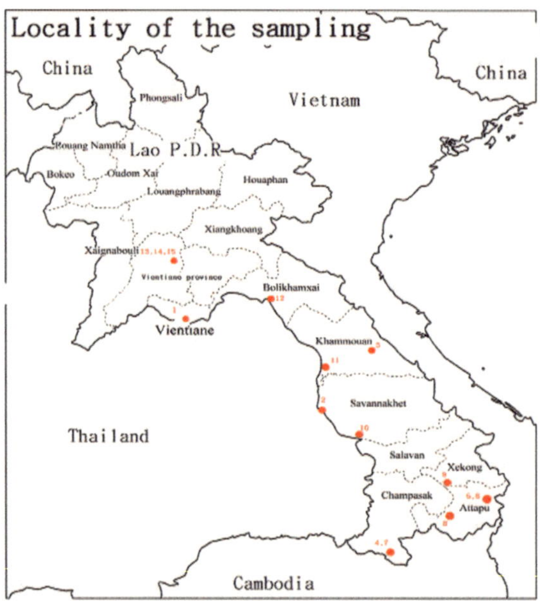

No.	**Locality by GPS**
1	N17.58.33.96, E102.38.54.70
2	N16.33.34.9, E104.45.07.4
3	N17.41.23.4, E105.13.24.7
4	N14.6.55.12, E105.51.18.65
5	-
6	N14.48.05.2, E106.50.03.8
7	N14.5.29.33, E105.50.31.29
8	N14.48.4.77, E106.50.6.86
9	N15.13.39.24, E106.44.41.18
10	N16.5.56.14, E105.22.31.01
11	N17.23.39.52, E104.48.12.05
12	N18.19.24.59, E103.59.53.02
13	N19.06.39.9, E102.22.21.3
14	N18.54.39.8, E102.26.34.0
15	N18.54.34.21, E102.26.34.74

Fig. 7. Locality of the water sampling.

Water sample collection was performed with a sterile plastic container. Before collecting the sample, a conventional on-site coliform test using filter-paper (Sancoli, Tokyo, Japan) was conducted. In 2006, 20L of the raw water was condensed by DEAE to adsorb the microbes and about 1/200 of the volume was analyzed by PCR. During years 2009-2010, about 50 ml of the sample was collected to detect the target organisms by PCR. Common bacterial culture using TCBS (Eiken Kagaku, Tokyo, Japan) and DHL (Eiken Kagaku, Tokyo, Japan) media was also performed to detect vibrios and related enteropathogens as described in section II, except in 2006. Identification of bacteria was performed by API 20e system (BioMerieu, France). PCR analysis of a cultured sample using 10 ml of peptone water was also performed in 2011. All the samples were kept in cool and/or freezing conditions before analysis. PCR test for detection of the target organisms was as follows: DNA extraction from the water sample was performed on both the centrifuged pellet and the supernatant using commercial extraction kits. Target regions of PCR on *V. cholerae,* and *Entamoeba histolytica* and *E. dispar* were ompW (Nandy *et al.* 2000, Nakatsu *et al.* 2008) and mitochondorial rDNA 18s regions with the primers newly designed by us, respectively. The PCR tests were validated using a laboratory strain of *V. cholerae* 569B and both cultured strains of *E. histolytica* and *E. dispar* were used as controls. Nested-PCRs were performed in a DNA thermal cycler with initial denaturation at 95C for 5min, followed by 35 cycles of denaturation at 95C for 30sec, annealing at 55C for 30sec, extension at 72C for 45sec and a final elongation at 72C for 7min. Commercially-based sequencing of PCR products was also obtained to confirm homology analysis using DNA databases.

Results of PCR test for *V. cholerae, E. histolytica* and *E. dispar*: 25 water samples were collected from 15 sampling locations. The details are shown in Table 7. Although *V. cholerae* was detected in two locations, it was detected by the second PCR. Since these did not have a ctx gene, they were judged to be NAG vibrios. One of these strains was previously detected from three samplings of the Pa River at Xansay district, Attapeu province (Midorikawa *et al.*, 2010). The DNA sequence of this ompW was homologue to *V. cholerae* O21, which we reported (GenBank: AB441168). Although this sequence differed from the common one of Nandi *et al.*, (2000) it was reported also from the United States and detected even in Cambodia (Nakatsu *et al*, unpublished data). We have not detected corresponding NAG vibrios yet; however, it was thought that this DNA motif might be found widely over countries. Another was detected from the sample of the Pa Hom River in Vang Vieng, Vientiane province. This amplified DNA sequence was judged to be the usual NAG vibrios by the control and its DNA homology.

No.	Sample volume (ml)	Place/Locality of the sampling	Water	*E. histolytica*	*E. dispar*	*V. cholerae*
1	50-20000*	That Luang Swamp/Vientiane Capital	Sewage	-	(3/4)	-
2	20000*	Sewege ditch/Savannakhet	Sewage	-	-	-
3	50**	Namteun Lake/Khammouane	Lake	-	-	-
4	45	Guest house of Khong Island/Champasak	Public tap	-	-	-
5	45	Public Tube-well/Attapeu	Tube-well	(1/1)	-	-
6	50-20000*	Pa River/Attapeu	River	(1/3)	(1/3)	(1/3)
7	10-50	Mekong port of Khong Island/Champasak	River	-	(1/3)	-
8	50-20000*	Xe Kone / Attapeu	River	-	(1/3)	-
9	45	Xe Namnoi /Xekone	River	-	(1/1)	-
10	45	Xe Banhieng /Savannakhet	River	-	(1/1)	-
11	45-50	Mekhong /Khammouane	River	-	(2/2)	-
12	45	Nam Khading /Bolikhamxay	River	-	(2/2)	-
13	50**	Pa Hom River of Vangvieng/Vientiane Province	River	-	-	(1/1)
14	50**	Nam Som River of Vangvieng/Vientiane Province	River	-	-	-
15	1***	Nam Tam Chan of Vangvieng/Vientiane Province	River	-	-	-

* Concentrated sample by the method of adding DEAE (Yano et al 1993) to raw water was used for analysis.

** 10ml of the sample cultured with 1% of peptone water medium in 37C for overnight was also examined.

*** A filter paper sample containing 1 ml of the water cultured at 10 ml of 1% of peptone water in 37C overnight was used for the analysis.

Table 6. Frequency of PCR detection on en tamoeba and cholera vibrios in drinking water in Lao PRD

E. hystolytica which has pathogenicity in its genus was found only from the source of drinking water at Xansay district, Attapeu province. On the other hand, *E. dispar* was widely distributed over the rivers in the country. In particular, in this species, frequently detected in the sewers of Vientiane, it was thought that high-level fecal contamination of this water area was demonstrated.

Bacterial detection from sampled waters: Coliform bacteria was positive in all the samples except for the sample of well water from Xansay district, Attapeu province, and the tap water of Khong Island, Champasak province. 60 bacteria stocks were recovered from the samples through this research. A tentative classification of the strains was as follows: Enterobacteriaceae including *E. coli*, *Vibrionaceae* excluding cholera vibrios, and others such as *Pseudomonas* spp. were 42, 14, and 4, respectively. The major strains of this *Vibrionaceae* were *Aeromonas hydrophila*. No cholera vibrio was confirmed in this study.

In this study it is demonstrated that NAG vibrios and two species of *Entamoeba* were genetically confirmed in water for the first time in Lao PDR.

6. Conclusion

Details of the cholera epidemic from 1993-1996 in Laos which were previously unknown have now been brought to light through records and, in particular, cases in remote mountainous areas. As a result, we now know that the cholera strain primarily responsible for the outbreak was *Vibrio cholera* O1, serotype Ogawa, biotype El Tor.

The existence of other NAG vibrios was also confirmed through research during that period, with the exception of 0139, the cause of Bengal cholera. Furthermore, it was discovered that among these vibrio bacteria, there were some strains such as O169 and O21 with a likelihood of diarrheal pathogenisis. Also, from investigations in recent years, NAG vibrios were identified over an extended period of time as contaminant strains in food available in markets in towns and cities, as well as in the water environment at a molecular level.

The NAG strains within Laos may cause new occurrences of cholera outbreaks in the future and become vehicles for drug-resistance transposons. Continued surveillance and coordinated research among neighboring countries is required to enable further surveys and studies on human and animal hosts, sewage and leftover water and food at markets.

Needless to say, water and sewer service infrastructure is of vital importance in long-term prevention of diarrhea including cholera (Watanabe *et al.*, 2006). Laos has already experienced cholera epidemics. As for the prospect of prevention in the future, improvements can be seen in the habitat and infrastructure within Laos following rapid improvements in the country's economic conditions in recent years. In particular, the mountainous areas where fatality rates were high during the epidemic period from 1993-96 have been designated as focus regions in the implementation of poverty countermeasures as part of the 7th National Socio-Economic Development Plan (NSEDP) for 2011-2015. Improvements are anticipated in the installation of clean water facilities following dam construction, as well as in transportation, communication, medical care, living conditions and educational attainment. Furthermore, by training people as qualified medical technicians and introducing them to these regions, the overall standards of PHC policy implementation will be raised and consequently disease countermeasures should be considerably improved.

However, in relation to citizens' hygiene education, differences in language culture lead to problems in communicating and understanding information and knowledge on practical disease prevention. In order to effectively promote hygiene education, we recommend the proactive introduction and utilization of IEC computer terminals making full use of information technology (IT). In addition, the introduction of a cholera vaccine for Laos will require further improvements in relevant areas, such as establishing the logistics of EPI disease monitoring specimens, creating new regional laboratories and strengthening coordination between existing regional labs and the central lab in, for example, medical technology training, together with improvements in information technology.

7. Acknowledgements

We would like to express thanks to villagers and staff of health centres and hospitals of Nale district in Luangnamtha and of the surveyed districts in Oudomxay Province. We are thankful to Professor Boungnong Boupha, Professor Sithat Insisiengmay, Professor Michel Strobel, and Professor Masaaki Iwanaga who supported for the research in Lao PDR. We are grateful for the technical assistance provided by Mr. Lay Sisavath, and Mr. Khampheuy Mummalath, Dr. Kanpheng Choumlasack, Mr. Trykhouane Phoutavane, and Dr. Noy Khaseumsy at the Bacteriology Unit of the National Centre of Laboratory and Epidemiology, Vientiane. We also express thanks to Drs. Toshio Shimada and Eiji Arakawa of the National Institute of Infectious Diseases for identification of O antigen typing of NAG *V. cholerae* and their NAG ST assay by PCR, and to Dr. Paul Newton for his critical review of section 4. We express sincere thanks to Dr. Khamthan for help in performing the water-food sampling in the natural environment and the markets in Vientiane Capital. Special thanks are due to Drs. Lianne Kuppens, and Richard Nesbit, WHO Officers, for their help in active surveillance and for providing epidemic information, and to Prof Khammouliene Pholsena, former Director of the National Centre of Malariology, Parasitology and Entomology for providing national cholera information and the direction of the surveillance during 1993-1996.

This work was supported by a Grant-in-Aid from the Ministry of Education, Science, Culture and Sports of Japan (MEXT) in the project entitled "International Cooperation Research concerning water-borne diseases in relocated people and the development of related risk management techniques" (No. 22256003), by MEXT in the project entitled "Sustainable Co-existence of Human, Nature and the Earth" under Research Revolution 2002 (Prof. Tatsuo Omura), and by MEXT in the project entitled "A Transdisciplinary Study on the Regional Eco-History in Tropical Monsoon Asia: 1945-2005, under Research Institute for Humanity and Nature (Prof. Tomoya Akimichi).

8. References

Albert MJ, Siddique AK, Islam MS, Faruque AS, Ansaruzzaman M, Faruque SM, Sack RB. Large outbreak of clinical cholera due to Vibrio cholerae non-O1 in Bangladesh. Lancet. 1993 Mar 13;341(8846):704.

Anonymous: Summarized report of surveillance on 18 symptoms/diseases classification in 2002. The National Centre of Laboratory and Epidemiology, Ministry of Health., Lao PDR, 2003

Anonymous: Epidemic diarrhoea due to Vibrio cholerae non-O1. Weekly Epidemiol Rec 1993; 68: 141-2. World Health Organization

Anonymous: Cholera epidemic control in Lao People's Democratic Republic situation report No. 3, UN Department of Humanitarian Affairs, 1995 http://reliefweb.int/node/37880

Bag PK, Maiti S, Sharma C, Ghosh A, Basu A, Mitra R, Bhattacharya SK, Nakamura S, Yamasaki S, Takeda Y and Nair GB. Rapid spread of the new clone of *Vibrio cholerae* O1 biotype El Tor in cholera endemic areas in India. Epidemiol Infect 1998; 121: 245-251

Bodhidatta L, Echeverria P, Hoge CW, Pitarangsi C, Serichantalergs O, Henprasert-Tae N, HARIKUL S and Kitpoka P. Vibrio cholerae 0139 in Thailand in 1994. Epidemiol Infect 1995; 114: 71-3.

Chongsa-nguan M, Chaicumpa W, Moolasart P, Kandhasingha P, Shimada T, Kurazono H, and Takeda Y. *Vibrio cholerae* 0139 Bengal in Bangkok. Lancet 1993; 342: 430-1.

Dalsgaard A., Forslund A, Tam NV, Vinh DS, and Cam PD. Cholera in Vietnam: Changes in genotypes and emergence of class I integron containing aminoglycoside resistance gene cassettes in *Vibrio cholerae* O1 strains isolated from 1979 to 1996.

Dalsgaard, A, Forslund A, Serichantalergs O, Sandvang D. Distribution and content of Class 1 integrons in different Vibrio cholera O-serotype strains isolated in Thailand. Antimicrobial Agents and Chemotherapy. 44 (5): 1315-1321, 2000 Thailand

Echeverria P, Hoge CW, Bodhidatta L, Serichantalergs O, Dalsgaard A, Eampokalap B, Perrault J, Pazzaglia G, O'Hanley P, English A. Molecular characterization of Vibrio cholerae 0139 isolates from Asia. Am J Trop Med Hyg 1995; 52: 124-7.

Global Task Force on Cholera Control, Cholera Country Profile: Laos. World Health Organization. 9 December 2008

Halpern, JM. Traditional medicine and the role of the phi in Laos. The Eastern Anthropologist, 16: 191-200, 1996

Hoge, CW., Bodhidatta L, Echeverria P, Deesuwan M, Kitporka P. Epidemiologic study of Vibrio cholerae O1 and O139 in Thailand: at the advancing edge of the eighth pandemic. Am J Epidemiol. 1996 Feb 1;143(3):263-8.

Iwanaga M, Toma C, Miyazato T, Insisiengmay S, Nakasone N and Ehara M: Antibiotic resistance conferred by a class I integron and SXT constin in *Vibrio cholerae* O1 strains isolated in Laos. Antimicrob. Agents Chemother. 48, 2364-2369, 2004

Kabir, S. Cholera vaccines: the current status and problems. Reviews in Medial Microbiology 2005, 16: 101-116

Keast A and Riley TV. Identification of *Vibrio* spp. with the 'string' test. Letters in Applied Microbiology 25(2), 106–108, 1997

Klose KE, Mekalanos JJ. Differential regulation of multiple flagellins in Vibrio cholerae. J Bacteriol.1998 Jan; 180(2):303-16.

Lenglet A, Khamphaphongphane B, Thebvongsa P, Vongprachanh P, Sithivong N, Chantavisouk C, Tsuyuoka R. A cholera epidemic in Sekong Province, Lao People's Democratic Republic, December 2007-January 2008. Jpn J Infect Dis. 2010 May;63(3):204-7.

Mata L, Vives M, and Vicente G. Extinction of *Vibrio cholerae* in acidic substrata: contaminated fish marinated with lime juice (ceviche). Revista de Biologica Tropical. 42, 479-485, 1994.

Midorikawa Y, Nakamura S, Iwade Y, Sugiyama A, Sisavath L, Phakhounthong R. Bacterial diarrhoea in Laos, a region where cholera was endemic. Southeast Asian J Trop Med Public Health 1996; 27: 724-727

Midorikawa Y, Midorikawa K, Phethsouvanh RP, Phoutavane T, Newton P, Boupha B, Nakamura S. Establishment of a simple method for the detection of non-typhoidal *Salmonella* serovars and its application to samples from human and foods in Lao PDR. In: Proceedings of 3rd International Symposium of Southeast Asian Water Environment, 65-71, AIT, Bangkok, Thailand, 7th, December, 2006

Midorikawa Y, Midorikawa K, Sangsomsack B, Phoutavane T, Choumlasack K, Watanabe T, Vannavong N, Habe S, Masami N, Kosaka Y, Akkhavong K, Strobel M, Boupha B, Nakamura S. Water, livelihood and health in Attapeu province in Lao PDR. Southeast Asian Studies 47(4), 478-498, 2010

Monnais-Rousselot L. Medecine et colonization L' aventure indochinoise 1860-1939. Paris, CNRS Editions, 1999

Nakamura S, Sisavath L, Midorikawa Y, Higa N, Mummalath K, Sithivong N, Khampheng, Sisoulath P, Phanthouamath B and Insisengmay S. Epidemic features and characterization of *Vibrio cholerae* O1 in Lao P.D.R. 14th International Congress for Tropical Medicine and Malaria, Nagasaki, Japan. November, 1996

Nakamura S and Marui E. *Korera taisaku jirei wo tsuujite mita Raosu no kannsennsho yobou gyousei no ichi sokumen.* [An aspect of health administration on epidemic control in Laos: Case study of cholera epidemic in remote area and central area.] *Ryukyu-daigaku Igakukai-shi* [Ryukyu Med J], 2000; 19: 155-158

Nakamura S, Midorikawa Y, Midorikawa K, Sano K, Bouopha B. Distribution of food-borne bacteria in Lao People's Democratic Republic: frequent observations at market places in Vientiane City. Forum 8, Mexico City, 2004, www.globalforumhealth.org/Forum8/Forum8-CDROM/Posters.html

Nakamura S. *Raosu no yakuzai taisei korera to wakuchin kouka ni kannsuru ekigaku kenkyu.* [Epidemiological study on drug resistant strains of cholera, and vaccine efficacy on cholera in Lao PDR.] *Heisei 16 nendo Kousei-roudou sho kokusaiiryou kyouryoku kennkyu itaku hi kenkyu houkokusho.* [Proceedings of the international cooperation study of grant-in-aid of Ministry of Health, Labor and Welfare in Japan in 2003], 301-307, 2004

Nakamura S, Midorikawa Y, Sugiyama A, Akachi S, Midorikawa K, Khampheng C, Phouthavane T, Sano K, Shioda C, Ishikawa S, Kurokura H, and Boupha B. Study on enteropathogenic bacteria in Lao PDR. - Recent observation on human and foods at Vientiane capital area- In: 2nd International Symposium on the Development of Water Resource Management System in Mekong Watershed, 92-96, AIT Conference Center, Bangkok, Thailand, December 7th, 2005

Nakamura S, Ajisaka T, Fujita Y, Midorikawa Y, Habe S, Akimichi T, Takenaka C, and Tomokawa S. *Shoku, Mizu, Shintai* [Food, Water, and Body], *Asia monsoon no seitai-shi.* In: Akimichi T ed. "Eco-history of Asia monsoon vol. 3", 65-83, *Kobundo*, Tokyo, 2008. ISBN 978-4-335-52013-6

Nakamura S. *Kindai-iryo no shinto to rekishi* [Permeation and history of modern health care in Laos], *Asia monsoon no seitai-shi.* In: Daniels C ed. "Eco-history of Asia monsoon vol. 2", 229-246, *Kobundo*, Tokyo, 2008. ISBN 978-4-335-52012-9

Nandi B, Nandy RK, Mukhopadhyay S, Nair GB, Shimada T, Ghose AC. Rapid method for species-specific identification of Vibrio cholerae using primers targeted to the gene of outer membrane protein OmpW. J Clin Microbiol. 2000 Nov;38(11):4145-51.

Phetsouvanh R, Nakatsu M, Arakawa E, Davong V, Vongsouvath M, Lattana O, Moore CE, Nakamura S, and Newton PN. Fatal bacteremia due to immotile *Vibrio cholerae* serogroup O21 in Vientiane, Laos - a case report. Annals of Clinical Microbiology and Antimicrobials, 7(10), 2008. http://www.ann-clinmicrob.com/content/pdf/1476-0711-7-10.pdf

Phetsouvanh R, Midorikawa Y and Nakamura S. The seasonal variation in the microbial agents implicated in the etiology of diarrheal diseases among children in Lao People's Democratic Republic. Southeast Asian J. Trop. Med. Public Health vol. 30, 1999, pp. 319-323

Ramamurthy T, Garg S, Sharma R, et al. Emergence of novel strain of Vibrio cholerae with epidemic potential in southern and eastern India. Lancet 1993; 341: 703-4.

St. Louis ME, Porter JD, Helal A, Drame K, Hargrette-Bean N, Wells JG, and Tauxe RV. Epidemic cholera in West Africa: The role of food handling and high-risk foods. American Journal of Epidemiology. 131, 719-728, 1990

Sano, K, Nakamura S, Ishikawa S, Midorikawa Y, Phomsouvanh A and Kurokura H. Risk assessment of food-borne disease relating with marine products consumption in Vientiane, Lao P.D.R. The Second Symposium on Southeast Asian Water Environment. 2004

Sharma C, Thungapathra M, Ghosh A, Mukhopadhyay AK., Basu A, Mitra R, Basu I, Bhattacharya SK, Shimada T, Ramamurthy T, Takeda T, Yamasaki S, Takeda Y, Nair GB. Molecular analysis of non-O1, non-O139 Vibrio cholerae associated with an unusual upsurge in the incidence of cholera-like disease in Calcutta, India. J Clin Microbiol 1998; 36: 756-763

Toma C, Sisavath L, Higa N, and Iwanaga M. Characterization of *Vibrio cholerae* O1 isolated in Lao People's Democratic Republic. Jpn J. Trop Med. Hyg. 1997; 25: 85-87

Watanabe T, Miura T, Sasaki T, Nakamura S and Omura T. *Mekong ryu-iki ni okeru mizu-kyokyu sisutemu nichakumoku shita suikei-kansensho no risuku-hyoka.* [Risk evaluation for waterborne infectious diseases in the Mekong watershed considering water supply system] *Kankyo-Kogaku Kenkyu Ronbun-shu* [Environmental Engineering Research], 2006; 43: 245-254

Yamai S, Okitsu T, Shimada T, and Katube Y. Distribution of serogroups of *Vibrio cholerae* non-O1 non-O139 with specific reference to their ability to produce cholera toxin and addition of novel serogroups. *Kansenshogaku Zasshi* 1997; 10: 1037-1045

Yamamoto K, Ichinose Y, Nakasone N, Tanabe M, Nagahama M, Sakurai J, and Iwanaga M. Identity of hemolysins produced by *Vibrio cholerae* Non-O1 and *V. cholerae* O1, biotype El Tor. Infection and Immunity 1986; 51: 927-931

Part 2

Biology of *Vibrio Cholera*

4

Vibrio cholerae Flagellar Synthesis and Virulence

Anastasia R. Rugel[1,2] and Karl E. Klose[1]
[1]*South Texas Center for Emerging Infectious Diseases, Department of Biology, University of Texas at San Antonio, San Antonio, Texas*
[2]*Department of Microbiology and Immunology, University of Texas Health Science Center at San Antonio, San Antonio, Texas*
USA

1. Introduction

Vibrio cholerae is a Gram-negative bacterium with a single sheathed polar flagellum (Fig. 1.). *V. cholerae* causes the severe diarrheal disease cholera in humans when it colonizes the small intestine and expresses various virulence factors, including cholera toxin (CT) and toxin co-regulated pilus (TCP). *V. cholerae* is also a natural inhabitant of the marine environment, where it forms biofilms on chitinous surfaces. Motility contributes to both aspects of the *V. cholerae* lifecycle. The flagellum facilitates chemotactic-directed movement toward the preferred colonization site within the intestine (Camilli and Mekalanos 1995; Butler and Camilli 2004), and also contributes to biofilm formation within the environment (Watnick and Kolter 1999). *V. cholerae* strains defective for motility are less virulent than motile strains (Guentzel and Berry 1975; Freter and O'Brien 1981; Richardson 1991). As flagellar synthesis, motility, and chemotaxis have become better understood in *V. cholerae*, it has also become clear that motility is intimately integrated into all aspects of the lifestyle of this bacterium.

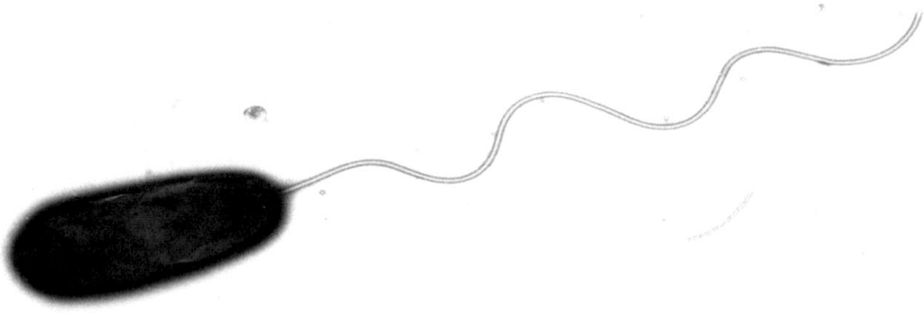

Fig. 1. Vibrio cholerae

2. Structure

The flagellum is a motor-driven organelle present in many bacteria. Different flagellar placement and quantity are seen in different bacteria. Monotrichous bacteria have a single polar flagellum (e.g. *V. cholerae*), lofotrichous bacteria have multiple flagella at a single pole (e.g. *Helicobacter pylori*), amphitrichous bacteria have flagella at two poles (e.g. *Campylobacter jejuni*), and peritrichous bacteria have multiple flagella emanating from the cell in all directions (e.g. *Escherichia coli*).

The base of the bacterial flagellum is composed of a secretion system related to the Type III secretion system, which facilitates export of flagellar components from the cytoplasm to the periplasm and the exterior of the cell. The basic components of the flagellum are the basal body, which extends from the cytoplasmic membrane through the periplasm and into the outer membrane (OM), connected to the flexible hook (composed of FliE) found exterior to the cell, which in turn is connected to the flagellar filament (Kojima and Blair 2004; Terashima, Kojima et al. 2008). The motor components that drive flagellar rotation are found in the cytoplasmic membrane, and the switch components (FliG, FliM, FliN) that interact with the chemotaxis signaling system and the motor (Francis, Sosinsky et al. 1994) extend into the cytoplasm from the basal body (Fig. 2.).

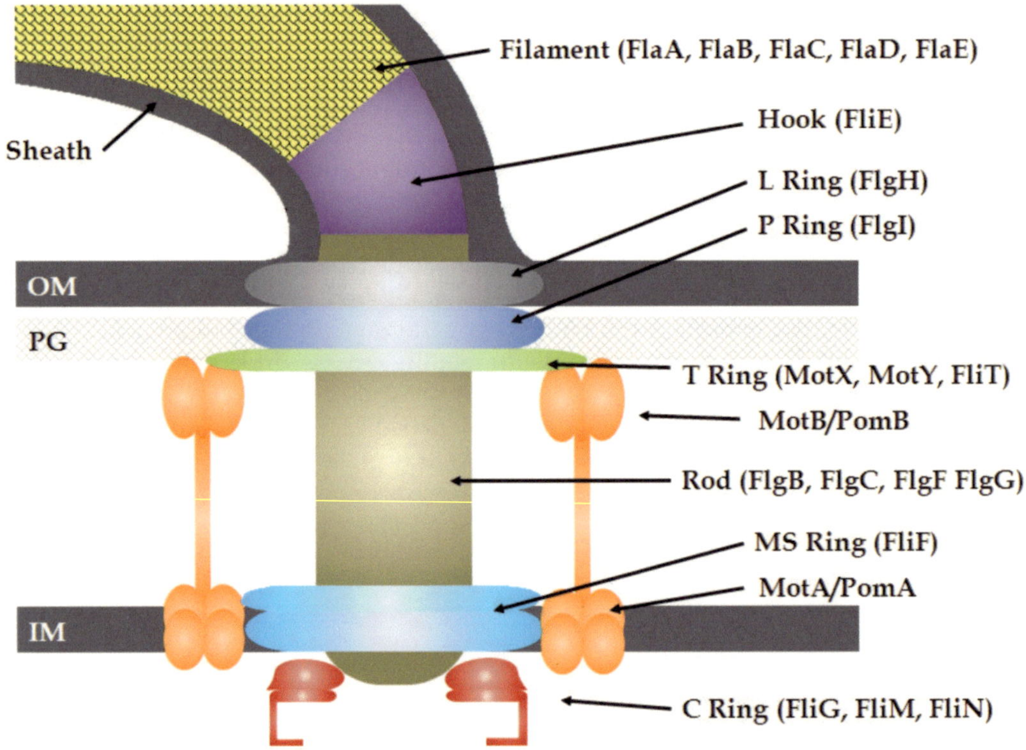

Fig. 2. Flagellar Motor Complex

Unlike most other bacterial flagella, the *V. cholerae* flagellum has a sheath composed of OM that coats the entire filament (Allen and Baumann 1971; Sjoblad, Emala et al. 1983; Fuerst and Perry 1988). Sheathed flagella are found in *Vibrio spp.* and a few other Gram-negative bacteria (e.g. *H. pylori*). It is hypothesized that the sheath acts as a protective covering that shields the antigenic flagellins from recognition by the host's immune response (Yoon and Mekalanos 2008). The mechanism whereby the OM is extended to cover the filament during

V. cholerae flagellar synthesis rather than the filament protruding through the OM as in other bacterial flagella is not understood.

The bacterial flagellar filament is made up of thousands of flagellin subunits, with a cap protein (FliD) at the distal end (Ikeda, Asakura et al. 1985; Ikeda, Homma et al. 1987; Homma, DeRosier et al. 1990). The structure of the *Salmonella typhimurium* flagellin FliC has been solved by cryomicroscopy. FliC is composed of domains at its N- and C-termini that interact with each other: D0 (aa 1-45 and 456-495), D1 (aa 46-180 and 408-455), and D2 (aa 181-190 and 285-407). The D2 domains, along with the D3 domain (aa 191-284) form the antigenic variable region that are present on the filament surface, (Yonekura, Maki-Yonekura et al. 2003). Interaction of the D0 and D1 domains allows the flagellins to polymerize under the cap (FliD) protein into a hollow helical filament at the growing tip of the flagellum as they are being secreted.

In contrast to most other bacteria which have filaments composed of a single flagellin subunit, *V. cholerae* has a filament composed of 5 different flagellins, FlaABCDE. These flagellins share a high degree of homology, yet only FlaA is essential for flagellar synthesis; the other four flagellins are not required for the synthesis of the filament (Klose and Mekalanos 1998). Alignment of FlaA with the other four *V. cholerae* flagellins, as well as with *S. typhimurium* FliC, reveals that the D0 and D1 domains are well-conserved, whereas the variable regions D2 and D3 are more divergent. Interestingly, the *V. cholerae* flagellins have a much shorter region corresponding to D2 and D3 (129 aa shorter) when compared to *S. typhimurium* FliC. Because this antigenic portion of the flagellins extends out from the hollow filament core, it may be that the presence of the flagellar sheath over the *V. cholerae* filament restricts the size of the antigenic region protruding from the filament.

The basal body contains the rod structure (FlgB, FlgC, FlgF and FlgG) with L (FlgH), P (FlgI), and MS rings (FliF) localized to the OM, periplasm (peptidoglycan), and cytoplasmic membranes, respectively. In *Vibrio* spp. an additional T ring is located immediately below the P ring, which is composed of the *Vibrio*-specific components MotX, MotY, and FlgT . The C-ring, which extends into the cytoplasm from the MS ring and is made up of FliG, FliM, and FliN, is difficult to preserve during microscopy and has not been visualized in its entirety in *Vibrio* spp.(Aizawa, Dean et al. 1985; Homma, Aizawa et al. 1987; Homma, Ohnishi et al. 1987; Homma, DeRosier et al. 1990; Homma, Kutsukake et al. 1990; Ueno, Oosawa et al. 1992; Francis, Sosinsky et al. 1994; Schoenhals and Macnab 1996; Terashima, Koike et al. 2010). The chemotaxis protein CheY relays information from the chemotaxis sensory system by binding to the C ring (FliM), causing the flagellum to switch rotation from counterclockwise to clockwise.

In *S. typhimurium* and *E. coli* MotA and MotB are membrane proteins that compose the motor that utilizes H+ motive force to drive flagellar rotation (Lloyd, Tang et al. 1996; Zhou, Lloyd et al. 1998; Zhou, Sharp et al. 1998; Braun, Poulson et al. 1999; Blair 2003). *Vibrio spp.* contain MotA and MotB homologues, alternately referred to as PomA and PomB (Dean, Macnab et al. 1984; Stader, Matsumura et al. 1986; Blair and Berg 1990; Stolz and Berg 1991; Asai, Kojima et al. 1997; Sato and Homma 2000; Sato and Homma 2000; Yorimitsu, Asai et al. 2000; Fukuoka, Yakushi et al. 2005), but they also contain *Vibrio*- specific motor proteins MotX and MotY, localized in the T ring (McCarter 1994; McCarter 1994; Okunishi, Kawagishi et al. 1996; Okabe, Yakushi et al. 2001; Okabe, Yakushi et al. 2002; Okabe,

Yakushi et al. 2005; Koerdt, Paulick et al. 2009). The *Vibrio* MotA and MotB form a membrane complex that utilizes a Na+ gradient (instead of H+ gradient) to drive flagellar rotation. A Na+ gradient is required to allow MotA/MotB to associate with the flagellum (through MotX/MotY) and open the Na+ channel; flux of Na+ through the channel provides the torque to generate flagellar rotation (McCarter 1994; McCarter 1994; Yorimitsu, Kojima et al. 2004; Terashima, Fukuoka et al. 2006).

Two additional proteins control flagellar number and placement in *Vibrio* spp. FlhG contains an ATPase motif and controls flagellar number; *Vibrio* cells without *flhG* synthesize multiple polar flagella, instead of a single polar flagellum (Correa, Peng et al. 2005; Kusumoto, Kamisaka et al. 2006; Kusumoto, Shinohara et al. 2008). FlhF contains a GTP binding motif and localizes to the cell pole, thus dictating polar localization of the flagellum. *Vibrio* cells without *flhF* are largely non-flagellated; however a few cells will synthesize a flagellum at a site away from the pole (Carpenter, Hanlon et al. 1992; Zanen, Antelmann et al. 2004; Salvetti, Ghelardi et al. 2007; Green, Kahramanoglou et al. 2009; Kusumoto, Nishioka et al. 2009). FlhG interacts with FlhF, and a current model suggests that FlhG interacts with FlhF to prevent additional FlhF deposition at the pole (Kusumoto, Shinohara et al. 2008). A *V. alginolyticus* strain lacking both FlhF and FlhG is mostly lacking flagella (Kojima, Nishioka et al. 2011), but a few cells possess multiple peritrichous flagella (similar to *S. typhimurium*). An unidentified suppressor mutation can lead to virtually all *flhFG V. alginolyticus* cells possessing peritrichous flagella and being able to swim; the identification of this suppressor mutation should lead to greater insights into control of polar flagellar synthesis in *Vibrio* spp.

Two additional outer membrane proteins, FlgO and FlgP, contribute to flagellar stability. FlgP homologues are restricted to *Vibrio*, *Helicobacter*, and *Campylobacter* spp. *V. cholerae* FlgP is a lipoprotein that affects flagellar stability; *flgP* mutants synthesize fragile flagella and appear non-motile in motility agar, presumably due to breakage of flagella during swimming (Morris, Peng et al. 2008; Martinez, Dharmasena et al. 2009). FlgO homologues are only found in *Vibrio* spp. *V. cholerae* strains lacking *flgO* have a similar phenotype as *flgP* strains, namely they produce fragile flagella that break easily while swimming (Morris, Peng et al. 2008; Martinez, Dharmasena et al. 2009).

3. Regulation

Transcription of the *V. cholerae* flagellar genes is controlled by a four-tiered transcription hierarchy (Fig. 3.) (Prouty, Correa et al. 2001). The *V. cholerae* flagellar transcription hierarchy is similar to that which controls flagellar transcription in *Pseudomonas aeruginosa*, another bacterium with a single polar flagellum (Dasgupta, Wolfgang et al. 2003). The master regulator, FlrA, is a σ^{54}-dependent transcriptional activator. FlrA represents the sole Class I gene product, and it activates transcription of Class II flagellar genes (Klose and Mekalanos 1998). It is not clear whether environmental conditions regulate transcription of *flrA*, but *flhG* (which controls flagellar number) also negatively regulates *flrA* transcription (Correa, Peng et al. 2005).

The *P. aeruginosa* FlrA homologue, FleQ, has been shown to bind to cyclic-di-GMP (cdGMP)(Hickman and Harwood 2008). Binding of cdGMP to FleQ prevents DNA binding, resulting in the absence of flagellar synthesis and de-repression in *P. aeruginosa* of genes involved in biofilm formation normally repressed by FleQ. Interestingly, cdGMP binds to

FleQ lacking the N-terminus, indicating it binds to the transcriptional activation/DNA binding domain, which shares high homology (63% identity) with *V. cholerae* FlrA. It is not yet known whether FlrA binds to and is modulated by cdGMP. *P. aeruginosa* FleQ also binds to FleN, the homologue of FlhG (Dasgupta and Ramphal 2001). FleN binding to FleQ does not inhibit DNA binding, but downregulates FleQ-dependent transcription, resulting in reduced (single) flagellar number. As mentioned above, FlhG has a negative effect on *flrA* transcription in *V. cholerae*, but it is not known whether it also binds to FlrA and negatively affects its activity.

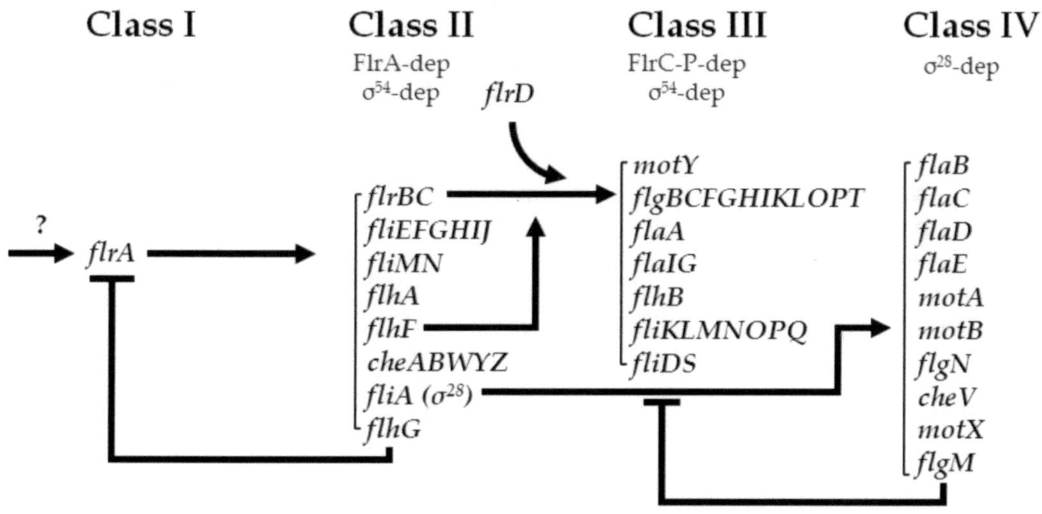

Fig. 3. Flagellar Transcription Regulatory Hierarchy

FlrA positively regulates Class II flagellar genes. Both FlrA and σ^{54}-containing RNA polymerase are required to activate transcription of the Class II flagellar genes (Klose and Mekalanos 1998; Klose, Novik et al. 1998; Prouty, Correa et al. 2001). The class II genes encode components of the MS ring-switch-export apparatus as well as chemotaxis and regulatory proteins. Two large flagellar operons (*fliEFGHIJ* and the *flhA* operon, which contains *flhFG*, mentioned above, as well as *fliA* (σ^{28}) and a number of chemotaxis genes), and the regulatory genes *flrBC*, are activated by FlrA. The Class II flagellar genes are predicted to encode an export apparatus-basal body intermediate; it seems likely that this structure is required to be assembled prior to progression to Class III gene expression, as is the case in *Campylobacter jejuni* and *Helicobacter pylori*, which have similar classes of flagellar genes (Hendrixson and DiRita 2003; Niehus, Gressmann et al. 2004).

The regulatory proteins FlrBC are a two-component system that controls Class III gene transcription (Prouty, Correa et al. 2001). FlrB undergoes autophosphorylation, and then activates FlrC activity by transferring a phosphate to the conserved aspartate-54 (D54) residue in the amino terminus of FlrC (FlrC-P) allowing it to activate the σ^{54}-dependent transcription of Class III genes (Correa, Lauriano et al. 2000; Correa and Klose 2005). The class III genes encode the rest of the components of the hook-basal body, as well as the flagellin FlaA and the OM proteins FlgOP. FlrC binds to enhancer sites downstream of the σ^{54}-dependent Class III promoters (Correa, Lauriano et al. 2000; Correa and Klose 2005).

Most of the Class III gene products are only required in small amounts, but the FlaA flagellin is transcribed at very high levels. One mechanism for achieving these different levels of expression is the relative binding strength of the FlrC sites, which bind FlrC strongly at the *flaA* promoter, but only weakly at other Class III promoters, e.g. the *flgK* promoter (Correa and Klose 2005).

FlrC must be phosphorylated to activate σ^{54}-dependent transcription, so presumably FlrB only phosphorylates FlrC upon assembly (not function) of the Class II export apparatus-basal body intermediate; a similar event controls expression of σ^{54}-dependent Class III genes in *C. jejuni* (Joslin and Hendrixson 2009). Detection of an intermediate that is not secretion competent may explain why the genes encoding some of the components presumably required for secretion (e.g. *fliOPQ*) are Class III (i.e. activated by FlrC) rather than Class II genes. FlrB is a soluble protein and could thus directly interact with the apparatus intermediate in the cytoplasmic membrane and phosphorylate FlrC upon assembly. Deletion of *flhF* in *V. cholerae* specifically downregulates Class III gene expression (Correa, Peng et al. 2005), suggesting that FlhF regulates FlrC-dependent transcription in addition to regulating polar flagellar placement (as discussed above). An inner membrane protein, FlrD, is also a positive regulator of class III genes. Expression of FlrD is not regulated by the flagellar transcription hierarchy, but the protein possesses a HAMP domain, so it may interact with FlrB or FlrC to influence phosphorylation and Class III transcription (Moisi, Jenul et al. 2009)

The Class II gene *fliA* encodes σ^{28}, which is required for transcription of Class IV flagellar genes (Klose and Mekalanos 1998). Similar to the checkpoint in *S. typhimurium* (Karlinsey, Tanaka et al. 2000; Chevance and Hughes 2008), the *V. cholerae* anti-sigma factor FlgM prevents σ^{28} transcriptional activity until it is secreted through a functional hook-basal body complex (Correa, Barker et al. 2004). The secretion of FlgM through the sheathed flagellum indicates that the sheath does not completely enclose the flagellum, at least at the tip. Secretion of FlgM frees σ^{28} to interact with RNA polymerase and activate Class IV flagellar genes, which encode the other four flagellins, FlaBCDE, as well as motor components (MotABX) and chemotaxis proteins (Klose and Mekalanos 1998). *V. cholerae* lacking *fliA* are non-motile and synthesize a truncated flagellum. The lack of expression of the four additional Class IV (σ^{28}-dependent) flagellins (FlaBCDE) in the *fliA* strain is likely not the reason for the truncated flagellum and lack of motility, since strains lacking *flaBCDE* are still motile and synthesize a full length flagellum, whereas a strain lacking the Class III FlaA flagellin is non-motile and aflagellate (Klose and Mekalanos 1998). Rather, the lack of expression of other Class IV genes (e.g. motor genes) likely contributes to the *fliA* phenotype. The contribution of the four Class IV flagellins to flagellar synthesis and motility is mysterious, considering that only the Class III FlaA flagellin is essential for flagellar synthesis, but perhaps the other flagellins impart subtle differences to the flagellum and thus swimming behavior that are not obvious under laboratory growth conditions.

4. Motility and virulence

V. cholerae virulence has been linked to motility. Spontaneous non-motile *V. cholerae* strains were characterized as less virulent than motile strains in several *in vivo* and *in vitro* rabbit models of cholera. Mutations that adversely affect flagellar synthesis and motility generally lead to decreased intestinal colonization in infant mice (Guentzel and Berry 1975; Montie,

Doyle-Huntzinger et al. 1982; Carsiotis, Weinstein et al. 1984; Weinstein, Carsiotis et al. 1984; Schmitt, Darnell et al. 1994; Kennedy, Rosey et al. 1997; Watnick, Lauriano et al. 2001; Syed, Beyhan et al. 2009). Non-motile live attenuated *V. cholerae* vaccine strains exhibit reduced reactogenicity (disease symptoms) in human volunteers, when compared to motile isogenic strains. (Coster, Killeen et al. 1995; Kenner, Coster et al. 1995). Using a newly-developed infant rabbit model of cholera, Rui *et al.* demonstrated that flagellin expression (whether in motile or non-motile vaccine strains) causes reactogenicity in rabbits by inducing proinflammatory cytokines in the intestine (Rui, Ritchie et al. 2010).

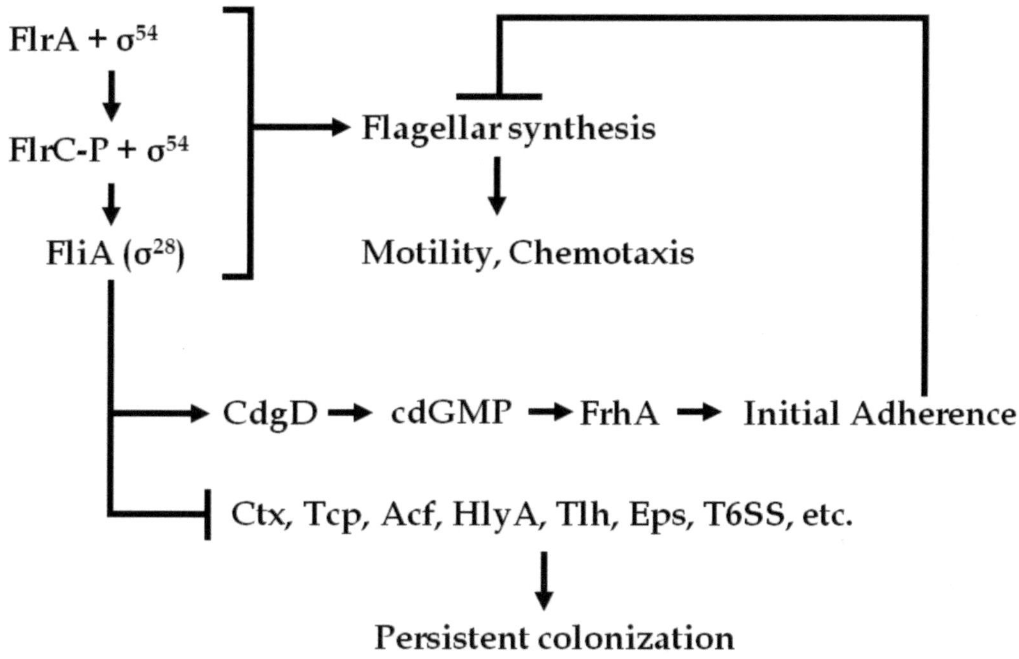

Fig. 4. Proposed Model of Flagellar-dependent Virulence Modulation

An inverse relationship between motility and virulence had been suggested by the observation that spontaneous hypermotile mutants express almost no CT or TCP, while spontaneous non-motile mutants express increased levels of CT and TCP (Gardel and Mekalanos 1996). Utilizing whole genome transcription profiling of *V. cholerae* strains with mutations in the key flagellar regulatory genes (*rpoN, flrA, flrC,* and *fliA*), it was observed that non-flagellated strains exhibit increased transcription of known (CT, TCP) and putative virulence factors (T6SS, hemolysins, etc)(Syed, Beyhan et al. 2009). The results suggest coordinate regulation by the flagellar regulatory hierarchy over a variety of virulence factors whose regulation was previously thought to be unlinked (Syed, Beyhan et al. 2009).

It had been known that non-motile *V. cholerae* mutants exhibited enhanced hemagglutinating activity and decreased hemolytic activity, but the identity of the respective factors was unknown (Gardel and Mekalanos 1996). The transcriptional profiling of the flagellar regulatory mutants identified the flagellar-regulated hemolysin as TLH, which is encoded adjacent to HlyA, the "El Tor" hemolysin (Syed, Beyhan et al. 2009). Also identified was the flagellar-regulated hemagglutinin, FrhA, which is a large cadherincontaining protein that enhances binding to epithelial cells *in vitro* and intestinal colonization in both infant and adult mice. The flagellar regulatory hierarchy positively regulates *frhA* transcription and negatively regulates *tlh* transcription. Regulation of *frhA* transcription by the flagellar hierarchy is mediated through an intermediate, CdgD, a cdGMP synthase. cdGMP is an important signaling molecule that modulates complex behaviors in bacteria, most notably biofilm formation (discussed below). The results demonstrate that the flagellar hierarchy controls the transcription of non-flagellar genes that contribute to other aspects of the *V. cholerae* lifecycle besides motility (Syed, Beyhan et al. 2009).

5. Chemotaxis and virulence

Chemotaxis controls flagellar rotation in response to environmental factors, and thus is intimately tied to motility. Chemoattractants stimulate the chemotaxis machinery to cause increased clockwise (CW) rotation of the flagellum, while chemorepellants enable increased counter-clockwise (CCW) rotation (Armitage 1999; Butler and Camilli 2005). The net result of these effects on flagellar rotation is net swimming towards chemoattractants and away from chemorepellants (Falke, Bass et al. 1997; Armitage 1999). *V. cholerae* encodes three clusters of chemotaxis proteins (Heidelberg, Eisen et al. 2000), but the cluster that is embedded within the flagellar gene cluster (within the Class II *flhA* operon: *cheY3, cheZ, cheA2, cheB2,* and *cheW1*) appears to be the major chemotaxis machinery that controls flagellar rotation under most conditions (Camilli and Mekalanos 1995; Hyakutake, Homma et al. 2005). Methyl-accepting chemotaxis proteins (MCPs) in the cytoplasmic membrane interact with chemoattractant/repellants and the signal is transmitted through CheA to CheY via phosphorylation. Phospho-CheY then interacts with the C-ring of the flagellum, which causes a reversion from CCW to CW rotation, resulting in a change of swimming direction. CheB and CheW are involved in modulating the signal transduction pathway (Freter and O'Brien 1981; Alm and Manning 1990; Everiss, Hughes et al. 1994; Harkey, Everiss et al. 1994; Lee, Butler et al. 2001; Banerjee, Das et al. 2002; Hyakutake, Homma et al. 2005).

Interestingly, *V. cholerae* in stool exhibit a transient hyper-infectious phenotype predicted to facilitate epidemic spread of cholera, and transcription profiling revealed a transient repression of chemotaxis genes (specifically *cheW*) in these bacteria (Merrell, Butler et al. 2002). In the infant mouse model, non-chemotactic *V. cholerae* are able to outcompete chemotactic *V. cholerae* for intestinal colonization, indicating that the repression of chemotaxis in stool bacteria enhances epidemic spread (Butler and Camilli 2004; Butler, Nelson et al. 2006). Preventing phosphorylation of CheY prevents chemotactic signal transduction to the flagellum and biases it toward CCW flagellar rotation (and hence longer periods of swimming in a straight direction). The flagellum can also be biased toward CW flagellar rotation (and shorter periods of swimming in a straight direction) by the introduction of mutations into CheY that inhibit its dephosphorylation. Within the intestine, only the CCW-biased *V. cholerae* dramatically outcompete chemotactic *V. cholerae,* whereas the CW-biased bacteria are defective for intestinal colonization (Butler and Camilli 2004). Chemotactic *V. cholerae* colonize the distal end of the small intestine, whereas the CCW-biased non-chemotactic *V. cholerae* colonize the entire length of the small intestine. These results suggest that chemotaxis normally facilitates the recognition of chemoattractants within the distal small intestine or, alternatively, the recognition of chemorepellants within the proximal small intestine.

6. Biofilm formation

V. cholerae readily forms biofilms in the laboratory, and it is generally thought that *V. cholerae* predominantly exists as biofilms associated with various surfaces in the aquatic environment, including close associations with shellfish and zooplankton (Costerton, Lewandowski et al. 1995; Watnick and Kolter 1999; Faruque, Biswas et al. 2006; Yildiz and Visick 2009). Biofilm growth on chitinous surfaces induces competence in *V. cholerae,* facilitating horizontal gene transfer and rapid evolution in the marine environment (Blokesch and Schoolnik 2007). *V. cholerae* biofilms are more resistant to environmental stresses such as antibiotics, chlorine, protozoan grazing, and bacteriophage infection (Vess, Anderson et al. 1993; Faruque, Albert et al. 1998; Watnick and Kolter 1999; Matz, McDougald et al. 2005). A significant amount of study has gone into understanding *V. cholerae* biofilm formation.

Biofilm formation requires an initial phase where the bacterium associates with a solid surface, followed by attachment, formation of microcolonies, and finally the formation of the mature three-dimensional biofilm structure with characteristic pillars and water channels (Costerton, Lewandowski et al. 1995; Watnick and Kolter 1999). Formation of the mature biofilm requires the expression of the *Vibrio* exopolysaccharide (VPS), which is the polysaccharide matrix that holds the structure together (Yildiz and Schoolnik 1999; Watnick, Lauriano et al. 2001; Lauriano, Ghosh et al. 2004). *V. cholerae* expressing the VPS results in obviously wrinkled ("rugose") colony morphology, and *V. cholerae* undergoes phase variation that leads to the rugose colony phenotype and enhanced biofilm formation (Yildiz and Schoolnik 1999; Watnick, Lauriano et al. 2001; Lim, Beyhan et al. 2007). A number of regulatory factors are involved in VPS expression and biofilm formation, and one of the driving signals behind biofilm formation is increased expression of the signaling molecule c-di-GMP (Tischler and Camilli 2004; Beyhan, Tischler et al. 2006; Beyhan, Bilecen et al. 2007; Lim, Beyhan et al. 2007; Beyhan, Odell et al. 2008; Hickman and Harwood 2008; Syed, Beyhan et al. 2009; Yildiz and Visick 2009).

In an initial screen for *V. cholerae* mutants unable to form biofilms, Watnick and Kolter identified motility as a major contributor to biofilm formation (Watnick and Kolter 1999). These results suggested that flagellar-mediated motility was important to approach and colonize a surface, and also to facilitate microcolony formation. Subsequently, it was determined that the flagellar motor itself controls VPS expression, at least in some *V. cholerae* strains, because non-flagellated mutants switch to the rugose phenotype, and this is dependent on a functional motor, suggesting that the motor acts as a sensor to induce mature biofilm formation (Lauriano, Ghosh et al. 2004). The *Vibrio* Na+-driven motor functioning to sense environmental conditions and drive altered gene expression is not unprecedented; the *V. parahaemolyticus* Na+-driven polar flagellar motor functions as a sensor to drive lateral flagellar synthesis (McCarter, Hilmen et al. 1988; Kawagishi, Imagawa et al. 1996).

In general, elevated levels of cdGMP drive *V. cholerae* toward enhanced VPS expression and down-regulate motility and virulence gene expression (Tischler and Camilli 2004; Yildiz and Visick 2009). Elevated cdGMP levels cause a decrease in Class III and IV flagellar transcription, and noticeable decreases in motility in soft agar assays(Beyhan, Tischler et al. 2006). These results suggest that activity of the Class III regulator FlrC may be responsive to elevated cdGMP levels. The effect of specific cdGMP synthases/phosphodiesterases on motility is complicated by the presence of multiple paralogs of both types of enzymes in *V. cholerae* (Lim, Beyhan et al. 2006; Beyhan, Odell et al. 2008). Moreover, the flagellar hierarchy also regulates the expression of cdGMP modulating enzymes (mentioned above), so the effect of cdGMP on flagellar synthesis and motility is likely extremely complex, involving a large number of counteracting enzymes that regulate and are regulated by the flagellar hierarchy.

7. Conclusion

The single polar flagellum of *V. cholerae* is assembled in a stepwise fashion of components that are tightly regulated by a flagellar transcriptional hierarchy. The study of some of the unique aspects of this flagellum are likely to yield further insight into the role of flagellar synthesis, motility, and chemotaxis on the virulence and environmental persistence of this important human pathogen. One of the most unique aspects is the sheath surrounding the flagellum, which is still mysterious. The presence and function of the multiple flagellins still needs to be elucidated. Regulation of the flagellar transcriptional hierarchy is still not understood, nor how this hierarchy regulates non-flagellar genes that influence virulence and biofilm formation. Clearly much remains to be illuminated in the study of the contribution of flagellar synthesis and motility to the lifecycle of *V. cholerae*.

8. Acknowledgement

Funded by NIH AI43486

9. References

Aizawa, S. I., G. E. Dean, et al. (1985). "Purification and characterization of the flagellar hook-basal body complex of Salmonella typhimurium." J Bacteriol 161(3): 836-849.
Allen, R. D. and P. Baumann (1971). "Structure and arrangement of flagella in species of the genus Beneckea and Photobacterium fischeri." J Bacteriol 107(1): 295-302.
Alm, R. A. and P. A. Manning (1990). "Characterization of the hlyB gene and its role in the production of the El Tor haemolysin of Vibrio cholerae O1." Mol Microbiol 4(3): 413-425.
Armitage, J. P. (1999). "Bacterial tactic responses." Adv Microb Physiol 41: 229-289.
Asai, Y., S. Kojima, et al. (1997). "Putative channel components for the fast-rotating sodium-driven flagellar motor of a marine bacterium." J Bacteriol 179(16): 5104-5110.
Banerjee, R., S. Das, et al. (2002). "Involvement of in vivo induced cheY-4 gene of Vibrio cholerae in motility, early adherence to intestinal epithelial cells and regulation of virulence factors." FEBS Lett 532(1-2): 221-226.
Beyhan, S., K. Bilecen, et al. (2007). "Regulation of rugosity and biofilm formation in Vibrio cholerae: comparison of VpsT and VpsR regulons and epistasis analysis of vpsT, vpsR, and hapR." J Bacteriol 189(2): 388-402.
Beyhan, S., L. S. Odell, et al. (2008). "Identification and characterization of cyclic diguanylate signaling systems controlling rugosity in Vibrio cholerae." J Bacteriol 190(22): 7392-7405.
Beyhan, S., A. D. Tischler, et al. (2006). "Transcriptome and phenotypic responses of Vibrio cholerae to increased cyclic di-GMP level." J Bacteriol 188(10): 3600-3613.

Blair, D. F. (2003). "Flagellar movement driven by proton translocation." FEBS Lett 545(1): 86-95.

Blair, D. F. and H. C. Berg (1990). "The MotA protein of E. coli is a proton-conducting component of the flagellar motor." Cell 60(3): 439-449.

Blokesch, M. and G. K. Schoolnik (2007). "Serogroup conversion of Vibrio cholerae in aquatic reservoirs." PLoS Pathog 3(6): e81.

Braun, T. F., S. Poulson, et al. (1999). "Function of proline residues of MotA in torque generation by the flagellar motor of Escherichia coli." J Bacteriol 181(11): 3542-3551.

Butler, S. M. and A. Camilli (2004). "Both chemotaxis and net motility greatly influence the infectivity of Vibrio cholerae." Proc Natl Acad Sci U S A 101(14): 5018-5023.

Butler, S. M. and A. Camilli (2005). "Going against the grain: chemotaxis and infection in Vibrio cholerae." Nat Rev Microbiol 3(8): 611-620.

Butler, S. M., E. J. Nelson, et al. (2006). "Cholera stool bacteria repress chemotaxis to increase infectivity." Mol Microbiol 60(2): 417-426.

Camilli, A. and J. J. Mekalanos (1995). "Use of recombinase gene fusions to identify Vibrio cholerae genes induced during infection." Mol Microbiol 18(4): 671-683.

Carpenter, P. B., D. W. Hanlon, et al. (1992). "flhF, a Bacillus subtilis flagellar gene that encodes a putative GTP-binding protein." Mol Microbiol 6(18): 2705-2713.

Carsiotis, M., D. L. Weinstein, et al. (1984). "Flagella of Salmonella typhimurium are a virulence factor in infected C57BL/6J mice." Infect Immun 46(3): 814-818.

Chevance, F. F. and K. T. Hughes (2008). "Coordinating assembly of a bacterial macromolecular machine." Nat Rev Microbiol 6(6): 455-465.

Correa, N. E., J. R. Barker, et al. (2004). "The Vibrio cholerae FlgM homologue is an anti-sigma28 factor that is secreted through the sheathed polar flagellum." J Bacteriol 186(14): 4613-4619.

Correa, N. E. and K. E. Klose (2005). "Characterization of enhancer binding by the Vibrio cholerae flagellar regulatory protein FlrC." J Bacteriol 187(9): 3158-3170.

Correa, N. E., C. M. Lauriano, et al. (2000). "Phosphorylation of the flagellar regulatory protein FlrC is necessary for Vibrio cholerae motility and enhanced colonization." Mol Microbiol 35(4): 743-755.

Correa, N. E., F. Peng, et al. (2005). "Roles of the regulatory proteins FlhF and FlhG in the Vibrio cholerae flagellar transcription hierarchy." J Bacteriol 187(18): 6324-6332.

Coster, T. S., K. P. Killeen, et al. (1995). "Safety, immunogenicity, and efficacy of live attenuated Vibrio cholerae O139 vaccine prototype." Lancet 345(8955): 949-952.

Costerton, J. W., Z. Lewandowski, et al. (1995). "Microbial biofilms." Annu Rev Microbiol 49: 711-745.

Dasgupta, N. and R. Ramphal (2001). "Interaction of the antiactivator FleN with the transcriptional activator FleQ regulates flagellar number in Pseudomonas aeruginosa." J Bacteriol 183(22): 6636-6644.

Dasgupta, N., M. C. Wolfgang, et al. (2003). "A four-tiered transcriptional regulatory circuit controls flagellar biogenesis in Pseudomonas aeruginosa." Mol Microbiol 50(3): 809-824.

Dean, G. E., R. M. Macnab, et al. (1984). "Gene sequence and predicted amino acid sequence of the motA protein, a membrane-associated protein required for flagellar rotation in Escherichia coli." J Bacteriol 159(3): 991-999.

Everiss, K. D., K. J. Hughes, et al. (1994). "The accessory colonization factor and toxin-coregulated pilus gene clusters are physically linked on the Vibrio cholerae 0395 chromosome." DNA Seq 5(1): 51-55.

Falke, J. J., R. B. Bass, et al. (1997). "The two-component signaling pathway of bacterial chemotaxis: a molecular view of signal transduction by receptors, kinases, and adaptation enzymes." Annu Rev Cell Dev Biol 13: 457-512.

Faruque, S. M., M. J. Albert, et al. (1998). "Epidemiology, genetics, and ecology of toxigenic Vibrio cholerae." Microbiol Mol Biol Rev 62(4): 1301-1314.

Faruque, S. M., K. Biswas, et al. (2006). "Transmissibility of cholera: in vivo-formed biofilms and their relationship to infectivity and persistence in the environment." Proc Natl Acad Sci U S A 103(16): 6350-6355.

Francis, N. R., G. E. Sosinsky, et al. (1994). "Isolation, characterization and structure of bacterial flagellar motors containing the switch complex." J Mol Biol 235(4): 1261-1270.

Freter, R. and P. C. O'Brien (1981). "Role of chemotaxis in the association of motile bacteria with intestinal mucosa: fitness and virulence of nonchemotactic Vibrio cholerae mutants in infant mice." Infect Immun 34(1): 222-233.

Fuerst, J. A. and J. W. Perry (1988). "Demonstration of lipopolysaccharide on sheathed flagella of Vibrio cholerae O:1 by protein A-gold immunoelectron microscopy." J Bacteriol 170(4): 1488-1494.

Fukuoka, H., T. Yakushi, et al. (2005). "Assembly of motor proteins, PomA and PomB, in the Na+-driven stator of the flagellar motor." J Mol Biol 351(4): 707-717.

Gardel, C. L. and J. J. Mekalanos (1996). "Alterations in Vibrio cholerae motility phenotypes correlate with changes in virulence factor expression." Infect Immun 64(6): 2246-2255.

Green, J. C., C. Kahramanoglou, et al. (2009). "Recruitment of the earliest component of the bacterial flagellum to the old cell division pole by a membrane-associated signal recognition particle family GTP-binding protein." J Mol Biol 391(4): 679-690.

Guentzel, M. N. and L. J. Berry (1975). "Motility as a virulence factor for Vibrio cholerae." Infect Immun 11(5): 890-897.

Harkey, C. W., K. D. Everiss, et al. (1994). "The Vibrio cholerae toxin-coregulated-pilus gene tcpI encodes a homolog of methyl-accepting chemotaxis proteins." Infect Immun 62(7): 2669-2678.

Heidelberg, J. F., J. A. Eisen, et al. (2000). "DNA sequence of both chromosomes of the cholera pathogen Vibrio cholerae." Nature 406(6795): 477-483.

Hendrixson, D. R. and V. J. DiRita (2003). "Transcription of sigma54-dependent but not sigma28-dependent flagellar genes in Campylobacter jejuni is associated with formation of the flagellar secretory apparatus." Mol Microbiol 50(2): 687-702.

Hickman, J. W. and C. S. Harwood (2008). "Identification of FleQ from Pseudomonas aeruginosa as a c-di-GMP-responsive transcription factor." Mol Microbiol 69(2): 376-389.

Homma, M., S. Aizawa, et al. (1987). "Identification of the M-ring protein of the flagellar motor of Salmonella typhimurium." Proc Natl Acad Sci U S A 84(21): 7483-7487.

Homma, M., D. J. DeRosier, et al. (1990). "Flagellar hook and hook-associated proteins of Salmonella typhimurium and their relationship to other axial components of the flagellum." J Mol Biol 213(4): 819-832.

Homma, M., K. Kutsukake, et al. (1990). "FlgB, FlgC, FlgF and FlgG. A family of structurally related proteins in the flagellar basal body of Salmonella typhimurium." J Mol Biol 211(2): 465-477.

Homma, M., K. Ohnishi, et al. (1987). "Identification of flagellar hook and basal body gene products (FlaFV, FlaFVI, FlaFVII and FlaFVIII) in Salmonella typhimurium." J Bacteriol 169(8): 3617-3624.

Hyakutake, A., M. Homma, et al. (2005). "Only one of the five CheY homologs in Vibrio cholerae directly switches flagellar rotation." J Bacteriol 187(24): 8403-8410.

Ikeda, T., S. Asakura, et al. (1985). ""Cap" on the tip of Salmonella flagella." J Mol Biol 184(4): 735-737.

Ikeda, T., M. Homma, et al. (1987). "Localization and stoichiometry of hook-associated proteins within Salmonella typhimurium flagella." J Bacteriol 169(3): 1168-1173.

Jobling, M. G. and R. K. Holmes (1997). "Characterization of hapR, a positive regulator of the Vibrio cholerae HA/protease gene hap, and its identification as a functional homologue of the Vibrio harveyi luxR gene." Mol Microbiol 26(5): 1023-1034.

Joslin, S. N. and D. R. Hendrixson (2009). "Activation of the Campylobacter jejuni FlgSR two-component system is linked to the flagellar export apparatus." J Bacteriol 191(8): 2656-2667.

Karlinsey, J. E., S. Tanaka, et al. (2000). "Completion of the hook-basal body complex of the Salmonella typhimurium flagellum is coupled to FlgM secretion and fliC transcription." Mol Microbiol 37(5): 1220-1231.

Kawagishi, I., M. Imagawa, et al. (1996). "The sodium-driven polar flagellar motor of marine Vibrio as the mechanosensor that regulates lateral flagellar expression." Mol Microbiol 20(4): 693-699.

Kennedy, M. J., E. L. Rosey, et al. (1997). "Characterization of flaA- and flaB- mutants of Serpulina hyodysenteriae: both flagellin subunits, FlaA and FlaB, are necessary for full motility and intestinal colonization." FEMS Microbiol Lett 153(1): 119-128.

Kenner, J. R., T. S. Coster, et al. (1995). "Peru-15, an improved live attenuated oral vaccine candidate for Vibrio cholerae O1." J Infect Dis 172(4): 1126-1129.

Klose, K. E. and J. J. Mekalanos (1998). "Differential regulation of multiple flagellins in Vibrio cholerae." J Bacteriol 180(2): 303-316.

Klose, K. E. and J. J. Mekalanos (1998). "Distinct roles of an alternative sigma factor during both free-swimming and colonizing phases of the Vibrio cholerae pathogenic cycle." Mol Microbiol 28(3): 501-520.

Klose, K. E., V. Novik, et al. (1998). "Identification of multiple sigma54-dependent transcriptional activators in Vibrio cholerae." J Bacteriol 180(19): 5256-5259.

Koerdt, A., A. Paulick, et al. (2009). "MotX and MotY are required for flagellar rotation in Shewanella oneidensis MR-1." J Bacteriol 191(16): 5085-5093.

Kojima, M., N. Nishioka, et al. (2011). "Conversion of mono-polar to peritrichous flagellation in Vibrio alginolyticus." Microbiol Immunol 55(2): 76-83.

Kojima, S. and D. F. Blair (2004). "The bacterial flagellar motor: structure and function of a complex molecular machine." Int Rev Cytol 233: 93-134.

Kusumoto, A., K. Kamisaka, et al. (2006). "Regulation of polar flagellar number by the flhF and flhG genes in Vibrio alginolyticus." J Biochem 139(1): 113-121.

Kusumoto, A., N. Nishioka, et al. (2009). "Mutational analysis of the GTP-binding motif of FlhF which regulates the number and placement of the polar flagellum in Vibrio alginolyticus." J Biochem 146(5): 643-650.

Kusumoto, A., A. Shinohara, et al. (2008). "Collaboration of FlhF and FlhG to regulate polar-flagella number and localization in Vibrio alginolyticus." Microbiology 154(Pt 5): 1390-1399.

Lauriano, C. M., C. Ghosh, et al. (2004). "The sodium-driven flagellar motor controls exopolysaccharide expression in Vibrio cholerae." J Bacteriol 186(15): 4864-4874.

Lee, S. H., S. M. Butler, et al. (2001). "Selection for in vivo regulators of bacterial virulence." Proc Natl Acad Sci U S A 98(12): 6889-6894.

Lim, B., S. Beyhan, et al. (2006). "Cyclic-diGMP signal transduction systems in Vibrio cholerae: modulation of rugosity and biofilm formation." Mol Microbiol 60(2): 331-348.

Lim, B., S. Beyhan, et al. (2007). "Regulation of Vibrio polysaccharide synthesis and virulence factor production by CdgC, a GGDEF-EAL domain protein, in Vibrio cholerae." J Bacteriol 189(3): 717-729.

Lloyd, S. A., H. Tang, et al. (1996). "Torque generation in the flagellar motor of Escherichia coli: evidence of a direct role for FliG but not for FliM or FliN." J Bacteriol 178(1): 223-231.

Martinez, R. M., M. N. Dharmasena, et al. (2009). "Characterization of two outer membrane proteins, FlgO and FlgP, that influence vibrio cholerae motility." J Bacteriol 191(18): 5669-5679.

Matz, C., D. McDougald, et al. (2005). "Biofilm formation and phenotypic variation enhance predation-driven persistence of Vibrio cholerae." Proc Natl Acad Sci U S A 102(46): 16819-16824.

McCarter, L., M. Hilmen, et al. (1988). "Flagellar dynamometer controls swarmer cell differentiation of V. parahaemolyticus." Cell 54(3): 345-351.

McCarter, L. L. (1994). "MotX, the channel component of the sodium-type flagellar motor." J Bacteriol 176(19): 5988-5998.

McCarter, L. L. (1994). "MotY, a component of the sodium-type flagellar motor." J Bacteriol 176(14): 4219-4225.

Merrell, D. S., S. M. Butler, et al. (2002). "Host-induced epidemic spread of the cholera bacterium." Nature 417(6889): 642-645.

Moisi, M., C. Jenul, et al. (2009). "A novel regulatory protein involved in motility of Vibrio cholerae." J Bacteriol 191(22): 7027-7038.

Montie, T. C., D. Doyle-Huntzinger, et al. (1982). "Loss of virulence associated with absence of flagellum in an isogenic mutant of Pseudomonas aeruginosa in the burned-mouse model." Infect Immun 38(3): 1296-1298.

Morris, D. C., F. Peng, et al. (2008). "Lipidation of an FlrC-dependent protein is required for enhanced intestinal colonization by Vibrio cholerae." J Bacteriol 190(1): 231-239.

Niehus, E., H. Gressmann, et al. (2004). "Genome-wide analysis of transcriptional hierarchy and feedback regulation in the flagellar system of Helicobacter pylori." Mol Microbiol 52(4): 947-961.

Okabe, M., T. Yakushi, et al. (2001). "Cloning and characterization of motX, a Vibrio alginolyticus sodium-driven flagellar motor gene." J Biochem 130(6): 879-884.

Okabe, M., T. Yakushi, et al. (2005). "Interactions of MotX with MotY and with the PomA/PomB sodium ion channel complex of the Vibrio alginolyticus polar flagellum." J Biol Chem 280(27): 25659-25664.

Okabe, M., T. Yakushi, et al. (2002). "MotX and MotY, specific components of the sodium-driven flagellar motor, colocalize to the outer membrane in Vibrio alginolyticus." Mol Microbiol 46(1): 125-134.

Okunishi, I., I. Kawagishi, et al. (1996). "Cloning and characterization of motY, a gene coding for a component of the sodium-driven flagellar motor in Vibrio alginolyticus." J Bacteriol 178(8): 2409-2415.

Prouty, M. G., N. E. Correa, et al. (2001). "The novel sigma54- and sigma28-dependent flagellar gene transcription hierarchy of Vibrio cholerae." Mol Microbiol 39(6): 1595-1609.

Richardson, K. (1991). "Roles of motility and flagellar structure in pathogenicity of Vibrio cholerae: analysis of motility mutants in three animal models." Infect Immun 59(8): 2727-2736.

Rui, H., J. M. Ritchie, et al. (2010). "Reactogenicity of live-attenuated Vibrio cholerae vaccines is dependent on flagellins." Proc Natl Acad Sci U S A 107(9): 4359-4364.

Salvetti, S., E. Ghelardi, et al. (2007). "FlhF, a signal recognition particle-like GTPase, is involved in the regulation of flagellar arrangement, motility behaviour and protein secretion in Bacillus cereus." Microbiology 153(Pt 8): 2541-2552.

Sato, K. and M. Homma (2000). "Functional reconstitution of the Na(+)-driven polar flagellar motor component of Vibrio alginolyticus." J Biol Chem 275(8): 5718-5722.

Sato, K. and M. Homma (2000). "Multimeric structure of PomA, a component of the Na+-driven polar flagellar motor of vibrio alginolyticus." J Biol Chem 275(26): 20223-20228.

Schmitt, C. K., S. C. Darnell, et al. (1994). "Mutation of flgM attenuates virulence of Salmonella typhimurium, and mutation of fliA represses the attenuated phenotype." J Bacteriol 176(2): 368-377.

Schoenhals, G. J. and R. M. Macnab (1996). "Physiological and biochemical analyses of FlgH, a lipoprotein forming the outer membrane L ring of the flagellar basal body of Salmonella typhimurium." J Bacteriol 178(14): 4200-4207.

Sjoblad, R. D., C. W. Emala, et al. (1983). "Invited review: bacterial flagellar sheaths: structures in search of a function." Cell Motil 3(1): 93-103.

Stader, J., P. Matsumura, et al. (1986). "Nucleotide sequence of the Escherichia coli motB gene and site-limited incorporation of its product into the cytoplasmic membrane." J Bacteriol 166(1): 244-252.

Stolz, B. and H. C. Berg (1991). "Evidence for interactions between MotA and MotB, torque-generating elements of the flagellar motor of Escherichia coli." J Bacteriol 173(21): 7033-7037.

Syed, K. A., S. Beyhan, et al. (2009). "The Vibrio cholerae flagellar regulatory hierarchy controls expression of virulence factors." J Bacteriol 191(21): 6555-6570.

Terashima, H., H. Fukuoka, et al. (2006). "The Vibrio motor proteins, MotX and MotY, are associated with the basal body of Na-driven flagella and required for stator formation." Mol Microbiol 62(4): 1170-1180.

Terashima, H., M. Koike, et al. (2010). "The flagellar basal body-associated protein FlgT is essential for a novel ring structure in the sodium-driven Vibrio motor." J Bacteriol 192(21): 5609-5615.

Terashima, H., S. Kojima, et al. (2008). "Flagellar motility in bacteria structure and function of flagellar motor." Int Rev Cell Mol Biol 270: 39-85.

Tischler, A. D. and A. Camilli (2004). "Cyclic diguanylate (c-di-GMP) regulates Vibrio cholerae biofilm formation." Mol Microbiol 53(3): 857-869.

Ueno, T., K. Oosawa, et al. (1992). "M ring, S ring and proximal rod of the flagellar basal body of Salmonella typhimurium are composed of subunits of a single protein, FliF." J Mol Biol 227(3): 672-677.

Vess, R. W., R. L. Anderson, et al. (1993). "The colonization of solid PVC surfaces and the acquisition of resistance to germicides by water micro-organisms." J Appl Bacteriol 74(2): 215-221.

Watnick, P. I. and R. Kolter (1999). "Steps in the development of a Vibrio cholerae El Tor biofilm." Mol Microbiol 34(3): 586-595.

Watnick, P. I., C. M. Lauriano, et al. (2001). "The absence of a flagellum leads to altered colony morphology, biofilm development and virulence in Vibrio cholerae O139." Mol Microbiol 39(2): 223-235.

Weinstein, D. L., M. Carsiotis, et al. (1984). "Flagella help Salmonella typhimurium survive within murine macrophages." Infect Immun 46(3): 819-825.

Yildiz, F. H. and G. K. Schoolnik (1999). "Vibrio cholerae O1 El Tor: identification of a gene cluster required for the rugose colony type, exopolysaccharide production, chlorine resistance, and biofilm formation." Proc Natl Acad Sci U S A 96(7): 4028-4033.

Yildiz, F. H. and K. L. Visick (2009). "Vibrio biofilms: so much the same yet so different." Trends Microbiol 17(3): 109-118.

Yonekura, K., S. Maki-Yonekura, et al. (2003). "Complete atomic model of the bacterial flagellar filament by electron cryomicroscopy." Nature 424(6949): 643-650.

Yoon, S. S. and J. J. Mekalanos (2008). "Decreased potency of the Vibrio cholerae sheathed flagellum to trigger host innate immunity." Infect Immun 76(3): 1282-1288.

Yorimitsu, T., Y. Asai, et al. (2000). "Intermolecular cross-linking between the periplasmic Loop3-4 regions of PomA, a component of the Na+-driven flagellar motor of Vibrio alginolyticus." J Biol Chem 275(40): 31387-31391.

Yorimitsu, T., M. Kojima, et al. (2004). "Multimeric structure of the PomA/PomB channel complex in the Na+-driven flagellar motor of Vibrio alginolyticus." J Biochem 135(1): 43-51.

Zanen, G., H. Antelmann, et al. (2004). "FlhF, the third signal recognition particle-GTPase of Bacillus subtilis, is dispensable for protein secretion." J Bacteriol 186(17): 5956-5960.

Zhou, J., S. A. Lloyd, et al. (1998). "Electrostatic interactions between rotor and stator in the bacterial flagellar motor." Proc Natl Acad Sci U S A 95(11): 6436-6441.

Zhou, J., L. L. Sharp, et al. (1998). "Function of protonatable residues in the flagellar motor of Escherichia coli: a critical role for Asp 32 of MotB." J Bacteriol 180(10): 2729-2735.

5

Genetic Analysis of CTX Prophage and Antibiotic Resistance Determinants in *Vibrio cholerae* O1 Belonging to the Atypical El Tor Biotype from Kelantan, Malaysia

Choo Yee Yu, Geik Yong Ang and Chan Yean Yean
Department of Medical Microbiology and Parasitology, School of Medical Sciences, Health Campus, Universiti Sains Malaysia, Kelantan, Malaysia

1. Introduction

Epidemic and global pandemic cholera have claimed millions of lives since the first pandemic in 1817 and it continues to exact a huge annual toll, with endemics established in approximately 50 countries worldwide (Ryan, 2011). More than 200 serogroups have been reported to date (Safa et al., 2009), but only two serogroups of *Vibrio cholerae*, the O1 and O139 serogroups, are known to have the potential for unleashing epidemic and pandemic cholera. The O1 serogroup of *V. cholerae* can be further divided into the classical or El Tor biotypes based on a number of phenotypic and genotypic characteristics (Sack et al., 2004). Seven pandemics of cholera have been recorded to date, where the first six pandemics were associated with *V. cholerae* serogroup O1 of the classical biotype, whereas the current ongoing seventh pandemic (1961 until present day) is caused by *V. cholerae* serogroup O1 of the El Tor biotype (Faruque et al., 1998). In 1992, the emergence and rapid spread of *V. cholerae* serogroup O139 from the Indian subcontinent to neighbouring countries was viewed as a possible threat that might initiate an eighth cholera pandemic. At the height of the O139 outbreak, the Indian subcontinent saw a dramatic displacement of the *V. cholerae* O1 El Tor as the dominant strain. However, rather than being driven to gradual extinction like the classical biotype, an unprecedented turn of events in 1994 saw *V. cholerae* O1 El Tor regain its predominance over the O139 serogroup and both serogroups continue to cause disease on the Indian subcontinent (Faruque et al., 2003).

The current seventh pandemic rein has reached its half a century mark, but several variants of the *V. cholerae* O1 El Tor biotype emerged cryptically during the late 1990s. These variants were untypable according to the conventional biotyping classification, because they possessed traits of both classical and El Tor biotypes (Nair et al., 2002; Ansaruzzaman et al., 2004). Given this dilemma, Safa et al. (2009) proposed the designation 'atypical El Tor' as an umbrella term to encompass all variants of the El Tor biotype. One such atypical El Tor was collectively known as the Matlab variants isolated from hospitalized patients in Matlab, Bangladesh between 1991 and 1994. Chronologically, the Matlab variants were the first to be characterized as having attributes of both the classical and El Tor biotypes, which meant that they could not be differentiated into a specific biotype based on their phenotypic traits (Nair et al., 2002). In 2004, a second variant, designated as the Mozambique variant, was found to have typical El Tor phenotypic traits but it genetically harboured a tandem repeat of the classical CTX prophage on the small chromosome (Ansaruzzaman et al., 2004). The third, and perhaps the most significant atypical El Tor, was the altered El Tor that is uniquely recognized as carrying the classical cholera toxin while retaining almost all aspects of the prototypic seventh pandemic El Tor strain.

This altered El Tor was initially reported in Bangladesh and growing evidence suggests the wide spread of this variant around the world in recent years (Nguyen et al., 2009; Okada et al., 2010; Morita et al., 2010; Sithivong et al., 2010; Ceccarelli et al., 2011). The altered El Tor was reported to have fully displaced prototypic seventh pandemic El Tor strains in several countries, including India and Bangladesh (Nair et al., 2006; Raychoudhuri et al., 2009). Two different conjectures have been proposed for the emergence and global transmission of atypical El Tor (Alam et al., 2010). The emergence of altered El Tor was postulated to be the result of either clonal expansion of a single ancestral El Tor which had acquired the classical *ctxB* gene in a cholera endemic region or a multiclonal event occurring independently in each region from co-existing El Tor and classical strains. Transnational transmission of altered El Tor was exemplify by the recent 2010 Haiti outbreak which was thought to be introduced by human activity from South Asian countries (Chin et al., 2011) and subsequently spread to United States, Canada and Dominican Republic via importation by travellers from Haiti (CDC, 2010; Gilmour et al., 2011).

The emergence of atypical El Tor marks a significant event in the evolution of *V. cholerae* and the epidemiology of cholera. The 2009 cholera outbreak strain from Kelantan state on the east coast of peninsular Malaysia was characterized as belonging to the altered El Tor biotype and it carried the classical cholera toxin (*ctxB*) gene (Ang et al., 2010). The present study further investigated genetic aspects of the Kelantan altered El Tor strain using multiple PCR analysis to elucidate the structure of the CTX prophage and to detect the presence of class I integron and SXT element antibiotic determinants.

2. Materials and methods

2.1 *V. cholerae* strains

A total of 20 *V. cholerae* isolates belonging to serogroup O1 of the altered El Tor biotype were collected during the 2009 cholera outbreak in Kelantan, Malaysia as described earlier (Ang et al., 2010). All the *V. cholerae* isolates were revived from glycerol stock and identification was performed using standard biochemical methods (Kay et al., 1994). Serotyping was conducted using slide agglutination tests with polyvalent O1 and monospecific Ogawa and Inaba antisera (Denka Seikan, Japan). All isolates were routinely grown on Luria-Bertani (LB) agar throughout the study.

2.2 Genomic DNA preparation

The genomic DNA template for genetic analysis was purified using a NucleoSpin Tissue kit (Macherey-Nagel, Germany), according to the manufacturer's instructions. The purity and concentration of purified genomic DNA was determined using a Biophotometer (Eppendorf, Germany).

2.3 *rstR* typing

The type of *rstR* gene in each isolate was determined using a set of allele-specific forward primers (*rstR*$^{El\ Tor}$, *rstR*^{Classical}, *rstR*^{Calcutta} and *rstR*^{Environment}) and a common reverse primer, *rstRR* (Nusrin et al., 2004; Bhattacharya et al., 2006). A list of all primers used in this study is presented in Table 1.

Primer	Nucleotide sequence (5′ to 3′)	References
rstR^{Classical}	CTTCTCATCAGCAAAGCCTCCATC	Bhattacharya et al., 2006
rstR$^{El\ Tor}$	GCACCATGATTTAAGATGCTC	Bhattacharya et al., 2006
rstR^{Calcutta}	CTGTAAATCTCTTCAATCCTAGG	Bhattacharya et al., 2006
rstR^{Environment}	GTTAACGCTTCAAGCCTG	Nusrin et al., 2004
rstRR	TCGAGTTGTAATTCATCAAGAGTG	Bhattacharya et al., 2006
Ch1F	GACCACTCAGGCCGCTGAAAT	Nguyen et al., 2009
Ch1R	CCGCGCTCAAGTGGTTATCGG	Nguyen et al., 2009
Ch2F	AACAACAGGTTGCAAGAGAGCATT	Nguyen et al., 2009
Ch2R	TATTGCTTTTTTAATGGCCGTT	Nguyen et al., 2009
rstAR	CCGTGAAAGTCATCAACG	Nguyen et al., 2009
rstCF	GATGTTTACGATAGCCTAGAAGACTT	Nguyen et al., 2009
rstCR	TACAGTGATGGCTCAGTCAATGC	Nguyen et al., 2009
ctxBF	AGATATTTTCGTATACAGAATCTCTAG	Nguyen et al., 2009
cepR	AAACAGCAAGAAAACCCCGAGT	Nguyen et al., 2009
rstCF4	AAATCCGCAACTCAAGGCATTGA	Nguyen et al., 2009
rstCR4	TAAGCGCCTGAACGCAGATATAAAG	Nguyen et al., 2009
rtxC-F	CGACGAAGATCATTGACGAC	Chow et al., 2001
rtxC-R	CATCGTCGTTATGTGGTTGC	Chow et al., 2001
inDS-F	CGGAATGGCCGAGCAGAT C	Dalsgaard et al., 2001
inDS-B	CAAGGTTCTGGACCAGTTGCG	Dalsgaard et al., 2001
qacEΔ1-F	ATCGCAATAGTTGGCGAAGT	Dalsgaard et al., 2001
su1-B	GCAAGGCGGAAACCCGCGCGG	Dalsgaard et al., 2001
in-F	GGCATCCAAGCAGCAAGC	Dalsgaard et al., 2001
in-B	AAGCAGACT TGACCTGAT	Dalsgaard et al., 2001
aadA-B	ATTGCCCAGTCGGCAGCG	Dalsgaard et al., 2001
INT1	GCTGGATAGGTTAAGGGCAG	Hochhnut et al., 2001
INT2	CTCTATGGGCACTGTCCACATTG	Hochhnut et al., 2001
Sul2-F	AGG GGG CAG ATG TGATCGAC	Hochhnut et al., 2001
Sul2-B	TGTGCGGATGAAGTCAGCTCC	Hochhnut et al., 2001
FLOR-F	TTATCTCCCTGTCGTTCCAGCG	Hochhnut et al., 2001
FLOR-2	CCTATG AGCACACGGGGAGC	Iwanaga et al., 2004
strB-F	GGCACCCATAAGCGTACGCC	Iwanaga et al., 2004
strB-R	TGCCGAGCACGGCGACTACC	Iwanaga et al., 2004
DFR1-F	CGAAGAATGGAGTTATCGGG	Iwanaga et al., 2004
DFR1-B	TGCTGGGGATTTCAGGAAAG	Iwanaga et al., 2004

Table 1. Primers used in this study

2.4 Genetic analysis of CTX prophage array

Genetic analysis of CTX prophage array was performed using several combinations of primer pairs, as described by Nguyen et al. (2009). The presence of a RS1 element was determined using the primer pair rstCF/rstCR. Investigations of the arrays for RS1 and CTX prophage were performed using two primer pairs: ctxBF/rstCR for the CTX prophage-RS1 array and rstCF4/rstAR for the RS1-CTX prophage array. The presence of tandem repeats of the RS1 element or CTX prophage was determined using the primer pair rstCF4/rstCR4 and ctxBF/cepR, respectively. The chromosomal localization of RS1 and CTX prophage was confirmed using the primer pairs Ch1F/rstRR and ctxBF/Ch1R for the large chromosome and Ch2F/Ch2R for the small chromosome.

2.5 *rtxC* PCR

Detection of the *rtxC* gene was performed using the primer pair *rtxC-F/rtxC-R* (Chow et al., 2001).

2.6 PCR detection of class I integrons

Detection of class I integrons was performed using a set of primers described by Dalsgaard et al. (2001). Briefly, the primer pairs inDS-F/inDS-B and qacEΔ1-F/su1-B were used for the amplification of the 5′-CS and 3′-CS of the class I integron. The primer pair in-F/in-B was used to amplify gene cassettes inserted in the integron, while the primer pair in-F/aadA-B was used for the amplification of the gene cassette *aad1A* that encodes streptomycin resistance.

2.7 PCR detection of SXT constins

The isolates were screened for the presence of SXT constins (large conjugative elements) using the primer pair INT1/INT2. Presence of the antibiotic resistance genes *floR* that encodes resistance to chloramphenicol, *sulII* for resistance to sulfamethoxazole, *strB* for resistance to streptomycin, and *dfrA1* for resistance to trimethoprim, were determined using the primer pairs FLOR-F/FLOR-2, Sul2-F/Sul2-B, strB-F/strB-R, and DFR1-F/DFR1-B, respectively (Hochhut et al., 2001).

2.8 Sequencing of tandem repeats of RS1 elements and upstream regions of the CTX prophage

The DNA sequence spanning tandem repeats of RS1 elements and upstream regions of the CTX prophage (~8.5 kb) was generated with the primer pairs Ch1F/rstCR, rstCF4/rstCR4, and rstCF/cepR. Amplicons from each PCR reaction were cloned into the pCR4-TOPO vector (Invitrogen, CA) and sequenced by First Base Laboratories Sdn. Bhd. (Malaysia). The sequencing data was assembled and complete nucleotide sequences of the RS1-RS1-CTX prophage arrays for isolates 03/09-KB and 27/09-KB were deposited in GenBank under the accession numbers JN545744 and JN545745.

2.9 Sequencing of PCR amplicons

The nucleotide sequences of the PCR amplicons generated by each of the primer pairs Ch2F/Ch2R, INT1/INT2, Sul2-F/Sul2-B, strB-F/strB-R, DFR1-F/DFR1-B, and *rtxC-F/rtxC-*

R were confirmed by sequencing reactions. Prior to being sequenced, all amplicons from positive PCR reactions were purified using Wizard SV Gel and PCR Clean-up System (Promega, Australia), according to the manufacturer's instructions. The complete nucleotide sequences of *Sui1* gene amplified using the primer pair Ch2F/Ch2R for isolates 03/09-KB and 27/09-KB were assigned the GenBank accession numbers JN545747 and JN545748. The partial nucleotide sequences of *rtxC*, SXT element, *SulII*, *strB*, and *dfrA1* for isolate 03/09-KB were deposited under accession numbers JN545752, JN545751, JN545754, JN545753, and JN545750, respectively.

3. Results

All the revived isolates were identified as *V. cholerae* biotype El Tor using standard biochemical tests and slide agglutination tests showed they belonged to serogroup O1 of the Ogawa serotype.

3.1 *rstR* typing

The *rstR* typing by PCR amplification of the 501 bp amplicon using the primer pair *rstR*$^{El\ Tor}$/*rstRR* showed that all isolates possessed only the El Tor type *rstR* (Fig. 1). No amplicon was produced for other allele-specific primers among all isolates analyzed, which indicated the absence of classical, Calcutta, and environmental type *rstR*.

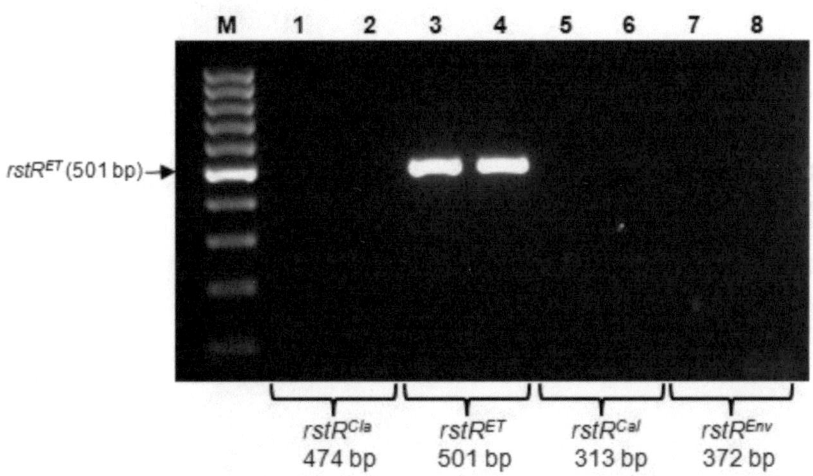

Fig. 1. Agarose gel electrophoresis products of *rstR* typing. The expected product size and types of *rstR* targeted by specific primer pairs are indicated below the gel. Lane M: 100 bp DNA ladder; lanes 1, 3, 5, and 7: representative isolate 03/09-KB; lanes 2, 4, 6, and 8: representative isolate 27/09-KB. *rstR*^{Cla}: classical type *rstR*; *rstR*^{ET}: El Tor type *rstR*; *rst*^{Cal}: Calcutta type *rstR*; *rstR*^{Env}: environmental type *rstR*.

3.2 Genetic analysis of the CTX prophage array

The presence of RS1 element was confirmed using the primer pair rstCF/rstCR to amplify a 197 bp region of *rstC* gene from all the isolates (Fig. 2a). The CTX prophage and RS1 element in each isolate was found to be arranged in the form of a RS1-CTX prophage array, as shown by the positive amplification of a 1551 bp amplicon with the primer pair rstCF4/rstAR (Fig. 2b). However, no additional RS1 element was found downstream of the CTX prophage because no amplicon was generated by the primer pair ctxBF/rstCR. The primer pair rstCF4/rstCR4 indicated the tandem arrangement of the RS1 element through the amplification of a 2629 bp amplicon, whereas no amplicon was produced for the primer pair ctxBF/cepR which indicated the presence of only a single CTX prophage. The location of the RS1-RS1-CTX prophage array on the large chromosome was verified using the primer pairs Ch1F/rstRR and ctxBF/Ch1R which amplify fragments corresponding to the upstream and downstream regions of the RS1-RS1-CTX prophage array found on the large chromosome. The absence of an RS1 element or CTX prophage on the small chromosome was confirmed through the amplification of a 910 bp amplicon using the primer pair Ch2F/Ch2R.

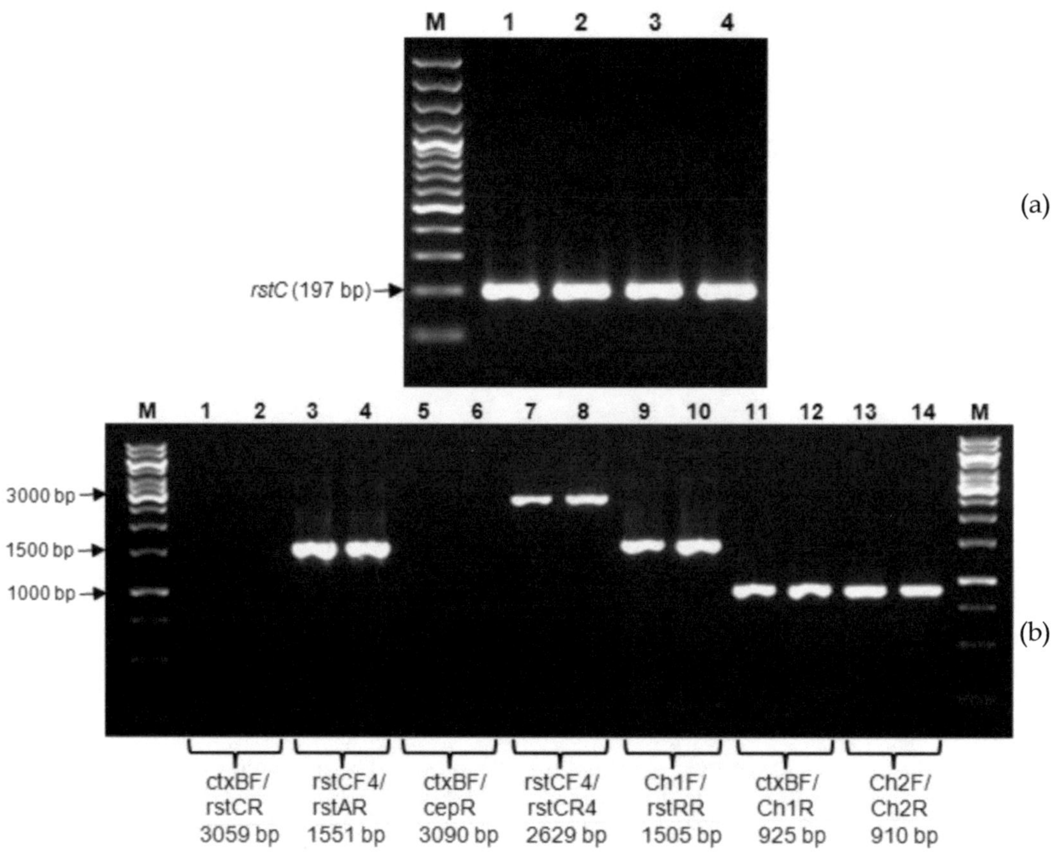

Fig. 2. (a) Agarose gel electrophoresis products in the detection of RS1 elements from representative isolates. Lane M: 100 bp Plus DNA ladder; lane 1: isolate 03/09-KB; lane 2: isolate 11/09-KB; lane 3: isolate 27/09-KB; lane 4: isolate 29/09-KB. (b) Agarose gel electrophoresis products from the analysis of the CTX prophage array. The combinations of different primer pairs and their expected product sizes are indicated below the gel. Lane M: 1 kb DNA ladder; lanes 1, 3, 5, 7, 9, 11, and 13: representative isolate 03/09-KB; lanes 2, 4, 6, 8, 10, 12, and 14: representative isolate 27/09-KB.

3.3 *rtxC* PCR

PCR analysis of *rtxC* showed that all the isolates yielded a 263 bp amplicon of the *rtxC* gene (Fig. 3).

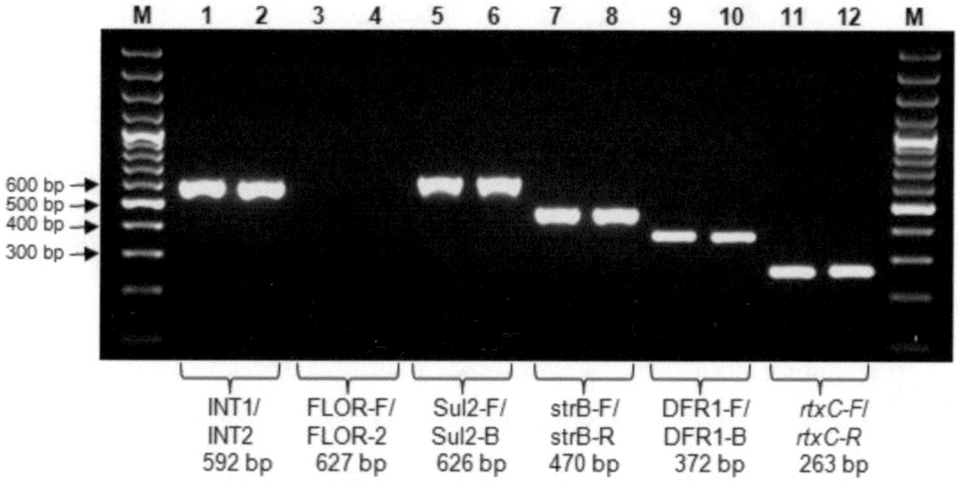

Fig. 3. Agarose gel electrophoresis products from the detection of the *rtxC* gene and the analysis of the SXT constin. The combinations of different primer pairs and their expected product sizes are indicated below the gel. Lane M: 100 bp Plus DNA ladder; lanes 1, 3, 5, 7, 9, and 11: representative isolate 03/09-KB; lanes 2, 4, 6, 8, 10, and 12: representative isolate 27/09-KB.

3.4 PCR detection of class I integrons

None of the isolates were positive for class I integrons, because no PCR amplicons were obtained with all the primer pairs tested.

3.5 PCR detection of SXT constins

All the isolates were shown to be positive for SXT element by the amplification of a 592 bp amplicon with the primer pair INT1/INT2 (Fig. 3). These isolates also had positive PCR results for the *SulII, strB,* and *dfrA1* genes, because 626 bp, 470 bp, and 372 bp amplicons were generated for the respective genes. None of the isolates were positive for *floR* genes.

4. Discussion

In November 2009, Kelantan was struck by a cholera outbreak that marked the re-emergence of this secretory diarrheal disease in the eastern state after years of absence. The aetiological agent was later found to be *V. cholerae* O1 of the altered El Tor biotype and this discovery indicated the first reported appearance of the atypical El Tor strain on Malaysian soil (Ang et al., 2010). Various genetic studies have been undertaken to gain insights into the evolution of this predominant atypical strain and research into the altered El Tor strain has primarily been directed towards the CTX prophage encoding the classical cholera toxin gene (Nguyen et al., 2009; Lee et al., 2009).

The CTX prophage found in the genome of pathogenic *V. cholerae* strains is actually an integrated form of a lysogenic filamentous bacteriophage known as the CTX phage (CTXΦ). CTXΦ is approximately 7 kb in length and it is composed of a 4.6 kb core region with a 2.4 kb RS2 region (Waldor & Mekalanos, 1996). The core region contains genes that encode for proteins involved in phage morphogenesis, specifically the core-encoded pilin (*cep*), $pIII^{CTX}$ (previously known as *orfU*), accessory cholera enterotoxin (*ace*), and zonula occludens (*zot*) genes. This core region also contains genes encoding for cholera toxin, so the acquisition of CTXΦ is viewed as virulence acquisition by a host cell. The RS2 region complements the core, because it contains genes that enable the replication (*rstA*), integration (*rstB*), and regulation (*rstR*) of CTXΦ. The RS1 element is another RS2-like element that is frequently found adjacent to the CTX prophage. The RS1 element is a 2.7 kb satellite phage that only differs from RS2 by an additional gene designated *rstC*, which encodes for a novel antirepressor to the RstR protein (Waldor et al., 1997; Heilpern & Waldor, 2003). The RS1 element provides a dual function by promoting the transcription of phage genes via an interaction between RstC and RstR, as well as enabling the replication of an adjacent CTX prophage to produce infective phage particles (Davis et al., 2002).

The *rstR* regulatory gene sequence found in the RS2 region also determined the type of CTX prophage carried by a *V. cholerae* strain. Three types of CTX prophage has been established to date, i.e., the classical CTX prophage and El Tor CTX prophage that were first detected in the *V. cholerae* serogroup O1 of the respective biotypes, and the Calcutta CTX prophage from the epidemic-causing serogroup O139 (Kimsey et al., 1998). A fourth type, the Mozambique CTX prophage, was proposed by Choi et al. (2010) and described based on the inclusion of other genetic features of the CTX prophage, including intergenic sequences and the *rstA* gene, although the CTX prophage contained a classical *rstR* gene. In the present study, the CTX prophage from the 2009 Kelantan cholera outbreak strain was found to be regulated by an El Tor type *rstR* repressor gene, but it carried a classical type *ctxB* gene. A CTX prophage with this combination of El Tor type *rstR* and classical cholera toxin gene was also designated as a hybrid CTX prophage by Grim et al. (2010). Further genetic analysis of the CTX prophage structure revealed that all isolates harboured a RS1-RS1-CTX prophage array, which was integrated on the large chromosome. As found in the prototypic seventh pandemic El Tor strains, no RS1 element or CTX prophage was integrated on the small chromosome. The RS1-RS1-CTX prophage array of the Kelantan variant represents a novel arrangement for these genetic elements among atypical El Tor strains. To the best of our knowledge, no RS1-RS1-CTX prophage array with an El Tor type *rstR* on the large chromosome has been demonstrated or reported elsewhere among the altered El Tor biotypes.

In 2009, Nguyen et al. were the first to characterize and report the CTX prophage array of altered El Tor strains isolated during cholera outbreaks that occurred in Vietnam between 2007 and 2008. All the Vietnamese isolates were found to contain the RS1-CTX prophage array with an El Tor type *rstR* on the large chromosome. Similarly, 400 *V. cholerae* isolates obtained between 2003 and 2007 from Kolkata, India were also characterized as having the RS1-CTX prophage array (Nguyen et al., 2009). Recently, the same RS1-CTX prophage array was identified in the altered El Tor isolates from Angola, Africa in 2006 (Ceccarelli et al., 2011) and from Hyderabad, India in 2009 (Goel et al., 2011). A study conducted by Goel et al. (2011) found that one of the altered El Tor isolates (VCH35) from Hyderabad, India harboured a tandem repeat of the CTX prophage in the small chromosome in addition to a RS1-CTX

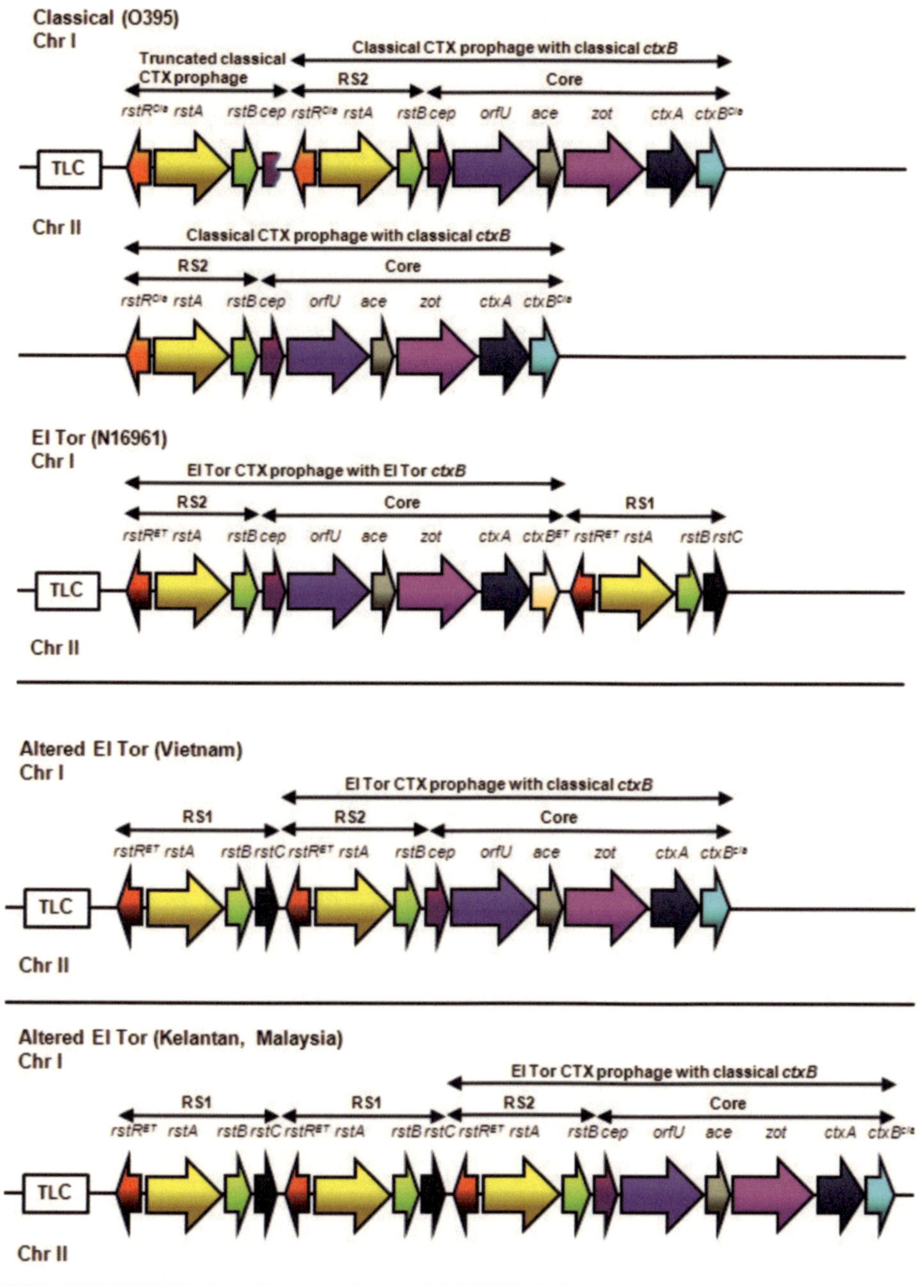

Fig. 4. Genetic map comparison of the CTX prophage arrays found in the classical reference strain (O395), El Tor reference strain (N16961), Vietnam altered El Tor, and the Kelantan altered El Tor characterized in this study. The transcription direction of each gene is indicated by arrows and each gene is shaded in different colours. Chr I: chromosome I; Chr II: chromosome II; *rstR^ET^*: El Tor type *rstR*; *rstR^Cla^*: classical type *rstR*; *ctxB^ET^*: El Tor type *ctxB*; *ctxB^Cla^*: classical type *ctxB*, TLC: toxin-linked cryptic. The map is not drawn to scale.

prophage array in the large chromosome. Although *rstR* typing of VCH35 revealed the presence of both El Tor and classical type *rstR*, the localization of these *rstR* alleles in the multiple CTX prophages was not confirmed. Various combinations of CTX prophage arrays have been documented, but the RS1-CTX prophage array appears to be the most frequently reported arrangement in altered El Tor strains associated with cholera outbreaks (Lee et al., 2009). Fig. 4 provides a diagrammatic comparison of various CTX prophage arrays, including the classical, prototypic seventh pandemic El Tor, and altered El Tor.

One of the main issues accompanying the emergence of atypical El Tor is standardization of the nomenclature and the classification scheme used when referring to these variants. This is further complicated by the fact that the current genotypic and phenotypic diversity reported among atypical El Tor strains is only the tip of the iceberg, because there are frequent new reports. In 2009, Lee et al. proposed the classification of atypical El Tor strains into two groups based on genetic differences in their RS1 element and the CTX prophage structure on each chromosome. Group I represents atypical El Tor strains with a tandem repeat of classical CTX prophage on the small chromosome, while Group II represents those possessing the RS1 and CTX prophage with El Tor type *rstR* and classical *ctxB* on the large chromosome. Based on these criteria, the Matlab and Mozambique variants were classified into Group I, while altered El Tor, such as those described by Nguyen et al. (2009), fell into Group II. This classification system was also used by Goel et al. (2011) to categorize the VCH35 isolate from Hyderabad, India into Group I, because it carried a tandem repeat of CTX prophage on the small chromosome. The type of *rstR* gene determines the type of corresponding CTX prophage, so a minor discrepancy when adhering to this classification system arises when both El Tor and classical type *rstR* are present, as is the case with VCH35. Therefore, the exact nature of the CTX prophages in tandem arrangements needs to be elucidated to ascertain whether VCH35 truly belonged to Group I. The existence of VCH35 also questions the possible need for a subgroup within Group I, should further analysis of VCH35 reveal the presence of both an El Tor and classical type CTX prophage in a tandem arrangement. In-depth genetic analysis of VCH35 is highly warranted before any conclusions can be drawn on its classification. In contrast, only one array of the RS1-CTX prophage has been reported in Group II (Lee et al., 2009). Therefore, we were able to describe a new type of array belonging to Group II based on the findings of this study. An arrangement of RS1 in tandem repeats followed by CTX prophage with an El Tor type *rstR* and classical *ctxB* was characterized in this study. This suggests that more varieties of the CTX prophage array may exist among the altered El Tor than are currently known.

The current study revealed an El Tor type *rstR* in the CTX prophage, but we also reported in our previous study that the 2009 Kelantan outbreak strain carried the El Tor type *tcpA* gene allele. In order to substantiate the El Tor lineage of this strain, we performed additional PCR analysis on the repeat in the toxin (RTX) gene cluster. The RTX gene cluster in *V. cholerae* was first identified and characterized in 1999 and it was found to be physically linked to the downstream region of the CTX prophage. The RTX gene cluster consists of *rtxA*, *rtxB*, *rtxC*, and *rtxD* genes, and it is responsible for the cytotoxic activity of *V. cholerae* in mammalian cells *in vitro*. However, gene deletions in the RTX gene cluster (specifically the *rtxC* gene and the downstream region of the *rtxA* gene) were noted among the classical biotype of *V. cholerae* O1, which resulted in defective production of cytotoxic activity (Lin et al., 1999). Based on this observation, Chow et al. (2001) developed a PCR assay targeting the *rtxC* gene for biotyping *V. cholerae* serogroup O1. We used this biotyping assay and found that all the isolates possessed the *rtxC* gene. This provided further evidence that the El Tor genomic backbone was preserved in the Kelantan altered El Tor strain.

The emergence of multidrug-resistant *V. cholerae* strains has been documented frequently in recent years (Kiiru et al., 2009; Jain et al., 2011) and this phenomenon has led to repeated calls for the more prudent use of antibiotics by the global community. Multidrug-resistant *V. cholerae* have been reported from Malaysia and the antibiogram profile of the Kelantan outbreak strain showed that the isolates were resistant to various antibiotics, including, tetracycline, erythromycin, sulfamethoxazole-trimethoprim, streptomycin, penicillin G, and polymyxin B. However, they were susceptible to ciprofloxacin, norfloxacin, chloramphenicol, gentamicin, and kanamycin (Ang et al., 2010). Therefore, we investigated the phenotypes of the outbreak strain by characterizing the corresponding genes encoding for antibiotic resistance. Amita et al. (2003) studied antibiotic resistance genes in *V. cholerae* O1 and showed that the class I integron carrying the *aadA1* gene cassette was prevalent in strains isolated before 1992, whereas the SXT element was prevalent in strains isolated after 1992. Integrons are characterized by the presence of an integrase gene (*intI*) that mediates recombination between the *attI* site found on the integron and the *attC* site on the gene cassette. The insertion of a gene cassette into the integron results in the expression of functional proteins using a promoter found in the integron (Recchia & Hall, 1995). In agreement with Amita et al. (2003), PCR analysis of the Kelantan outbreak strain showed it was negative for the class I integron and the gene cassette *aadA1* encoding resistance to streptomycin and spectinomycin.

In one of the most remarkable events in the recorded history of cholera, a novel serogroup of *V. cholerae* emerged in 1992 that was designated O139 and it replaced the O1 El Tor biotype in Bangladesh and the Indian subcontinent where it became the dominant strain, although its reign was short-lived (Faruque et al., 2003). The *V. cholerae* serogroup O139 differed from serogroup O1 in having a different somatic antigen and it was also uniquely characterized by its antibiotic resistance to sulfamethoxazole, trimethoprim, chloramphenicol, and streptomycin. Interestingly, a distinctive pattern of antibiotic resistance was found after the re-emergence of serogroup O1 El Tor in 1994 where all the El Tor strains were found to be resistant to these four antibiotics, which strikingly resembled the profile of serogroup O139 (Waldor et al., 1996). The corresponding antibiotic resistance genes in serogroup O1 El Tor were collectively referred to as ICE*Vch*Ind1 (previously known as SXT^{ET}) and they were genetically closely related to the SXT^{MO10}, which encodes for antibiotic resistance to the same four antibiotics mentioned above by serogroup O139. Based on a comparative DNA analysis, both the ICE*Vch*Ind1 and the SXT^{MO10} elements were considered to be derived from a common precursor (Hochhut et al., 2001; Burrus et al., 2006). The results of PCR conducted on the SXT constin in this study showed that all the Kelantan outbreak strains contained the SXT element. Genes conferring resistance to sulfamethoxazole (*SulII*), trimethoprim (*dfrA1*), and streptomycin (*strB*) were detected in all isolates, with the exception of the chloramphenicol resistance gene (*floR*). The detection of the antibiotic genes was consistent with the findings in the phenotypic antibiotic susceptibility testing and the SXT constin detected in the present outbreak strain appeared to have a deletion of the *floR* gene, when compared with the STX^{ET} reported from elsewhere (Hochhut et al., 2001). The SXT constin without the *floR* gene represented a variant of the SXT^{ET} constin and, other than this study, the SXT variant has also been found among altered El Tor strains from India (Goel & Jiang, 2010). It was recently reported that an altered El Tor strain carrying both an integron and an SXT element had been identified among outbreak strains from Solapur, India (Jain et al., 2011). These findings are important, because the management of cholera patients usually entails fluid replacement therapy to replace the electrolytes lost during profuse diarrheal bouts. However, antibiotic therapy serves as an adjunct to fluid replacement therapy to reduce the duration of the disease and the excretion of the bacterium (Lindenbaum et al., 1967). Thus, continuous monitoring of changes in antibiotic resistance patterns is highly recommended, because the SXT constin harbouring various antibiotic resistance genes can be acquired easily via lateral gene transfer (Iwanaga et al., 2004).

5. Conclusion

Genetic analysis performed on the Kelantan altered El Tor strain isolated during a cholera outbreak in 2009 revealed a novel CTX prophage array where a tandem repeat of the RS1 element was found upstream of the CTX prophage on the large chromosome. This is the first report of a RS1-RS1-CTX prophage array among altered El Tor strains that fit into Group II according to the classification system of Lee et al. (2009). All isolates carried the SXT constin and we identified genes conferring resistance to sulfamethoxazole, trimethoprim and chloramphenicol, which correlated with their phenotypic expression in the antibiogram profile.

The emergence of the altered El Tor is viewed as an evolutionary optimization of *V. cholerae* strains in the development of a successor to the current cholera pandemic. The altered El Tor strains are poised to become epidemiologically dominant and they might hold the key to sustaining the current seventh pandemic. Equipped with the unique characteristics of the classical and El Tor biotypes, the altered El Tor has already been associated with more severe cases of cholera (Siddique et al., 2010) and it appears to be widely disseminated around the globe. The research community should actively unravel the wealth of knowledge that lies within these atypical El Tor strains and gain a better understanding that can be translated into measures to combat and conquer cholera.

6. Acknowledgements

This study was funded by USM Research University Grant 1001/PPSP/813045, Postgraduate Research Grant Schemes (1001/PPSP/8144014 and 1001/PPSP/8144013) and eScienceFund 305/PPSP/6113214. The first and second authors gratefully acknowledge the financial support provided by USM through the Vice-Chancellor Award and USM Fellowship Scheme, respectively.

7. References

Alam, M., Nusrin, S., Islam, A., Bhuiyan, N. A., Rahim, N., Delgado, G., Morales, R., Mendez, J. L., Navarro, A., Gil, A. I., Watanabe, H., Morita, M., Nair, G. B. & Cravioto, A. (2010). Cholera between 1991 and 1997 in Mexico was associated with infection by classical, El Tor, and El Tor variants of *Vibrio cholerae*. *J Clin Microbiol*, 48 (10), 3666-74.

Amita, Chowdhury, S. R., Thungapathra, M., Ramamurthy, T., Nair, G. B. & Ghosh, A. (2003). Class I integrons and SXT elements in El Tor strains isolated before and after 1992 *Vibrio cholerae* O139 outbreak, Calcutta, India. *Emerg Infect Dis,* 9 (4), 500-2.

Ang, G. Y., Yu, C. Y., Balqis, K., Elina, H. T., Azura, H., Hani, M. H. & Yean, C. Y. (2010). Molecular evidence of cholera outbreak caused by a toxigenic *Vibrio cholerae* O1 El tor variant strain in Kelantan, Malaysia. *J Clin Microbiol,* 48 (11), 3963-9.

Ansaruzzaman, M., Bhuiyan, N. A., Nair, B. G., Sack, D. A., Lucas, M., Deen, J. L., Ampuero, J. & Chaignat, C. L. (2004). Cholera in Mozambique, variant of *Vibrio cholerae. Emerg Infect Dis,* 10 (11), 2057-9.

Bhattacharya, T., Chatterjee, S., Maiti, D., Bhadra, R. K., Takeda, Y., Nair, G. B. & Nandy, R. K. (2006). Molecular analysis of the rstR and orfU genes of the CTX prophages integrated in the small chromosomes of environmental *Vibrio cholerae* non-O1, non-O139 strains. *Environ Microbiol,* 8 (3), 526-634.

Burrus, V., Marrero, J. & Waldor, M. K. (2006). The current ICE age: biology and evolution of SXT-related integrating conjugative elements. *Plasmid,* 55 (3), 173-83.

Ceccarelli, D., Spagnoletti, M., Bacciu, D., Cappuccinelli, P. & Colombo, M. M. (2011). New *V. cholerae* atypical El Tor variant emerged during the 2006 epidemic outbreak in Angola. *BMC Microbiol,* 11 130.

Center for Diseases Control and Prevention (2010). Update on cholera --- Haiti, Dominican Republic, and Florida, 2010. *MMWR Morb Mortal Wkly Rep,* 59 (50), 1637-41.

Chin, C. S., Sorenson, J., Harris, J. B., Robins, W. P., Charles, R. C., Jean-Charles, R. R., Bullard, J., Webster, D. R., Kasarskis, A., Peluso, P., Paxinos, E. E., Yamaichi, Y., Calderwood, S. B., Mekalanos, J. J., Schadt, E. E. & Waldor, M. K. (2011). The origin of the Haitian cholera outbreak strain. *N Engl J Med,* 364 (1), 33-42.

Choi, S. Y., Lee, J. H., Kim, E. J., Lee, H. R., Jeon, Y. S., von Seidlein, L., Deen, J., Ansaruzzaman, M., Lucas, G. M., Barreto, A., Songane, F. F., Mondlane, C., Nair, G. B., Czerkinsky, C., Clemens, J. D., Chun, J. & Kim, D. W. (2010). Classical RS1 and environmental RS1 elements in *Vibrio cholerae* O1 El Tor strains harbouring a tandem repeat of CTX prophage: revisiting Mozambique in 2005. *J Med Microbiol,* 59 (Pt 3), 302-8.

Chow, K. H., Ng, T. K., Yuen, K. Y. & Yam, W. C. (2001). Detection of RTX toxin gene in *Vibrio cholerae* by PCR. *J Clin Microbiol,* 39 (7), 2594-7.

Dalsgaard, A., Forslund, A., Sandvang, D., Arntzen, L. & Keddy, K. (2001). *Vibrio cholerae* O1 outbreak isolates in Mozambique and South Africa in 1998 are multiple-drug resistant, contain the SXT element and the aadA2 gene located on class 1 integrons. *J Antimicrob Chemother,* 48 (6), 827-38.

Davis, B. M., Kimsey, H. H., Kane, A. V. & Waldor, M. K. (2002). A satellite phage-encoded antirepressor induces repressor aggregation and cholera toxin gene transfer. *EMBO J,* 21 (16), 4240-9.

Faruque, S. M., Albert, M. J. & Mekalanos, J. J. (1998). Epidemiology, genetics, and ecology of toxigenic *Vibrio cholerae. Microbiol Mol Biol Rev,* 62 (4), 1301-14.

Faruque, S. M., Sack, D. A., Sack, R. B., Colwell, R. R., Takeda, Y. & Nair, G. B. (2003). Emergence and evolution of *Vibrio cholerae* O139. *Proc Natl Acad Sci U S A,* 100 (3), 1304-9.

Gilmour, M. W., Martel-Laferriere, V., Levesque, S., Gaudreau, C., Bekal, S., Nadon, C. & Bourgault, A. M. (2011). *Vibrio cholerae* in traveler from Haiti to Canada. *Emerg Infect Dis,* 17 (6), 1124-5.

Goel, A. K., Jain, M., Kumar, P., Sarguna, P., Bai, M., Ghosh, N. & Gopalan, N. (2011). Molecular characterization reveals involvement of altered El Tor biotype *Vibrio cholerae* O1 strains in cholera outbreak at Hyderabad, India. *J Microbiol,* 49 (2), 280-4.

Goel, A. K. & Jiang, S. C. (2010). Genetic determinants of virulence, antibiogram and altered biotype among the *Vibrio cholerae* O1 isolates from different cholera outbreaks in India. *Infect Genet Evol,* 10 (6), 815-9.

Grim, C. J., Hasan, N. A., Taviani, E., Haley, B., Chun, J., Brettin, T. S., Bruce, D. C., Detter, J. C., Han, C. S., Chertkov, O., Challacombe, J., Huq, A., Nair, G. B. & Colwell, R. R. (2010). Genome sequence of hybrid *Vibrio cholerae* O1 MJ-1236, B-33, and CIRS101 and comparative genomics with V. cholerae. *J Bacteriol,* 192 (13), 3524-33.

Heilpern, A. J. & Waldor, M. K. (2003). pIIICTX, a predicted CTXphi minor coat protein, can expand the host range of coliphage fd to include *Vibrio cholerae. J Bacteriol,* 185 (3), 1037-44.

Hochhut, B., Lotfi, Y., Mazel, D., Faruque, S. M., Woodgate, R. & Waldor, M. K. (2001). Molecular analysis of antibiotic resistance gene clusters in *Vibrio cholerae* O139 and O1 SXT constins. *Antimicrob Agents Chemother,* 45 (11), 2991-3000.

Iwanaga, M., Toma, C., Miyazato, T., Insisiengmay, S., Nakasone, N. & Ehara, M. (2004). Antibiotic resistance conferred by a class I integron and SXT constin in *Vibrio cholerae* O1 strains isolated in Laos. *Antimicrob Agents Chemother,* 48 (7), 2364-9.

Jain, M., Goel, A. K., Bhattacharya, P., Ghatole, M. & Kamboj, D. V. (2011). Multidrug resistant *Vibrio cholerae* O1 El Tor carrying classical ctxB allele involved in a cholera outbreak in South Western India. *Acta Trop,* 117 (2), 152-6.

Kay, B. A., Bopp, C. A. & Wells, J. G. (1994) Isolation and identification of *Vibrio cholerae* O1 from fecal specimens, ASM Press, Washinton, DC.

Kiiru, J. N., Saidi, S. M., Goddeeris, B. M., Wamae, N. C., Butaye, P. & Kariuki, S. M. (2009). Molecular characterisation of *Vibrio cholerae* O1 strains carrying an SXT/R391-like element from cholera outbreaks in Kenya: 1994-2007. *BMC Microbiol,* 9 275.

Kimsey, H. H., Nair, G. B., Ghosh, A. & Waldor, M. K. (1998). Diverse CTXphis and evolution of new pathogenic *Vibrio cholerae. Lancet,* 352 (9126), 457-8.

Lee, J. H., Choi, S. Y., Jeon, Y. S., Lee, H. R., Kim, E. J., Nguyen, B. M., Hien, N. T., Ansaruzzaman, M., Islam, M. S., Bhuiyan, N. A., Niyogi, S. K., Sarkar, B. L., Nair, G. B., Kim, D. S., Lopez, A. L., Czerkinsky, C., Clemens, J. D., Chun, J. & Kim, D. W. (2009). Classification of hybrid and altered *Vibrio cholerae* strains by CTX prophage and RS1 element structure. *J Microbiol,* 47 (6), 783-8.

Lin, W., Fullner, K. J., Clayton, R., Sexton, J. A., Rogers, M. B., Calia, K. E., Calderwood, S. B., Fraser, C. & Mekalanos, J. J. (1999). Identification of a *Vibrio cholerae* RTX toxin gene cluster that is tightly linked to the cholera toxin prophage. *Proc Natl Acad Sci U S A,* 96 (3), 1071-6.

Lindenbaum, J., Greenough, W. B. & Islam, M. R. (1967). Antibiotic therapy of cholera. *Bull World Health Organ,* 36 (6), 871-83.

Morita, M., Ohnishi, M., Arakawa, E., Yamamoto, S., Nair, G. B., Matsushita, S., Yokoyama, K., Kai, A., Seto, K., Watanabe, H. & Izumiya, H. (2010). Emergence and genetic diversity of El Tor *Vibrio cholerae* O1 that possess classical biotype ctxB among travel-associated cases of cholera in Japan. *J Med Microbiol,* 59 (Pt 6), 708-12.

Nair, G. B., Faruque, S. M., Bhuiyan, N. A., Kamruzzaman, M., Siddique, A. K. & Sack, D. A. (2002). New variants of *Vibrio cholerae* O1 biotype El Tor with attributes of the classical biotype from hospitalized patients with acute diarrhea in Bangladesh. *J Clin Microbiol,* 40 (9), 3296-9.

Nair, G. B., Qadri, F., Holmgren, J., Svennerholm, A. M., Safa, A., Bhuiyan, N. A., Ahmad, Q. S., Faruque, S. M., Faruque, A. S., Takeda, Y. & Sack, D. A. (2006). Cholera due to altered El Tor strains of *Vibrio cholerae* O1 in Bangladesh. *J Clin Microbiol,* 44 (11), 4211-3.

Nguyen, B. M., Lee, J. H., Cuong, N. T., Choi, S. Y., Hien, N. T., Anh, D. D., Lee, H. R., Ansaruzzaman, M., Endtz, H. P., Chun, J., Lopez, A. L., Czerkinsky, C., Clemens, J. D. & Kim, D. W. (2009). Cholera outbreaks caused by an altered *Vibrio cholerae* O1 El Tor biotype strain producing classical cholera toxin B in Vietnam in 2007 to 2008. *J Clin Microbiol,* 47 (5), 1568-71.

Nusrin, S., Khan, G. Y., Bhuiyan, N. A., Ansaruzzaman, M., Hossain, M. A., Safa, A., Khan, R., Faruque, S. M., Sack, D. A., Hamabata, T., Takeda, Y. & Nair, G. B. (2004). Diverse CTX phages among toxigenic *Vibrio cholerae* O1 and O139 strains isolated between 1994 and 2002 in an area where cholera is endemic in Bangladesh. *J Clin Microbiol,* 42 (12), 5854-6.

Okada, K., Chantaroj, S., Roobthaisong, A., Hamada, S. & Sawanpanyalert, P. (2010). A cholera outbreak of the *Vibrio cholerae* O1 El Tor variant carrying classical CtxB in northeastern Thailand in 2007. *Am J Trop Med Hyg,* 82 (5), 875-8.

Raychoudhuri, A., Patra, T., Ghosh, K., Ramamurthy, T., Nandy, R. K., Takeda, Y., Balakrish-Nair, G. & Mukhopadhyay, A. K. (2009). Classical ctxB in Vibrio cholerae O1, Kolkata, India. *Emerg Infect Dis,* 15 (1), 131-2.

Recchia, G. D. & Hall, R. M. (1995). Gene cassettes: a new class of mobile element. *Microbiology,* 141 (Pt 12) 3015-27.

Ryan, E. T. (2011). The cholera pandemic, still with us after half a century: time to rethink. *PLoS Negl Trop Dis,* 5 (1), e1003.

Sack, D. A., Sack, R. B., Nair, G. B. & Siddique, A. K. (2004). Cholera. *Lancet,* 363 (9404), 223-33.

Safa, A., Nair, G. B. & Kong, R. Y. (2009). Evolution of new variants of *Vibrio cholerae* O1. *Trends Microbiol,* 18 (1), 46-54.

Siddique, A. K., Nair, G. B., Alam, M., Sack, D. A., Huq, A., Nizam, A., Longini, I. M., Jr., Qadri, F., Faruque, S. M., Colwell, R. R., Ahmed, S., Iqbal, A., Bhuiyan, N. A. & Sack, R. B. (2010). El Tor cholera with severe disease: a new threat to Asia and beyond. *Epidemiol Infect,* 138 (3), 347-52.

Sithivong, N., Izumiya, H., Munnalath, K., Phouthavane, T., Chomlasak, K., Sisavath, L., Vongdouangchanh, A., Vongprachanh, P., Watanabe, H. & Ohinishi, M. (2010). Cholera outbreak, Laos, 2007. *Emerg Infect Dis,* 16 (4), 745-6.

Waldor, M. K. & Mekalanos, J. J. (1996). Lysogenic conversion by a filamentous phage encoding cholera toxin. *Science,* 272 (5270), 1910-4.

Waldor, M. K., Rubin, E. J., Pearson, G. D., Kimsey, H. & Mekalanos, J. J. (1997). Regulation, replication, and integration functions of the *Vibrio cholerae* CTXphi are encoded by region RS2. *Mol Microbiol,* 24 (5), 917-26.

Waldor, M. K., Tschape, H. & Mekalanos, J. J. (1996). A new type of conjugative transposon encodes resistance to sulfamethoxazole, trimethoprim, and streptomycin in *Vibrio cholerae* O139. *J Bacteriol,* 178 (14), 4157-65.

6

Integration of Global Regulatory Mechanisms Controlling *Vibrio Cholerae* Behavior

Jorge A. Benitez[1] and Anisia J. Silva[2]
[1]*Southern Research Institute Drug Discovery Division, Birmingham, Alabama*
[2]*Morehouse School of Medicine Department of Microbiology, Biochemistry & Immunology, Atlanta, Georgia*
USA

1. Introduction

Cholera is an acute water-borne diarrheal disease caused by the facultative Gram-negative bacterium *Vibrio cholerae* of serogroup O1 of the classical and El Tor biotypes and serogroup O139. Characteristics of this bacterium are its comma-shaped morphology, expression of a fast-rotating polar flagellum, and production of cholera toxin (CT). The O1 *V. cholerae* serogroup contains a common A antigen and can be subdivided in Ogawa and Inaba serotypes on the basis of serotype-specific antigens B and C, respectively (Kaper et al., 1995). Mankind has experienced seven recorded cholera pandemics. The seventh and current pandemic is characterized by the predominance of the O1 serogroup El Tor biotype, with periodic emergence of O139 strains, which exhibit a new lipopolysaccharide (LPS) and a capsule (Albert, 1994). Cholera, which continues to be a major public health concern in endemic areas of South Asia and Africa, is estimated to cause 5.5 million cases of disease and 130,000 deaths per year. The disease, which commonly occurs as rapidly spreading and difficult to contain outbreaks in low-income countries, is a common sequel of natural and human disasters. The typical cholera symptoms include a profuse rice-watery diarrhea and vomiting. If untreated, this condition can lead to severe dehydration, electrolyte imbalances, and death. Cholera infections can be effectively treated with oral rehydration and, in cases of severe illness, with antibiotics. Antibiotic treatment lessens the duration of illness and reduces the excretion of highly infective *Vibrios* (Nelson et al., 2011). The downside however, is the emergence of multiple-antibiotic resistant O1 and O139 strains (Das & Kaur, 2008; Roychowdhury et al., 2008; Okeke et al., 2007; Mwansa et al., 2007; Faruque et al., 2007).

As illustrated in Fig. 1, the cholera bacterium is fundamentally an organism adapted to the aquatic environment, which has evolved to maximize the benefit of being casually ingested by humans. The goal of this chapter is to examine the global regulatory mechanisms that assist the cholera bacterium in colonizing the small bowel of humans and persisting in the aquatic environment.

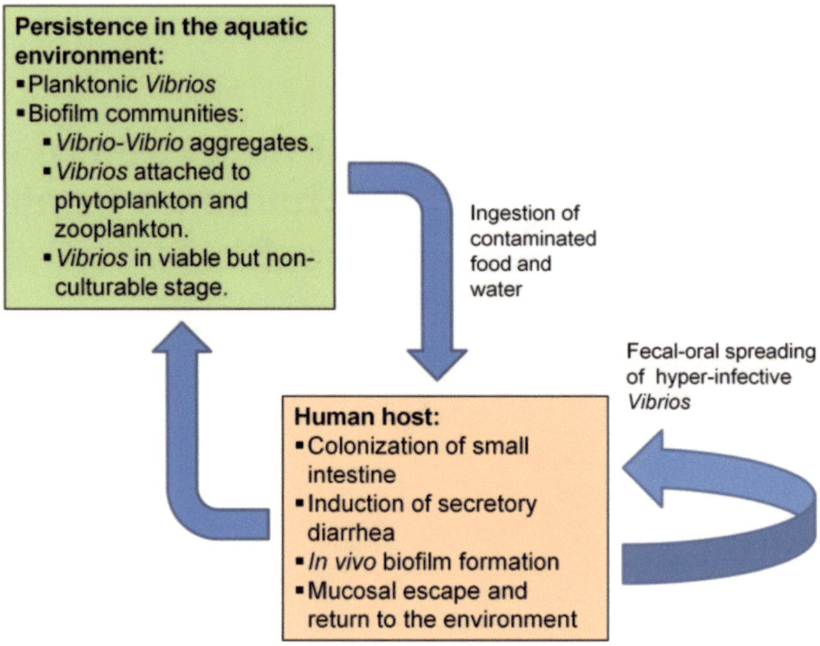

Fig. 1. The *V. cholerae* life cycle

2. The Vibrio cholerae dual life cycle

2.1 *Vibrio cholerae* persistence in the environment

V. cholerae occur globally in most estuaries and coastal ecosystems, where their concentrations range from 10^1 to 10^4 cells per mL and can reach 10^6 cells per g of sediment (Urakawa & Rivera, 2006). In nature, *Vibrios* are subject to various physical and chemical environmental stresses, which include nutrient limitation, extreme temperatures, and oxidative stress. The persistence of *Vibrios* in the aquatic environment is additionally challenged by protozoan grazing and bacteriophage infection (Matz et al., 2005; Jensen et al., 2006; Faruque et al. 2005, 2005a). The bacterium can be found in the form of planktonic free-swimming cells or as sessile biofilm communities associated with phytoplankton and zooplankton (Watnick & Kolter, 1999; Kierek & Watnick, 2003; Huq et al., 1983; Islam et al., 1990; Kaper et al., 1979). The capacity of *V. cholerae* to form biofilm communities has been proposed to be involved in bacterial survival in the aquatic environment (Faruque et al., 2006: Joelsson et al., 2006: Matz et al., 2005: Schoolnik & Yildiz, 2000). Biofilm formation and adoption of a rugose colonial morphology correlate with the production of *V. cholerae* exopolysaccharide (*vps*) (Yildiz & Schoolnik, 1999). The *V. cholerae* rugose colonial variant described by White (1938) is more resistant to chlorinated water (Morris et al., 1996: Rice et al., 1992) and to osmotic and oxidative stresses (Wai et al., 1998: Yildiz & Schoolnik, 1999). In aquatic ecosystems, *V. cholerae* can also be found in the form of large biofilm aggregates of partially dormant cells that resist cultivation in conventional media but can be recovered as virulent *Vibrios* by animal passage (Faruque et al., 2006). These biofilm aggregates, named conditionally viable environmental cells (CVEC), appear to be similar to previously described viable but not culturable cells (Xu et al. 1982). The role of these biofilm aggregates in infection is considered below.

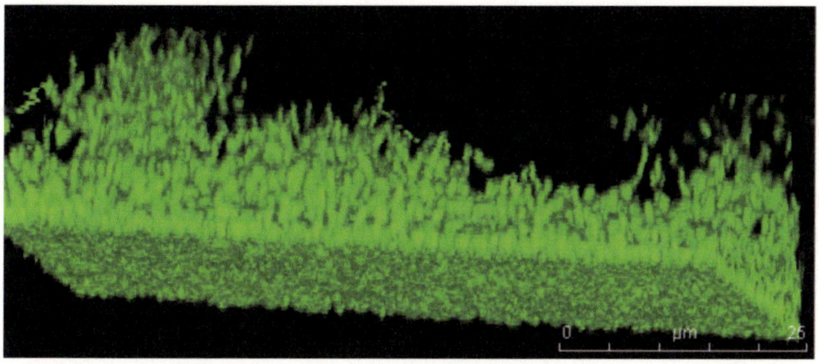

Fig. 2. Confocal microscopy three-dimensional image of a *V. cholerae* biofilm stained with the fluorescent dye, SYRO-9, and imaged using 485- and 498-nm excitation and emission wavelength, respectively. Biofilm developmental is initiated by a reversible surface attachment, followed by changes in gene expression patterns conducive to more permanent adherence, synthesis of exopolysaccharide matrix material, and building of three-dimensional columnar aggregates and channels.

2.2 Transition of Vibrio cholerae between the aquatic environment and the human intestine

A cholera infection starts with human ingestion of *V. cholerae* present in contaminated water or food (Fig. 1). Infecting *Vibrios* that survive passage through the acidic stomach compartment progress to the nutrient-rich environment of the human small intestine. It has been suggested that *V. cholerae* biofilm aggregates are more resistant to the initial low pH stress (Zhu & Mekalanos, 2003). Mutations in *vps* genes that block biofilm matrix exopolysaccharide biosynthesis impair colonization in the suckling mouse model (Fong et al., 2010). In addition, deletion of genes encoding the alternative stress-related sigma factors σ^S and σ^E inhibit bacterial colonization (Merrel et al., 2000; Kovacikova & Skorupski, 2002). *Vibrios* use their fast-rotating polar flagellum to swim toward and bind to the mucus layer through their LPS (Benitez et al., 1997), the GbpA adhesin (Bhowmick et al., 2008; Jude et al., 2009), and other factors. Subsequent colonization requires expression of the toxin co-regulated pilus (TCP) (Herrington et al., 1988). Intestinal fluid secretion results from production by colonizing *Vibrios* of CT, which acts by increasing the cAMP content of host cells. Dissemination of the infection throughout the small bowel most likely involves detachment of *Vibrios* in a motile stage that could swim toward and adhere to other sites along the small intestine. *Vibrio* detachment and adherence could create new infective foci and enhance the severity of the disease. In the course of this process, however, *Vibrios* that detach but fail to adhere and establish new infection foci can be cleared from the small intestine by peristalsis (Walker & Owen, 1990) and excreted in the rice-watery diarrhea. As the overall population of *Vibrios* increases, and nutrients become in short supply, detachment predominates over re-colonization, a process also known as mucosal escape (Nielsen et al., 2006). Late in infection and, in preparation for their extra-intestinal life, *Vibrios* associate into biofilm aggregates prior to exiting the host (Faruque et al., 2006). Such biofilms, formed *in vivo*, are in a stage of transient hyperinfectivity (Tamayo et al., 2010) that enhances their dissemination through the fecal-oral route (Merrel et al., 2002) (Fig. 1). This view of the time course of a cholera infection is consistent with the presence of highly motile planktonic *Vibrios* and biofilm aggregates in freshly shed cholera stools.

The timing of events that occur during infection is difficult to ascertain, since current models likely yield average data from *Vibrio* subpopulations at different stages of the infective process. A promising approach in this direction has been the development of a recombination-based *in vivo* expression technology (RIVET) (Camilli & Mekalanos, 1995; Lee et al., 1999). With this approach, it has been reported that *tcpA* and *ctxA* are expressed within the first 6 h of infection in the infant mouse intestine (Lee et al., 1999). Nevertheless, much remains to be learned about the events, occurring later in infection, that are involved in bacterial dissemination within the host and their exit to the environment.

3. Major virulence factors

V. cholerae O1 and O139 strains, which cause epidemic cholera, exhibit three major characteristics: (a) production of CT, (b) expression of TCP, and (c) expression of a sheathed polar flagellum. *V. cholerae* produces additional potentially toxic factors, such hemagglutinin (HA)/protease (Hase & Finkelstein, 1991), hemolysin (Nagamune et al., 1996), the repeat toxin (RTX) (Lin et al., 1999), the zonula occludens toxin (Fasano et al., 1991), and the accessory cholera enterotoxin (Trucksis et al., 1993). The potential contributions of these secondary factors to the infective process has been reviewed by Fullner (2003). The regulatory pathways that control virulence, motility, and biofilm formation have been extensively studied and reviewed elsewhere (Childers & Klose, 2007; Matson et al., 2007). In this chapter, we discuss how these regulatory pathways are interconnected.

3.1 Cholera toxin and the toxin co-regulated pilus

CT is an ADP-ribosyl transferase responsible for the profuse rice-watery diarrhea typical of this disease (Finkelstein, 1992; Kaper et al., 1995). It is composed of one A subunit (CTA) which catalyzes NAD-dependent ADP-ribosylation of host adenylate cyclase and five B subunits (CTB) that carry the ganglioside GM_1 receptor binding site (Finkelstein, 1992). The genes encoding CTA (*ctxA*) and CTB (*ctxB*) are located in the genome of the filamentous phage CTXΦ (Waldor & Mekalanos, 1996). The CTXΦ receptor is the type IV pilus and colonization factor TCP (Waldor & Mekalanos, 1996). The expression of CT and TCP is co-regulated by a complex regulatory network. At the top of the regulatory cascade, the regulator AphA enhances transcription of the transmembrane regulators TcpP and TcpH (Hase & Mekalanos, 1998; Kovacikova & Skorupski, 2001). AphA alone cannot activate transcription of *tcpPH,* but requires interaction with the LysR-type regulator, AphB which binds downstream of the AphA binding site to the *tcpPH* promoter (Kovacikova & Skorupski, 2001). TcpPH, in concert with the transmembrane regulators ToxR and ToxS (Miller & Mekalanos, 1985: Miller et al., 1989) (Fig. 3), activates expression of the soluble regulator, ToxT (DiRita et al., 1991). Finally, ToxT interacts with the *ctxA* and *tcpA* promoters to activate production of CT and TCP (DiRita et al., 1991).

3.2 Motility

Motility is necessary for *V. cholerae* to establish infections, for colonization of the small intestine, to detach and spread along the small intestine, and/or to exit the host and return to the environment (Butler & Camilli, 2004; Lee et al., 2001; Nielsen et al., 2006; Silva et al., 2006). In addition, shedding of *V. cholerae* flagellins induce an inflammatory response in the host by interacting with Toll-like receptor V to induce the production of pro-inflammatory interleukin-8 (Harrison et al., 2008; Rui et al., 2010; Xicohtencalt-Cortes, et al. 2006). Flagellar motility also influences the expression of CT and TCP (Gardel & Mekalanos, 1996; Hase, 2001; Hase & Mekalanos, 1999: Hase et al., 2001; Silva et al., 2006; Syed et al., 2009).

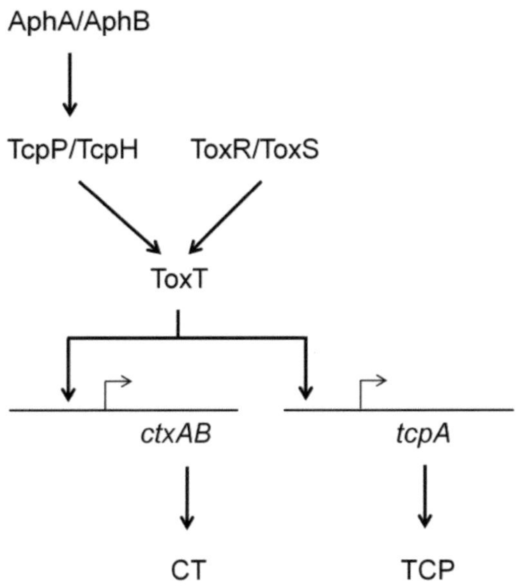

Fig. 3. Regulation of CT and TCP expression

Motility is a complex phenotype that requires (a) the synthesis and export of the flagellum and its motor, (b) coupling of the flagellum motor to an energy source and (c) coupling of flagellum rotation to numerous chemosensory pathways. The *V. cholerae* genome encodes multiple flagellin genes (*fllaABCDE*), but only flagellin mutants lacking FlaA are non-flagellated (Klose & Mekalanos, 1998; Klose et al., 1998; Klose & Mekalanos, 1998a). The expression of motility requires a hierarchical regulatory cascade involving the alternative RNA polymerase (RNAP) subunits, σ^{54} and σ^{28} and the σ^{54}-dependent transcriptional activators, FlrA and FlrC (Correa et al., 2004; Correa & Klose, 2005; Correa et al., 2000; Correa et al., 2005; Prouty et al., 2001; Syed et al., 2009).

The *V. cholerae* polar flagellum is powered by sodium motive force (Kojima et al., 1999). *V. cholerae* expresses Na^+ pumps such as the Na^+-translocating NADH: quinone oxidoreductase and multiple Na^+/H^+ antiporters responsible for maintaining the inward Na^+ gradient that drives flagellum rotation (Hase et al., 2001). Genes required for flagellum rotation include *pomA* (*motA*), *pomB* (*motB*), *motX, motY, fliG, fliM and fliN*. Inactivation of *motA motB, motY* or *motX* by mutation abolish motility but does not prevent flagellum assembly (Boles & McCarter, 2000; Kim & McCarter, 2000; McCarter, 2001). MotA and MotB translocate Na^+ by forming the Na^+ conducting channel; MotX and MotY are required for torque generation (Asai et al., 1997). FliG, FliM and FliN, also required for torque generation, form the switch complex at the base of the flagellum basal body (Boles & McCarter, 2000; McCarter, 2001). The direction of flagellum rotation (clockwise or counterclockwise) is dictated by the interaction between the response regulator CheY3 and the FliM component of the motor

(Berg, 2003; Boin et al., 2008; Hyakutake et al., 2005). The *V. cholerae* genome contains numerous chemotaxis-related genes, including multiple methyl-accepting chemotaxis proteins (MCP), methyltransferases (CheR), methylesterases (CheB), linker proteins (CheW), histidine kinases (CheA), and response regulators (CheY), mostly located in three clusters (Boin et al., 2008). Only a limited number of genes, however, have been demonstrated to be essential for chemotaxis. These genes include *cheA*-2 (Gosink et al., 2002), *cheR*-2 (Boin et al., 2004) and *cheY*-3 (Hyakutake et al., 2005). The function of other chemotaxis genes and the reason for their redundancy are not understood.

Transcription hierarchy class	Class I	Class II	Class III	Class IV
Upstream regulator	-	RpoN (σ^{54}) and FlrA	RpoN (σ^{54}) and FlrC	FliA (σ^{28})
Genes	*flrA*	*flrBC* *fliEFGHIJ* *flhA operon* *fliA*	*flgBCDEFGHIJ* *fliKLMNOPQ* *motY* *flaA* *flhB* *flgKLOPT*	*motAB* *motX* *flaBCDE*
Function	σ^{54}-dependent activator	Regulatory factors, MS ring-switch and export components	Basal body-hook, major flagellin, motor component	Alternative flagellins, anti-sigma factor FlgM, motor components

Table 1. Transcriptional organization of motility genes (adapted from Syed et al., 2009; Prouty et al., 2001).

We recently developed and validated a high-throughput screening assay for inhibitors of *V. cholerae* motility (Rasmussen et al., 2010). A new inhibitor consisting of a quinazoline 2,4-diamino analog (Q24DA) induced a flagellated, non-motile phenotype and was specific for the Na^+-dependent polar flagellum motor of pathogenic *Vibrios* (Rasmussen et al., 2010). While some motility mutants express more CT and TCP (Silva et al., 2006, Syed et al. 2009), blocking motility with Q24DA diminished CT and TCP expression. Thus, the relationship between motility and CT expression could be more complex than anticipated by genetic studies. Identification of the molecular target of Q24DA and other inhibitors is required to clarify the disconnection between the genetic and chemical approaches.

3.3 Hemagglutinin/protease

Numerous *V. cholerae* strains of the El Tor biotype express a Zn-dependent metalloprotease (mucinase) known as hemagglutinin (HA)/protease (Finkelstein et al., 1983; Hase & Finkelstein, 1991). HA/protease enhances enterotoxicity in the rabbit ileal loop model of cholera (Ichinose et al., 1994; Silva et al., 2006) and contributes to live vaccine candidates' reactogenicity in humans (Benitez et al., 1999; Garcia et al., 2005). In cell culture, HA/protease perturbs the paracellular barrier of intestinal epithelial cells (Mel et al., 2000: Wu et al., 1996) by acting on tight junction-associated proteins (Wu et al., 2000). A second proposed role for HA/protease is to facilitate *V. cholerae* detachment from the intestinal mucosa when infecting *Vibrios* reach a high cell density (Finkelstein et al., 1992; Benitez et al., 1997; Silva et al., 2003; Silva et al., 2006; Robert et al., 1996). Consistently, inactivation of *hapA* encoding HA/protease enhances adherence to mucin-coated polystyrene plates (Silva et al., 2006), adherence to mucin-secreting differentiated HT29-18N2 cultured cells (Benitez et al., 1997), and colonization of the suckling mouse intestine (Robert et al., 1996; Silva et al., 2006). The mucinase activity of HA/protease (Finkelstein et al., 1983), together with its capacity to cleave the mucin-binding adhesin GbpA (Jude et al., 2009) at high cell density, has provided a mechanism supporting the "detachase" function attributed to this protein. The high viscosity of the mucus layer promotes breakage and loss of the polar flagellum (Liu et al., 2008). We have proposed that production of extracellular proteases facilitates preservation of the flagellum of *V. cholerae* during detachment by decreasing the viscosity of the medium (Silva et al., 2003). This could result from HA/protease degradation of preexisting mucin (Finkelstein et al., 1983) and cleavage of the GbpA adhesin, which enhances the production of intestinal mucins (Bhowmick et al., 2008).

4. Global regulatory networks controlling *Vibrio cholerae* behavior

In a dynamic environment, the capacity of *V. cholerae* to switch between planktonic and sessile life styles or from virulence to detachment mode in response to environmental changes is essential. In the following sections, we discuss our current understanding of how *V. cholerae* integrates overlapping extracellular stimuli to adopt one or the other lifestyle.

4.1 Adenylate cyclase and cAMP signaling

Cyclic AMP (cAMP) is synthesized from ATP by the activity of adenylate cyclase. *V. cholerae* possesses only one adenylate cyclase, which belongs to the type-I (enterobacterial) class (Danchin, 1993: Baker et al., 2004). This enzyme is monomeric and consists of an N-terminal catalytic domain and a C-terminal regulatory domain. The C-terminal regulatory domain contains the His residue suggested to be phosphorylated by the phospho-EIIA^{glc} component of the phosphoenolpyruvate phosphotransferase system (PTS), leading to its activation (Baker et al., 2004). The PTS is a phosphoryl cascade that allows the transport and phosphorylation of sugars (Deutscher et al., 2006; Deutscher, 2008). It acts as sensory system, feeding information to adenylate cyclase to regulate bacterial behavior in response to the availability of sugars in the medium and the energy state of the cell (Lengeler et al., 2009). In the PTS, phosphate is transferred from phosphoenolpyruvate to a sugar by a pathway that sequentially involves enzyme I (EI), the protein HPr, and a sugar-specific enzyme II (EII) complex. The different EII complexes are characterized by their domains (A, B, C) present either on a single or distinct polypeptide chains. In the presence of a rapidly metabolizable sugar (i.e., D-glucose) phospho-EIIA^{glc} donates its phosphate to the sugar, leading to lower adenylate cyclase activity and lower intracellular concentrations of cAMP.

4.2 Cyclic diguanylate

In a broad spectrum of bacterial species, the second messenger, cyclic diguanylic acid (c-di-GMP), regulates the transition between sessile and motile lifestyle by activating biofilm formation and inhibiting motility (D'Argenio & Miller, 2004; Hengge 2009; Simm et al., 2004;

Tamayo et al., 2007). Cyclic di-GMP is synthesized from GTP by GGDEF domain family proteins that exhibit diguanylate cyclase (DGC) activity. On the other hand, proteins of the EAL and HD-GYP families exhibit a phosphodiesterase (PDE) activity degrading c-di-GMP to GMP (Galperin, 2004). The *V. cholerae* genome contains 31 genes encoding GGDEF domain family proteins; 10 genes encoding proteins with GGDEF and EAL domains; 12 genes encoding proteins with only EAL domains; and 9 genes encoding proteins with HD-GYP domains (Galperin, 2004). In *V. cholerae,* over-expression of the DGC, VCA0956, abolishes swimming, whereas expression of the PDE, VieA, enhances it (Tischler & Camilli, 2004). Transcriptional profiling has revealed that genes involved in flagellum biosynthesis, motility, and chemotaxis are repressed in response to an increase in intracellular c-di-GMP (Beyhan et al., 2006). The signaling pathways responsible for the phenotypic consequences of increasing the c-di-GMP pool are not fully understood. Potential c-di-GMP binding proteins include those containing the PilZ domain (Pratt et al., 2007). The *V. cholerae* genome contains five PilZ domain proteins (Pratt et al., 2007). Of these, PlzA and PlzE appear to be essential; PlzB, PlzC, and PlzD affect *V. cholerae* motility; and PlzC and PlzD bind to c-di-GMP *in vitro*. The positive regulator of biofilm formation, VpsT, can directly senses c-di-GMP to modulate motility and biofilm formation (Krasteva et al., 2010). Finally, there are two riboswitches responsive to c-di-GMP changes in the *V. cholerae* genome (Sudarsan et al., 2008). The function of these riboswitches in cholera infections is currently unknown.

4.3 Quorum sensing

Quorum sensing is a process by which bacteria communicate with one another by secreting extracellular signaling molecules termed autoinducers. In *V. cholerae,* two autoinducer/sensor systems have been identified. System 1 consists of cholera autoinducer 1 (CAI-1, 3-hydroxytridecane-4-one), synthesized by the activity of CqsA, and its cognate receptor, CqsS (Higgins et al., 2006: Miller et al., 2002). System 2 consists of an AI-2 molecule (a furanosyl borate diester), synthesized by the activity of LuxS, and its cognate receptor, LuxPQ (Chen et al., 2002; Miller et al., 2002). Sensory information is fed through a phosphorelay system to LuxO. At low cell density, the autokinase domains of CqsS and LuxPQ become phosphorylated, and phosphate is transferred to LuxU and then LuxO (Miller et al., 2002). Phospho-LuxO then activates expression of multiple, redundant small regulatory RNAs (sRNAs or *qrr*), which promotes translation of the mRNA encoding AphA and destabilize the *hapR* mRNA (Lenz et al., 2004; Rutherford et al., 2011). In addition, the global regulator, CsrA, and the small nucleoid protein factor for inversion stimulation (Fis) enhance phospho-LuxO activity to promote degradation of *hapR* mRNA at low cell density (Lenz et al., 2005; Lenz et al., 2007). When the amount of CAI-1 and AI-2 produced by growing bacteria reaches a threshold value, CqsS and LuxPQ switch from kinase activity to phosphatase. The flow of phosphate is reversed, and phospho-LuxO becomes de-phosphorylated and inactive (Miller et al., 2002). At this stage (high cell density), HapR is expressed (Zhu et al., 2002). The consequences of HapR expression include (a) diminished expression of CT and TCP due to transcriptional repression of *aphA* (Kovacikova and Skorupski, 2002a; Lin et al., 2007), (b) inhibition of *vps* expression (Waters et al., 2008), and (c) activation of *hapA* encoding HA/protease (Jobling & Holmes, 1997). The transition into or out from the quorum-sensing mode appears to be finely regulated by additional mechanisms. For instance, upon transiting into quorum-sensing mode (high cell density),

HapR binds to and represses its own promoter (Lin et al., 2005). Conversely, upon dilution of a high density culture, HapR activates the transcription of *qrr* sRNAs to promote rapid degradation of its own mRNA (Svenningsen et al., 2008). Further, at low cell density, the LuxR-type regulator, VqmA, enhances *hapR* transcription (Liu et al., 2006). In conclusion, at low cell density, *V. cholerae* expresses CT, TCP, and synthesizes matrix exopolysaccharide (*vps*); at high cell density, these functions are repressed, and production of HA/protease is activated (Fig. 4).

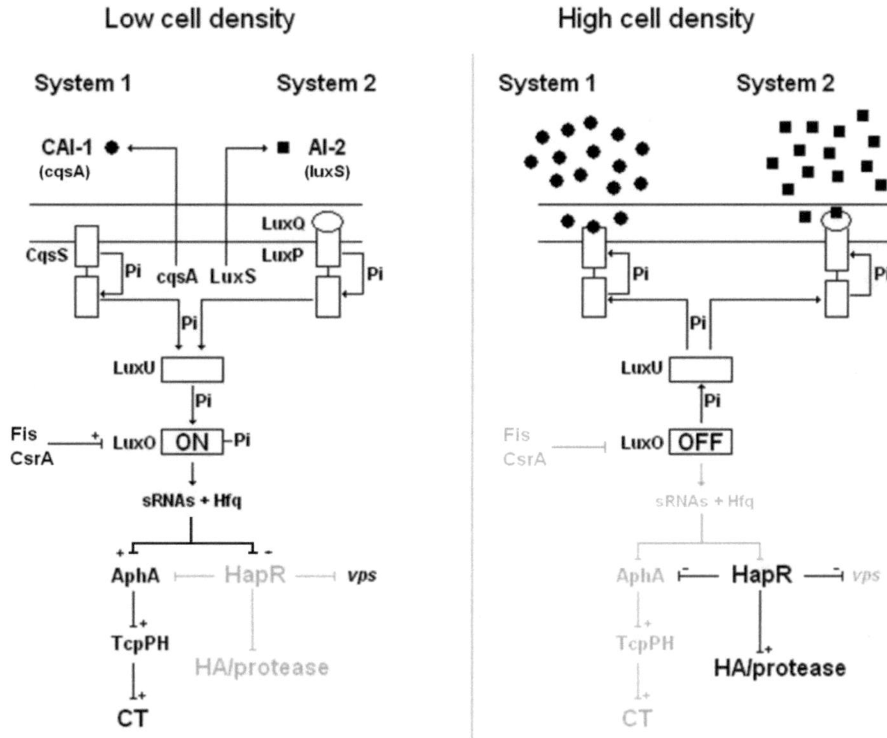

Fig. 4. Quorum sensing in *Vibrio cholerae*

4.4 Quorum sensing regulation of biofilm formation

The formation of a three-dimensional, mature biofilms involves a complex genetic program that includes the expression of motility and mannose-sensitive hemagglutinin for surface attachment and monolayer formation, as well as the biosynthesis of an exopolysaccharide matrix (Watnick & Kolter, 1999). Biofilm formation precedes adoption of the conditionally viable environmental cell stage described in section 1.3 (Kamruzzaman et al., 2010). In *V. cholerae*, biofilm formation is repressed by the master quorum sensing-regulator, HapR (Zhu & Mekalanos, 2003; Hammer & Bassler, 2003; Yildiz et al., 2004). The genes responsible for *vps* biosynthesis are clustered in two operons in which *vpsA* and *vpsL* are the first genes of operon I and II, respectively (Yildiz & Schoolnik, 1999). The expression of *vps* genes is regulated by a complex network involving a growing number of factors. For instance, the second messenger, c-di-GMP, enhances *vps* expression (Fong & Yildiz, 2008; Beyhan et al., 2006; Beyhan et al., 2007; Lim et al., 2006; Lim et al., 2007; Tischler & Camilli, 2004). Biofilm formation is also modulated by interplay between the positive transcription regulators, VpsT (Casper-Lindley & Yildiz, 2004) and VpsR (Yildiz et al., 2001), and the negative regulator, CytR (Haugo & Watnick, 2002). In addition, *vps* expression is modulated by the PhoBR two-component regulatory system (Pratts et al., 2009, 2010; Sultan et al., 2010) and by components of the PTS phosphoryl cascade (Houot et al., 2008; 2010, 2010a).

4.5 The cAMP receptor protein (CRP)

CRP is a member of the CRP/FNR family of transcriptional regulators known for its role in carbon catabolite repression, a process in which the presence of a favorable carbon source in the medium inhibits expression of enzymes involved in the catabolism of other carbon sources (Brückner & Titgemeyer, 2002; Stülke and Hillen, 1999). Activation of adenylate cyclase leads to high intracellular levels of cAMP. Then, cAMP binds to CRP to form a complex that acts at responsive promoters to activate or repress transcription (Brückner & Titgemeyer, 2002; Stülke & Hillen, 1999) The cAMP-CRP complex binds as a dimer to the consensus sequence TGTGA-(N_6)-TCACAA which can be found within, adjacent to or upstream from responsive promoters. The complex is believed to assist in binding of RNAP to the promoter by bending the DNA molecule. *V. cholerae crp* mutants form small colonies, are less motile, do not express *hapA* (Benitez et al., 2001) and are defective in colonization of the suckling mouse intestine (Skorupski and Taylor, 1997). The cAMP-CRP complex negatively affects CT and TCP expression by directly repressing the *tcpPH* promoter (Skorupski & Taylor, 1997; Kovacikova & Skorupski, 2001). The fact that *crp* mutants show reduced colonization in the suckling mouse, although expressing elevated TCP, suggests that CRP is required for the expression of additional colonization factors.

As a global regulator, CRP indirectly affects the expression of many genes by controlling the expression of a broad range of transcriptional factors. As an example, an isogenic Δ*crp* mutant of *V. cholerae* strain C7258 expressed elevated *fis* mRNA and lower levels of mRNAs encoding the general stress response regulator, RpoS, and the histone-like nucleoid structuring protein (H-NS) (Fig. 5) (Silva and Benitez, 2004; Liang et al., 2007). Gene expression profiling of a *crp* deletion mutant revealed 174 differentially expressed genes. With the exception of conserved hypothetical proteins, most differentially expressed genes fell into the functional categories of energy metabolism, transport and binding protein, and cellular processes (Fig. 6) (Liang et al., 2007). Furthermore, 77 % of the differentially expressed genes were down-regulated, suggesting that CRP most frequently acts as a positive regulator in *V. cholerae*. The *crp* mutant exhibited diminished expression of genes involved in motility and chemotaxis, outer membrane protein expression, genes specifically induced in rabbit ileal loops, and *rpoE* encoding σ^E (Liang et al., 2007). These data explain the colonization defect exhibited by *crp* mutants. Among the differentially expressed genes, *cqsA* (VCA0523) encoding CAI-1 synthase and *hapR*, encoding the master quorum sensing regulator, HapR, were diminished. Another gene (VC0291), annotated as coding for a NifR3/Smm1 family protein was up-regulated in the *crp* mutant. Tn5 insertions in this locus reduced the expression of the small nucleoid protein, Fis (Lenz & Bassler, 2007), a regulator that enhances degradation of *hapR* mRNA at low cell density (Lenz & Bassler, 2007). Since VC0291 and *fis* are predicted to be part of an operon (Osuna et al., 1995), this finding is consistent with CRP being a repressor of Fis (Fig. 5).

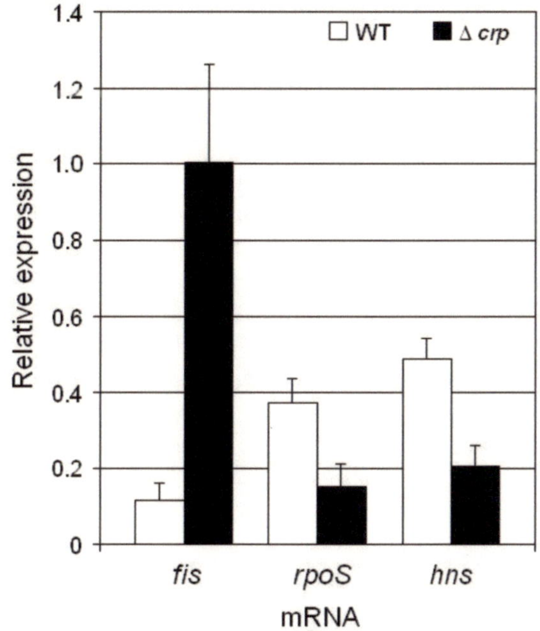

Fig. 5. Relative expression measured by quantitative, real-time reverse transcription PCR of global regulators *fis*, *rpoS*, and *hns* in a *V. cholerae crp* deletion mutant standardized by *recA* mRNA levels.

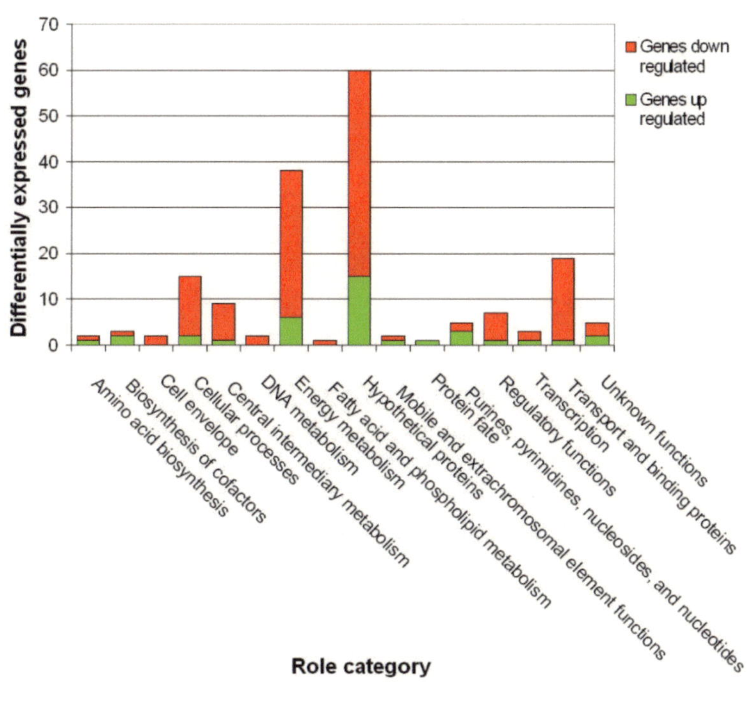

Fig. 6. Global regulation by the cAMP receptor protein.

4.6 Quorum modulation: Integration of cell density and carbon source sensory information

Since the *crp* mutant expresses reduced *cqsA* and *hapR* mRNA, we used a bioassay to compare the production of CAI-1 in wild-type and mutant backgrounds using a *V. cholerae* Δ*cqsA*Δ*luxP* reporter containing the *V. harveyi lux* operon on a cosmid (Miller et al., 2002). This reporter strain does not make its own CAI-1 nor does it respond to AI-2. Exogenous CAI-1 from a cell-free culture supernatant activates expression of HapR, which in turn induces the *lux* operon to make light. As shown in Fig. 7, no CAI-1 can be detected in culture supernatants of Δ*crp* and Δ*cya* (adenylate cyclase). The *crp*^{c} allele containing the amino acid substitutions T127L/S128A encodes a CRP protein that activates transcription in the absence of cAMP (Krueger et al., 1998; Shi et al., 1999; Wang et al., 2000). As shown in Fig. 7, introduction of this constitutive allele into a Δ*cya* mutant restored expression of HapR and light production. Furthermore, quorum sensing was restored in Δ*crp* and Δ*cya* mutants by introducing the corresponding genes on a plasmid vector and, in the case of a Δ*cya* mutant, by adding cAMP or the cAMP analog, 7-deaza-cAMP, to the culture medium (Liang et al., 2008). The mechanism by which the cAMP-CRP complex regulates *cqsA* expression is not known, although there is evidence suggesting a posttranscriptional regulation (Liang et al., 2008).

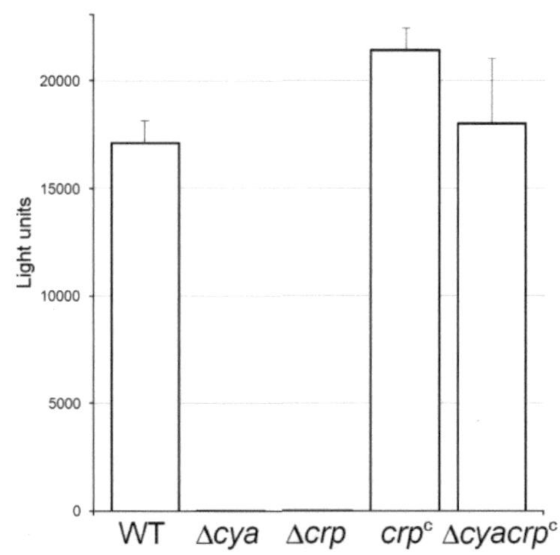

Fig. 7. The cAMP receptor protein is required for the biosynthesis of the *Vibrio cholerae* major autoinducer.

In section 4.5., we showed that cAMP-CRP controls quorum sensing by activating *cqsA* (Fig. 7) and repressing *fis* (Fig. 5). These findings suggest that the intensity of bacterial cell-to-cell communication is modulated by environmental signals other than population density, such as the type and availability of carbon sources. Thus, we propose a new level of regulation, termed quorum modulation, mediated in this case by cAMP. Quorum modulation functions in the following way. Under environmental conditions conducive to low intracellular cAMP levels (i.e., high glucose), the amount of CAI-1 produced per cell is diminished. The *V. cholerae* population would require a higher quorum (i.e., cells/ml) to activate HapR. Conversely, under conditions conducive to high cAMP levels (i.e., low glucose) the production of CAI-1 per cell is enhanced, and the bacterial population requires a lower quorum to activate HapR. Thus, quorum modulation controls the cell density at which *V.*

cholerae switches its metabolism to the quorum-sensing mode. As a consequence, commitment of the bacterial population to enter the quorum sensing-mode and turn on the HapR transcriptional program is placed in context with other features of the environment. This principle is illustrated in Fig. 8. Consistent with this scheme, the cell density at which *V. cholerae* enters the quorum-sensing mode is increased by addition of glucose to the medium (to lower the cAMP pool) and diminished by addition of cAMP (Liang et al., 2008).

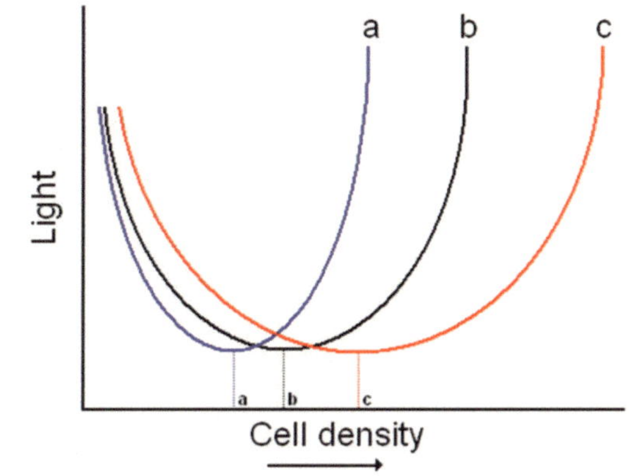

Fig. 8. Quorum modulation. When a culture at high cell density is diluted in broth, quorum sensing (i.e., light) is turned off. As the population increases, a threshold cell density is attained (quorum), at which quorum sensing is activated to generate a U-shape curve (b). The rate of autoinducer biosynthesis determines the cell density at which the bacterial population enters the quorum-sensing mode. A condition that enhances autoinducer biosynthesis lowers the threshold (a). A condition that inhibits autoinducer biosynthesis increases the threshold (c).

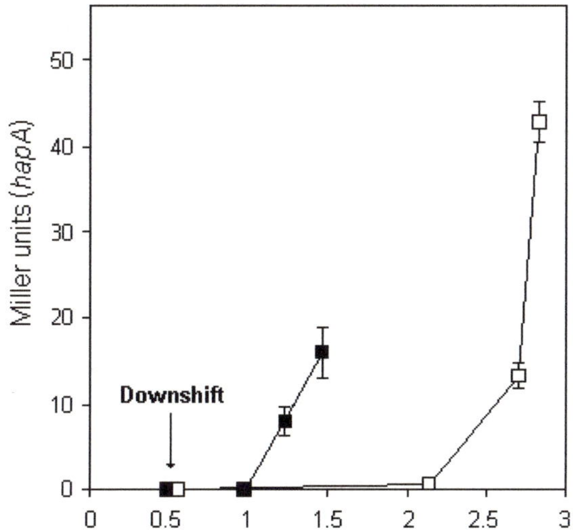

Fig. 9. Effect of a nutritional downshift on the cell density required for expression of a quorum sensing-regulated *hapA-lacZ* promoter fusion measured as β-galactosidase activity (Miller units) (Silva and Benitez, 2004).

A practical example of how quorum modulation works is provided in Fig. 9. In this case, a *V. cholerae* strain containing a chromosomally integrated *hapA-lacZ* promoter fusion is grown in rich medium, and, at an optical density of 0.5, half of the culture is nutritionally downshifted by centrifugation and reconstitution in a medium of diminished strength. This experiment shows that *hapA* expression can be detected at a lower cell density in nutritionally downshifted cells (Silva and Benitez, 2004). Quorum modulation is not restricted to carbon regulation of cellular cAMP levels, as other environmental conditions might influence autoinducer biosynthesis or even autoinducer stability in the medium.

4.7 Interplay between quorum sensing and cAMP in the fine regulation of matrix exopolysaccharide expression

Over-expression of *vps* in *hapR* mutants gives rise to the rugose colonial morphology (Yildiz et al., 2004). Although HapR is not detected in *crp* and *cya* mutants, these strains still produce the smooth colonial variant (Liang et al., 2007, 2007a). As shown in Fig. 10, the rugose colonial morphology of a *hapR* mutant is turned to smooth by deletion of *crp* or *cya,* and the resulting smooth strains can be converted back to rugose by introduction of the *crp* and *cya* genes on a plasmid vector. These results suggest that formation of the cAMP-CRP complex has a dual effect on *vps* expression by activating quorum sensing (a negative effect) and by enhancing the expression of a positive factor. In our strain, the positive factor was the regulator, VpsR (Liang et al., 2007a).

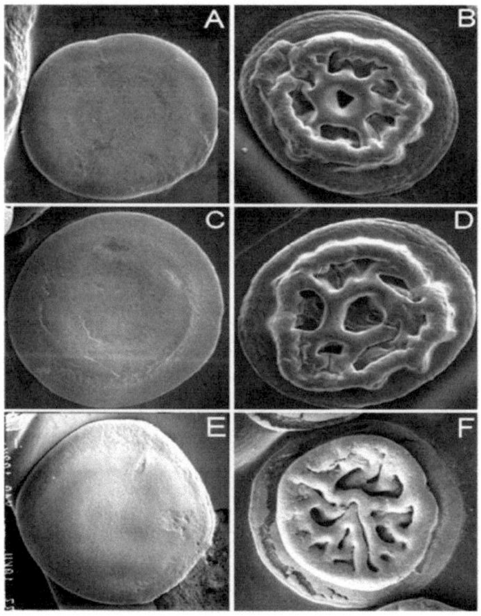

Fig. 10. Scanning electron microscopy of *V. cholerae* Δ*crp*, Δ*cya*, and Δ*hapR* colonies. A, Δ*crp*; B, Δ*hapR*; C, Δ*hapR*Δ*crp*; D, Δ*hapR*Δ*crp* transformed with *crp* plasmid; E, Δ*hapR*Δ*cya*; F, Δ*hapR*Δ*cya* transformed with *cya* plasmid

Fig. 11 schematically illustrates the dual input of adenylate cyclase and CRP on *V. cholerae* expression of *vps.* In this model, deletion of *crp* results in diminished expression of the positive regulator, VpsR, which is required for expression of rugose colonial morphology. This event, however, is partially compensated for by reduced expression of the negative regulator HapR. As a result, Δ*crp* mutants express elevated *vpsA* and *vpsL* compared to the wild-type strain, but this increase is not large enough to induce rugose colonial morphology. Maximal exopolysaccharide expression requires inactivation of HapR (repressor) but an active *crp* allele for enhancing VpsR (activator). In a different strain, however, CRP repressed VpsR, suggesting that there is strain variability in the regulation of this protein (Fong et al., 2008).

In addition to the abovementioned regulatory effects of *crp* and *cya* on *vps* expression, several components of the PTS that function upstream of adenylate cyclase have their own regulatory input on *vps* gene expression. For instance, in minimal medium, phosphoryl transfer from EI to HPr and FPr represses *vps* expression (Houot et al., 2008); in LB medium, glucose-specific $EIIA^{glc}$ and nitrogen-specific $EIIA^{Ntr1}$ and $EIIA^{Ntr2}$ activate and repress *vps* expression, respectively (Houot et al., 2010).

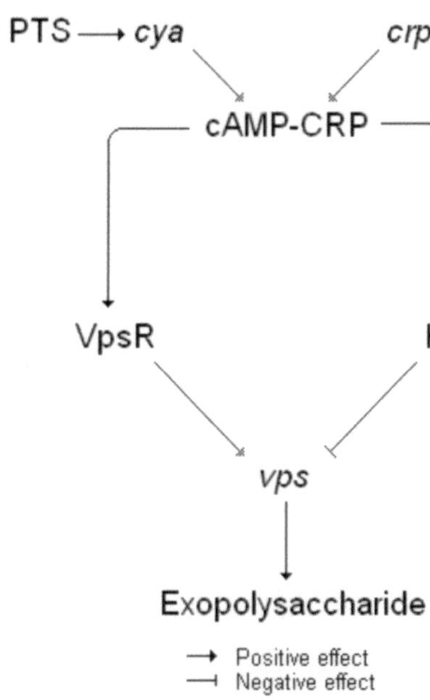

Fig. 11. Model for the dual regulatory input of the cAMP-CRP complex on biosynthesis of *V. cholerae* matrix exopolysaccharide.

4.8 Effect of extracellular phosphate on vps expression and biofilm formation

Since freshwater and estuarine ecosystems where *Vibrios* survive and persist outside the human host are limited in phosphate content (Benitez-Nelson, 2000; Correl, 1999), *V. cholerae* build stores of intracellular polyphosphate (poly-P) (Ogawa et al., 2000). The enzyme polyphosphate kinase (PPK) is responsible for the synthesis of poly-P from ATP (Ahn and Kornberg, 1990). A *V. cholerae ppk* mutant exhibits a reduced capacity to withstand conditions of low pH, high salinity, and oxidative stress in low- phosphate medium (Jahid et al., 2006). These findings underline the importance of phosphate homeostasis as well as sensing and responding to changes in extracellular phosphate in the *V. cholerae* life cycle. In *E. coli*, deprivation of phosphate induces the expression of the PhoB regulon (Lamarche et al., 2008). PhoB is part of the PhoR/PhoB two-component regulatory system. PhoR is an inner membrane histidine kinase that responds to periplasmic orthophosphate through its interaction with the phosphate transport system. Under conditions of phosphate limitation, phosphorus is transferred from phospho-PhoR to the response regulator PhoB. Phospho-PhoB then binds to DNA pho boxes to activate or repress the transcription of target genes (Lamarche et al., 2008). A proteomic comparison of wild-type and *phoB V. cholerae* strains revealed 140 differentially expressed proteins (von Kruger et al., 2006). A *V. cholerae phoB* mutant colonized rabbit ileal loops to a lesser extent suggesting a role for this regulator in intestinal colonization and pathogenesis (von Kruger et al., 1999). More recently, it was shown that PhoB negatively affects CT and TCP expression by repressing the *tcpPH* promoter (Pratt et al., 2010). In addition, PhoB negatively regulates biofilm formation in *V. cholerae* of classical and El Tor biotypes (Pratt et al., 2009; Sultan et al., 2010). A comparison of the levels of expression of known regulators of *vps* and biofilm between wild-type and Δ*phoB V. cholerae* of the El Tor biotype revealed that VpsR, is negatively regulated by PhoB (Sultan et al., 2010).

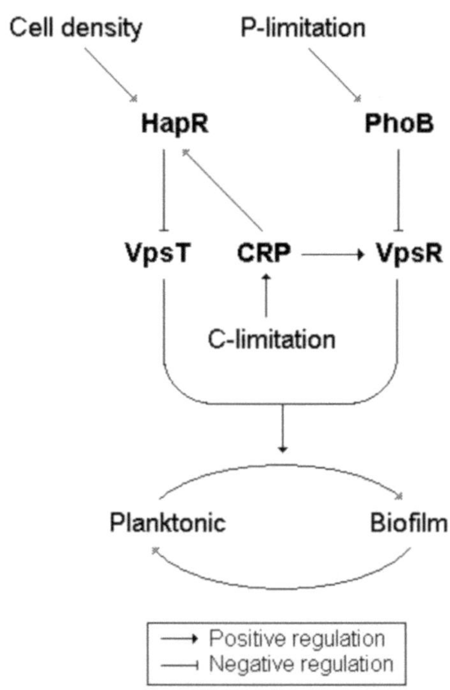

Fig. 12. Model for the integration of cell density, carbon and phosphorus sensory information in the regulation of biofilm formation.

Since VpsR is positively modulated by CRP (Fig. 11), we propose that VpsR has an essential function in biofilm formation by acting as a receiver of external carbon and phosphorus sensory information to modulate biosynthesis of the exopolysaccharide matrix. PhoB and CRP exhibit antagonistic effects on VpsR (Fig. 12). The parallel function of multiple signaling pathways with opposing and/or re-enforcing effects appears to be a common theme in metabolic regulation. We suggest that such a regulatory architecture allows bacteria to adjust their response quantitatively to chemical and physical changes in the extracellular milieu. For instance, in defined chemical media, maximal VpsR expression would be expected to occur under conditions of low glucose concentration (high cellular cAMP) and high phosphate (PhoB inactive). Furthermore, according to the scheme presented in Fig. 12, the regulator VpsT acts as a receiver of population density and carbon sensory information; VpsR acts as a receiver of carbon and phosphate sensory information to regulate the transition between the planktonic and biofilm life styles.

4.9 Enhancement of motility and detachment by the general stress response regulator, RpoS

As shown in Fig. 5, CRP enhances expression of the general response regulator, RpoS. The *rpoS* gene encodes the RNAP σ^S subunit, which regulates expression of more than 100 genes in response to starvation and other stresses such as osmotic shock, acid shock, and temperature changes (Hengge-Aronis, 2002). It is not clear what makes a given promoter selective for transcription by RpoS. Several promoter elements have been described including an upstream (UP) element, a more degenerate -35 region, a cytosine at -13, and a AT-rich region downstream from -10 (Hengge-Aronis, 2002a; Typas et al., 2007). It also has been suggested that histone-like proteins such as H-NS, the Leucine-responsive protein (Lrp), or the integration host factor (IHF) can contribute to σ^S promoter selectivity (Hengge-Aronis, 2002a; Hengge-Aronis, 1999; Typas et al., 2007). For instance, many σ^S-dependent genes are repressed by H-NS, and association of RNAP with σ^S on these promoters may overcome H-NS transcriptional repression (Barth et al., 1995; Bouvier et al., 1998; Hengge-Aronis, 1999). In *E. coli*, the intracellular level of σ^S is controlled at the levels of transcription, translation, and protein stability (Hengge-Aronis, 2002; Nogueira & Springer, 2000; Vicente et al., 1999). The regulation of RpoS expression in *V. cholerae* is less understood but, relative to *E. coli*, there are differences that likely reflect adaptation to distinct environments. In contrast to *E. coli*, *V. cholerae* mutants that produce diminished guanosine tetraphosphate (ppGpp) and poly-P are not affected in *rpoS* expression (Jahid et al., 2006, Silva and Benitez, 2006). Moreover, deletion of Hfq, a factor that enhances *rpoS* translation in *E. coli*, has no effect on expression of *V. cholerae* RpoS (Ding et al., 2005). Additionally, we have shown that H-NS, which negatively influences *rpoS* translation in *E. coli*, has the opposite effect in *V. cholerae* (Silva et al., 2008). We have constructed an RpoS reporter strain expressing an RpoS-FLAG protein from native *rpoS* transcription and translation signals (Wang et al., 2010). In rich tryptone soy broth, RpoS was detected in the late logarithmic phase and after the population entered quorum-sensing mode (Wang et al., 2010). The quorum-sensing regulator, HapR, enhanced RpoS expression.

Transcription hierarchy	Increase in c-di-GMP	Deletion of *rpoS*
Class II	*flhF, fliFGHIN, fliA* (σ28)	*flhAF, fliFGJ*
Class III	*flaAGI, flgBCDEFGI*	*flgBCDEFGHIJL, fliMNOPQ, flaA*
Class IV	*flaCD, flgM*	*flaBCDE*

Table 2. Comparison of motility genes differentially expressed in response to an increase in c-di-GMP and to deletion of *rpoS* (adapted from Beyhan et al., 2006; Nielsen et al., 2007).

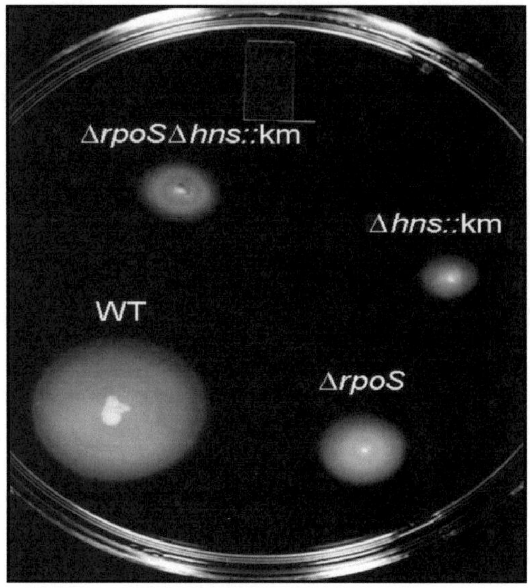

Fig. 13. Motility of *V. cholerae rpoS* and *hns* (Δ*hns*::km) mutants in swarm agar plates

V. cholerae rpoS mutants are more sensitive to starvation, high osmolarity, and oxidative stresses, are less motile than their wild-type precursors (Fig. 13), and do not express *hapA* (Nielsen et al., 2006; Silva et al., 2008; Yildiz & Schoolnik, 1998; Silva & Benitez, 2004). We have recently shown that, similar to HapR, expression of RpoS acts to diminish the c-di-GMP pool (Wang et al., 2011). Gene profiling experiments have shown that RpoS positively controls the expression of several proteins putatively identified as PDEs (Nielsen et al., 2006). As shown in Table 2, both deletion of *rpoS* and artificial enhancement of the c-di-GMP pool modulate the expression of class II through IV hierarchy motility genes. The data suggest that RpoS enhances motility by diminishing the c-di-GMP pool and by acting at an early step of the motility transcription hierarchy, such as RpoN and/or FlrA.

A common approach to investigate the phenotypic consequences of changes in intracellular c-di-GMP content is to increase or diminish the c-di-GMP pool by over-expressing a DGC or PDE, respectively. Using this method, we have investigated the effect of artificially altering the c-di-GMP pool on HapR and HA/protease expression. These studies revealed a complex interplay between c-di-GMP, HapR, VpsT, and RpoS that favors detachment of *V. cholerae* at high cell density (Fig. 13). Increasing the c-di-GMP pool enhances the expression of the c-di-GMP sensing protein, VpsT (Beyhan et al., 2006), which acts as a repressor of HapR (Yildiz et al., 2004). In the model shown in Fig. 14, expression of HapR at high cell density results in lower c-di-GMP content (Waters et al., 2008); lowering of c-di-GMP further enhances HapR, generating a double-negative regulatory loop that requires VpsT; HapR positively enhances RpoS expression (Joelsson et al., 2007); and the elevated expression of RpoS feeds into the regulatory loop by diminishing the intracellular concentration of c-di-GMP. The concurrent activation of HapR and RpoS results in elevated expression of HA/protease and motility, which promotes detachment. By promoting multiple cycles of detachment and re-colonization, the coordinate expression of HA/protease and motility could contribute to the dissemination of colonizing *Vibrios* along the small intestine.

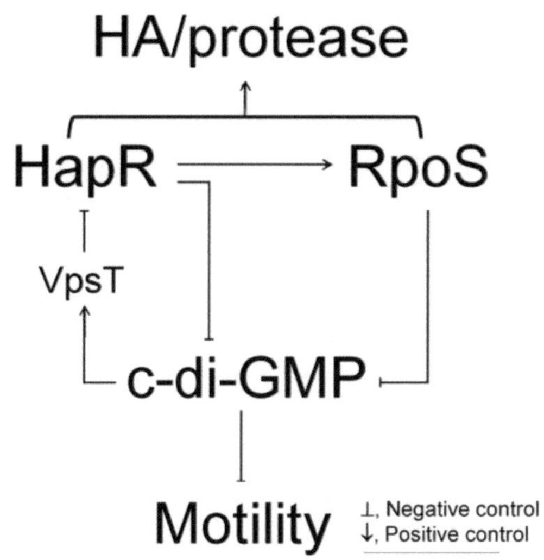

Fig. 14. Coordinate regulation of HA/protease and motility by c-di-GMP, HapR, VpsT and RpoS.

4.10 The histone-like nucleoid structuring protein (H-NS) represses the expression of virulence genes

H-NS belongs to a family of small nucleoid-associated proteins that include its paralog StpA; Fis, the heat-unstable protein (HU); and IHF (Dorman, 2004; Dorman & Deighan, 2003). In *E. coli,* H-NS is a 15-kDa, highly abundant protein present at about 20,000 copies per cell; it was initially characterized for its capacity to mediate DNA condensation (Dorman, 2004; Dorman & Deighan, 2003). Mutations that inactivate *hns* are pleiotropic, suggesting that H-NS influences a broad spectrum of physiological processes (Atlung & Hansen, 2002; Atlung & Ingmer, 1997; Hommais et al., 2001). The H-NS proteins of *E. coli* and *V. cholerae* contain an N-terminal oligomerization domain connected by a flexible linker to a nucleic acid binding domain (Atlung & Ingmer, 1997; Cerdan et al., 2003; Dorman, 2004; Nye & Taylor, 2003). Both oligomerization and DNA binding are essential for the biological activities of H-NS, which include DNA condensation and regulation of transcription (Dame et al., 2001; Spurio et al., 1997). In regulation of transcription, H-NS most commonly negatively affects gene expression by binding to promoters exhibiting AT-rich, highly curved DNA regions that contain clusters of the more conserved 10 bp motif, TCGATAAATT (Lang et al., 2007; Owen-Hughes et al., 1992; Uegushi & Mizuno, 1993). In *V. cholerae, hns* mutants form small colonies, are incapable of using β-glucosides as a carbon source, exhibit diminished motility (Fig. 12) and intestinal colonization capacity, and show altered responses to environmental stresses (Ghosh et al., 2006; Krishnan et al., 2004; Silva et al., 2008; Tending et al., 2000; Silva et al. 2008). An emerging function of H-NS is the transcriptional silencing of horizontally acquired genes (Lucchini et al., 2006; Navarre et al., 2006; Oshima et al., 2006). Consistent with this role, H-NS silences expression of virulence genes in *V. cholerae* by acting at different levels of the ToxR regulatory cascade (Fig. 3), which include the *toxT, tcpA* and *ctxA* promoters (Nye et al., 2000). Binding of H-NS to a promoter apparently inhibits transcription by a bridging mechanism consisting of cross-linking DNA segments in a manner that traps RNAP (Dorman & Kane, 2009). There is considerable evidence indicating that H-NS-mediated repression can be antagonized in response to environmental stimuli that activate the expression of other regulators whose binding sites overlap that of H-NS (anti-bridging) (Dorman & Kane, 2009). For instance, the small nucleoid protein, Fis opposes the repression activity of H-NS at a various promoters (Dorman & Kane, 2009). The IHF alleviates H-NS silencing of *S. enterica hilA* (Queiroz et al., 2011), *E. coli csgD* (Ogasawara et al., 2010), *Shigella flexneri vir* genes (Porter & Dorman, 1997), and bacteriophage Mu early promoter (Van Ulsen et al., 1996). In the case of *V. cholerae*, transcriptional silencing of the *tcpA* and *ctxA* promoters by H-NS is antagonized by the AraC-like transcriptional regulator, ToxT, and by IHF (Stonehouse et al., 2008, 2010; Yu & DiRita, 2002). In theory, other small nucleoid proteins, such as Lrp and HU, can exhibit the anti-bridging activity required to attenuate H-NS repression (Dorman & Kane, 2009).

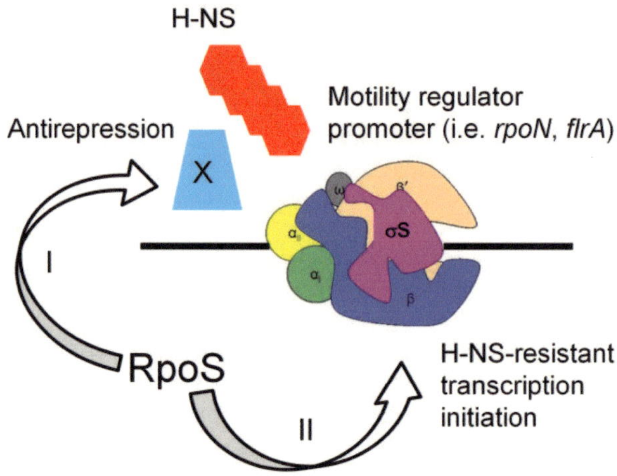

Fig. 15. Hypothetical model for the interaction of RpoS and H-NS in the regulation of *V. cholerae* motility. RpoS could enhance the transcription of motility by inducing the expression of an antirepressor (I), and by binding to core RNAP to promote transcription initiation that is H-NS-resistant.

The effect of H-NS on motility of *V. cholerae* is not fully understood. On one hand, H-NS could enhance motility by positively affecting the expression of RpoS (Silva et al., 2008). This effect, however, is modest compared to the reduction in motility observed for *hns* mutants (Fig. 13). Bright-field microscopy has revealed that *hns* mutants are flagellated nut non-motile. In *E. coli*, H-NS binds to the switch protein, FliG, to enhance motility, and *hns* mutants express a paralyzed flagellum (Donato & Kawula, 1998). A similar mechanism may function in *V. cholerae*. Moreover, in the absence of RpoS, H-NS appears to function as a repressor of the motility genes, *flaA*, *flaC* and *motY* (Silva et al., 2008). This suggests that, in addition to lowering the c-di-GMP pool, RpoS enhances motility by attenuating H-NS repression. A speculative model for the anti-repressor function of RpoS is shown in Fig. 15. Based on data derived by transcriptional profiling, we suggest that RpoS is most likely to act at the *rpoN* and/or *flrA* promoters to enhance expression of downstream class II-IV motility genes (Table 2). In the stationary phase, transcription initiation at the *rpoN* and *flrA* promoters by RNAP containing σ^S could be more resistant to H-NS repression (Barth et al., 1995; Bouvier et al., 1998; Hengge-Aronis, 1999). In addition, RpoS could enhance the expression of other nucleoid-associated proteins, such as IHF to attenuate H-NS repression by an anti-repressor (anti-bridging) mechanism (Dorman & Kane, 2009).

5. CRP as a master regulator of *V. cholerae* behavior

As described in the preceding sections, CRP acts as an upstream master regulator modulating quorum sensing, virulence, stress response, motility, and biofilm development. Thus, in Fig. 16, we provide an integrative model for CRP regulation of *V. cholerae* behavior. The CRP protein is activated when the intracellular concentration of cAMP is increased due to PTS activation of adenylate cyclase. Thus, the PTS system acts as the primary carbon source sensing mechanism. The state of activity of CRP controls the execution of secondary genetic programs mediated by HapR, RpoS and H-NS that modulate *V. cholerae* switching from planktonic to sessile life styles or from virulence to detachment. For instance, in its active state, CRP enhances the expression of (a) HapR by activating CAI-1 biosynthesis and repressing Fis, (b) RpoS, and (c) H-NS. The expression of HapR and RpoS enhances motility and activates HA/protease, favoring detachment. Simultaneous activation of HapR and H-NS leads to quorum-sensing repression of *aphA* and to H-NS-mediated transcriptional silencing of *toxT, ctxA,* and *tcpA* to diminish expression of virulence genes. By enhancing HapR, RpoS and H-NS, formation of the cAMP-CRP complex favors the motile planktonic stage; the opposite is true for biofilm formation.

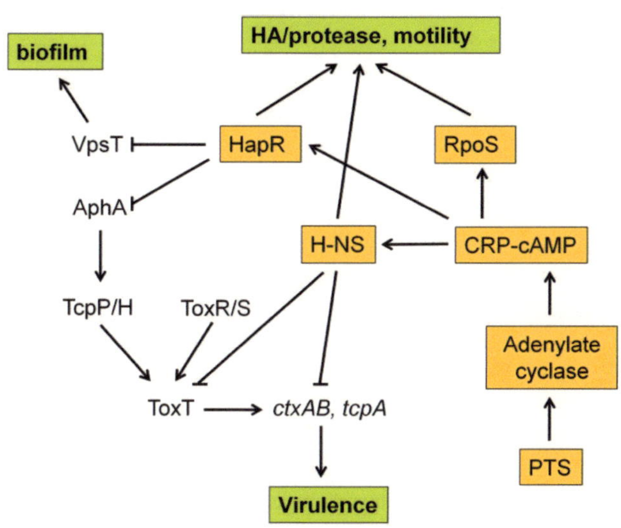

Fig. 16. Multilevel regulation of *V. cholerae* behavior by CRP.

6. Significance to anti-virulence drug discovery

The increase in our understanding of the regulatory pathways that control *V. cholerae* behavior creates the possibility of identifying new drugs to block infection and to prevent biofilm development. This is particularly relevant due to the emergence of antibiotic-resistant *V. cholerae* (Das & Kaur, 2008; Roychowdhury et al., 2008; Okeke et al., 2007; Mwansa et al., 2000). Consequently, development of anti-virulence drugs is proceeding

(Waldor, 2006). An example is the small molecule inhibitor of *V. cholerae* intestinal colonization, virstatin [N-(1, 8-(naphthalimide)-n-butyric acid], which was identified in a high-throughput phenotypic screen (Hung et al., 2005; Shakhnovich et al., 2007, 2007a). This molecule inhibits *ctxAB* and *tcpA* transcription by preventing dimerization of their positive regulator, ToxT (Shakhnovich et al., 2007a). Another example is the newly identified inhibitor of the Na^+-dependent flagellar motor, Q24DA, which could prevent infection dissemination by blocking motility and indirectly diminishing CT and TCP secretion (Rasmussen et al., 2010. An attractive target to block infection is the quorum- sensing phosphoryl cascade leading to the expression of HapR (Higgins et al., 2007). Pretreatment of mice with commensal bacteria engineered to express CAI-1 affords protection against a cholera challenge (Duan and March, 2010). A second set of attractive targets are the PTS components that modulate biofilm formation (Houot et al., 2008, 2010, 2010a). A comparative genomic analysis of 202 fully sequenced genomes (174 bacterial, 19 archaeal, and 9 eukaryotic) did not reveal components of the PTS system in eukaryotic cells (Barabote et al., 2005). A third potential target is CRP, whose cyclic nucleotide binding (CNB) domain is substantially different from eukaryotic cAMP binding proteins, with substitutions in highly conserved positions within the phosphate-binding cassette that determine ligand specificity (Kannan et al., 2007). These differences can be exploited to identify and/or synthesize CRP ligands selective for the bacterial CNB domain. Based on the results described in this chapter, CRP agonists would be expected to inhibit expression of virulence genes and biofilm formation while favoring motility and detachment. An advantage of targeting the PTS and CRP is their broad range. For instance, CRP modulates the expression of virulence factors in bacterial pathogens such as *V. vulnificus*, *Salmonella enterica* serovar Typhimurium, *Yersinia enterocolitica*, *Y. pestis*, and *Pseudomonas aeruginosa*. The genes encoding global regulators, such as CRP, and the virulence factors under its control are generally not essential. Thus, contrary to anti-bacterial drugs, inhibitors of expression of virulence genes are not expected to exert a high selective pressure for the dissemination of resistance or to impact the commensal flora. Finally, targeting global regulators such as CRP, RpoS and H-NS could significantly impair bacterial *in vivo* stress response allowing the host to clear the infection and diminish the use of antibiotics. The use of anti-virulence versus anti-bacterial therapies is still a matter of debate, particularly in regard to pathogens capable of long-term persistence in the host, which is not the case in cholera.

7. Conclusions

The bacterial pathogen *V. cholerae* has evolved to colonize the human small bowel efficiently and to persist in aquatic environments. A sophisticated regulatory network allows the cholera bacterium to modify its behavior in response to the environmental changes dictated by its dual life cycle. Studies conducted in the last few decades have revealed that:

a. *V. cholerae* can switch from virulence to detachment modes and from motile to sessile (biofilm) life styles to maximize fitness.
b. The cAMP receptor protein acts as an upstream master regulator of *V. cholerae* behavior by controlling the execution of secondary regulatory pathways, such as quorum sensing (HapR), RpoS, and H-NS.
c. Efficient regulation requires substantial molecular cross-talking between regulatory modules, as exemplified by the interplays between quorum sensing (HapR) and RpoS

expression as well as the interactions between RpoS and H-NS repression in the regulation of expression of motility genes.

d. A salient feature of this complex global regulatory network is the occurrence of parallel or overlapping regulatory outputs with opposing or re-enforcing effects to fine-tune bacterial responses to environmental stresses. In this chapter, this principle is illustrated by the dual effect of CRP on *vps* expression involving HapR and VpsR, and the opposing effects of CRP and PhoB on the expression of VpsR.
e. As we continue to develop a better understanding of the *V. cholerae* regulatory landscape, it should become possible to identify small molecules capable of shifting bacterial behavior from pathogenic to commensal.

8. Acknowledgements

We wish to acknowledge the contributions of postdoctoral associates Weili Liang, Zafar S. Sultan, Hongxia Wang and Julio C. Ayala to results included in this chapter. In addition, studies from our laboratory included in this chapter were supported by research grants from the National Institutes of Health (Bethesda, Maryland).

9. References

Ahn, K., &. Kornberg, A. (1990). Polyphosphate kinase from *Escherichia coli. J. Biol. Chem.* 265:11734–11739.

Albert, M.J. (1994). *Vibrio cholerae* O139 Bengal. *J. Clin. Microbiol.* 32: 2345-2349.

Asai, Y., Kojima, S., Kato, H., Nishioka, N., Kawagishi, I., & Homma, M. (1997). Putative channel components for the fast-rotating sodium-driven flagellar motor of a marine bacterium. *J. Bacteriol.* 179: 5104-5110.

Atlung, T., & Hansen, F.G. (2002). Effect of different concentrations of H-NS protein on chromosome replication and the cell cycle in *Escherichia coli. J. Bacteriol.* 184: 1843-1850.

Atlung, T., & Ingmer, H. (1997). H-NS: a modulator of environmentally regulated gene expression. Mol Microbiol 24: 7-17.

Baker, D.A., & Kelly, J.M. (2004). Structure, function and evolution of microbial adenylyl and guanylyl cyclases. *Mol. Microbiol.* 52: 1229-1242.

Barabote, R.D., and Saier Jr., M.H. (2005). Comparative genomic analysis of the bacterial phosphotransferase system. *Microbiol. Mol. Biol. Rev.* 69: 608-634.

Barth, M., Marschall, C., Muffler, A., Fischer, D & Hengge-Aronis, R. (1995). Role for the histone-like protein H-NS in growth phase-dependent and osmotic regulation of σ^S and many σ^S-dependent genes in *Escherichia coli. J. Bacteriol.* 177: 3455-3464.

Benitez, J. A., Garcia, L. Silva, A.J., Garcia, H., Fando, R., Cedre, B., Perez, A., Campos, J., Rodriguez, B.L., Perez, J.L., Valmaseda, T., Perez, O., Perez, A., Ramirez, M., Ledon, T., Diaz, M., Lastre, M., Bravo, L., & Sierra, G. (1999). Preliminary assessment of the safety and immunogenicity of a new CTX_- negative hemagglutinin/protease-defective El Tor strain as a cholera vaccine candidate. *Infect. Immun.* 67:539–545.

Benitez, J.A., Silva, A. & Finkelstein, R.A. (2001). Environmental signals controlling production of hemagglutinin/protease in *Vibrio cholerae. Infect. Immun.* 69: 6549-6553.

Benitez, J.A., Spelbrink, R.G., Silva, A.J., Phillips, T.E., Stanley, C.M., Boesman-Finkelstein, M., & Finkelstein, R.A. (1997). Adherence of *Vibrio cholerae* to cultured differentiated human intestinal cells: an *in vitro* colonization model. *Infect. Immun.* 65: 3474-3477.

Benitez-Nelson, C.R. (2000). The biogeochemical cycling of phosphorus in marine systems. *Earth-Science Reviews* 51: 109-135.

Berg, H.C. (2003). The rotator motor of bacterial flagella. *Ann Rev. Biochem.* 72: 19-54.

Beyhan, S., Bilecen, K., Salama, S.R., Casper-Lindley, C., & Yildiz, F.H. (2007). Regulation of Rugosity and Biofilm Formation in *Vibrio cholerae*: Comparison of VpsT and VpsR Regulons and Epistasis Analysis of *vpsT*, *vpsR*, and *hapR*. *J. Bacteriol.* 189: 388-402.

Beyhan, S., Tischler, A.D., Camilli, A., & Yildiz, F.H. (2006). Transcriptome and phenotypic responses of *Vibrio cholerae* to increased cyclic di-GMP level. *J. Bacteriol.* 188: 3600-3613.

Bhowmick, R., Ghosal, A., Das, B., Koley, H., Saha, D.R., Ganguly, S., Nandy, R.K., Bhadra, R.K., & Chatterjee, N.S. (2008). Intestinal adherence of *Vibrio cholerae* involves a coordinated interaction between colonization factor GbpA and mucin. *Infect. Immun.* 76:4968-4977.

Boin, M.A., Austin, M.J., & Hase, C.C. (2004). Chemotaxis in *Vibrio cholerae*. *FEMS Microbiol. Lett.* 239: 1-8.

Boles, B.R., & McCarter, L.L. (2000). Insertional inactivation of genes encoding components of the sodium-type flagellar motor and switch of *Vibrio parahaemolyticus*. *J. Bacteriol.* 182: 1035-1045.

Bouvier, J., Gordia, S., Kampmann, G., Lange, R., Hengge-Aronis, R., & Gutierrez, C. (1998). Interplay between global regulators of *Escherichia coli*: effect of RpoS, Lrp and H-NS on transcription of the gene *osmC*. *Mol. Microbiol.* 28: 971-980.

Brückner, R., & Titgemeyer, F. (2002). Carbon catabolite repression in bacteria: choice of the carbon source and autoregulatory limitation of sugar utilization. *FEMS Microbiol. Lett.* 209: 141-148.

Butler, S.M., & Camilli, A. (2004). Both chemotaxis and net motility greatly influence the infectivity of *Vibrio cholerae*. *Proc. Natl. Acad. Sci.* USA 101: 5018-5023.

Camilli, A., & Mekalanos, J.J. (1995). Use of recombinase gene fusions to identify *Vibrio cholerae* genes induced during infection. *Mol. Microbiol.* 18: 671-683.

Casper-Lindley, C. & Yildiz, F.H. (2004). VpsT is a transcriptional regulator required for expression of vps biosynthesis genes and the development of rugose colonial morphology in *Vibrio cholerae* O1 El Tor. *J. Bacteriol.* 186: 1574-1578.

Cerdan, R., Bloch, V., Yang, Y., Bertin, P., Dumas, C., Rimsky, S., Kochoyan, M., & Arold, S.T. (2003). Crystal structure of the N-terminal dimerization domain of VicH, the H-NS-like protein of *Vibrio cholerae*. *J. Mol. Biol.* 334: 179-185.

Chen, X., Schauder, S., Potier, N., Van Dorsselaer, A., Pelczer, I., Bassler, B.L., & Hughson, F.M. (2002). Structural identification of a bacterial quorum-sensing signal containing boron. *Nature* 415: 545-549.

Childers, B.M., & Klose, K.E. (2007). Regulation of virulence in *Vibrio cholerae*: the ToxR regulon. *Future Microbiol.* 3: 335-344.

Correa N.E., Barker, J.R. & Klose, K.E. (2004). The *Vibrio cholerae* FlgM homologue is an anti-σ^{28} factor that is secreted through the sheathed polar flagellum. *J. Bacteriol.* 186: 4613-4619.

Correa, N.E., & Klose, K.E. (2005). Characterization of enhancer binding by the *Vibrio cholerae* flagellar regulatory protein FlrC. *J. Bacteriol.* 187: 3158-3170.

Correa, N.E., Lauriano, C.M., McGee, R., & Klose, K.E. (2000). Phosphorylation of the flagellar regulatory protein FlrC is necessary for *Vibrio cholerae* motility and enhances colonization. *Mol. Microbiol.* 35: 743-755.

Correa, N.E., Peng, F., & Klose, K.E. (2005). Roles of the regulatory proteins FlhF and FlhG in the *Vibrio cholerae* flagellar transcription hierarchy. *J. Bacteriol.* 187: 6324-6332.

Correll, D.L. (1999). Phosphorus: a rate limiting nutrient in surface waters. *Poultry Sci.* 78: 674-682.

D'Argenio, D.A., & Miller, S.I. (2004). Cyclic di-GMP as a bacterial second messenger. *Microbiology* 150: 2497-2502.

Dame, R.T., Wyman, C., & Goosen, N. (2001). Structural basis for preferential binding of H-NS to curved DNA. *Biochimie* 83: 231-234.

Danchin, A. (1993). Phylogeny of adenylyl cyclases. *Adv. Second Messenger and Phosphoprotein Res.*, Shenoilikar, S. & Nairn, A.C. (Eds.), Raven Press, Ltd. New York, Volume 27, page 109.

Das, S., Saha, R., & Kaur, I.R. (2008). Trend of antibiotic resistance of *Vibrio cholerae* strains from east Delhi. *Indian. J. Med. Res.* 127: 478-482.

Deutscher, J. (2008). The mechanism of carbon catabolite repression in bacteria. *Current Opinion Microbiol.* 11: 87-93.

Deutscher, J., Francke, C., & Postma, P.W. (2006). How phosphotransferase system-related protein phosphorylation regulates carbohydrate metabolism in bacteria. *Microbiol. Mol. Biol. Rev.* 70: 939-1031.

Ding, Y., Davis, B.M., Waldor, M.K. (2004). Hfq is essential for *Vibrio cholerae* virulence and down regulates sigma expression. *Mol. Microbiol.* 53: 345-354.

DiRita, V.J., Parsot, C., Jander, G., & Mekalanos, J.J. (1991). Regulatory cascade controls virulence in *Vibrio cholerae. Proc. Natl. Acad. Sci.* USA. 88:5403-5307.

Donato, G.M., & Kawula, T.H. (1998). Enhanced binding of altered H-NS to flagellar rotor protein FliG causes increased flagellar rotation speed and hypermotility in *Escherichia coli. J. Biol. Chem.* 273: 24030-24036.

Dorman, C.J. (2004). H-NS: a universal regulator for a dynamic genome. *Nature Rev. Microbiol.* 2: 391-400.

Dorman, C.J., & Deighan, P. (2003). Regulation of gene expression by histone-like proteins in bacteria. *Curr. Opinion Genet.* Develop. 13: 179-184.

Dorman, C.J., & Kane, K.A. (2009). DNA bridging and antibridging: a role for bacterial nucleoid-associated proteins in regulating the expression of laterally acquired genes. *FEMS Microbiol. Rev.* 33: 587-592.

Duan, F., & March, J.C. (2010). Engineered bacterial communication prevents *Vibrio cholerae* virulence in an infant mouse model. *Proc. Natl. Acad. Sci.* USA 107: 11260-11264.

Faruque, A.S.G., Alam, K., Malek, M.A., Khan, M.G.Y., Ahmed, S., Saha, D., Khan, W.A., Nair, G.B. Salam, M.A., Luby, S.P., & Sack, D.A. (2007). Emergence of multidrug-resistant strains of *Vibrio cholerae* O1 in Bangladesh and reversal of their susceptibility to tetracycline after two years. *Health Popul. Nutr.*25: 241-243.

Faruque, S.M., Biswas, K., Nashir Udden, S.M., Ahmad, Q.S., Sack, D.A., Nair, G.B., & Mekalanos, J.J. (2006). Transmissibility of cholera: *in vivo* formed biofilms and their relationship to infectivity and persistence in the environment. *Proc. Natl. Acad. Sci. USA* 103:6350–6355

Faruque, S.M., Islam, M.J., Ahmad, Q.S., Faruque, A.S., Sack, D.A., Nair, G.B., & Mekalanos, J.J. (2005a). Self-limiting nature of seasonal cholera epidemics: role host-mediated amplification of phage. *Proc. Natl. acad. Sci*. USA 102: 6119-6124.

Faruque, S.M., Naser, I.B., Islam, M.J., Faruque, A.S., Ghosh, A.N., Nair, G.B., Sack, D.A., & Mekalanos, J.J. (2005). Seasonal epidemics of cholera inversely correlate with the prevalence of environmental cholera phages. *Proc. Natl. acad. Sci. USA 102: 1702 - 1707.*

Fasano, A., Baudry, B., Pumplin, D.W., Wasserman, S.S., Tall, B.D., Ketley, J.M., & Kaper, J.B. (1991). *Vibrio cholerae* produces a second enterotoxin, which affects intestinal tight junctions. *Proc Natl Acad Sci* USA 88:5242–5246

Finkelstein, R. A., Boesman-Finkelstein, M., Chang, Y. & Hase, C.C. (1992). *Vibrio cholerae* hemagglutinin/protease, colonial variation, virulence, and detachment. *Infect. Immun*. 60:472–478.

Finkelstein, R.A. (1992). Cholera enterotoxin (choleragen): a historical perspective, p. 155-187. In Barua, D. & Greenough, W.B. (Eds.), Cholera. Plenum Medical Book Company, New York.

Finkelstein, R.A., Boesman-Finkelstein, M., & Holt, P. (1983). *Vibrio cholerae* hemagglutinin/lectin/protease hydrolyzes fibronectin and ovomucin: F.M. Burnet revisited. *Proc. Natl. Acad. Sci*. USA 80: 1092-1095.

Fong, J.C., & Yildiz, F.H. (2008). Interplay between cyclic AMP-cyclic AMP receptor protein and cyclic di-GMP signaling in *Vibrio cholerae* biofilm formation. *J. Bacteriol*. 190: 6646-6659.

Fong, J.C.N., Syed, K.A., Klose, K.E., & Yildiz, F.H. (2010). Role of *Vibrio* polysaccharide (*vps*) genes in VPS production, biofilm formation and *Vibrio cholerae* pathogenesis. *Microbiology* 156: 2757-2769.

Fullner, K.J. (2003). Toxins of *Vibrio cholerae*: consensus and controversy. In: Hecht, G.A. (Ed) Microbial pathogenesis and the intestinal epithelial cell. ASM Press, Washington, DC.

Galperin, M.Y. (2004). Bacterial signal transduction network in a genomic perspective. *Environ. Microbiol*. 6: 552-567.

Garcia, L., Jidy, M.D., Garcia, H., Rodriguez, B.L. Fernandez, R., Ano, G., Cedre, B., Valmaseda, T., Suzarte, E., Ramirez, M., Pino, Y., Campos, J., Menendez, J., Valera, R., Gonzalez, D., Gonzalez, I., Perez, O., Serrano, T., Lastre, M., Miralles, F., Del Campo, J., Maestre, J.L., Perez, J.L., Talavera, A., Perez, A., Marrero, K., Ledon, T., & Fando, R. (2005). The vaccine candidate *Vibrio cholerae* 638 is protective against cholera in healthy volunteers. *Infect. Immun*. 73:3018–3024.

Gardel, C.L.,& Mekalanos, J.J. (1996). Alterations in *Vibrio cholerae* motility phenotype correlate with changes in virulence factor expression. *Infect. Immun*. 64: 2246-2255.

Ghosh, A., Paul, K., & Chowdhury, R. (2006). Role of the histone-like nucleoid structuring protein in colonization, motility, and bile-dependent repression of virulence gene expression in *Vibrio cholerae*. *Infect. Immun*. 74: 3060-3064.

Gosink, K.K., Kobayashi, R., Kawagishi, I., & Hase, C.C. (2002). Analysis of the role of the three *cheA* homologs in chemotaxis of *Vibrio cholerae*. *J. Bacteriol*. 184: 1767-1771.

Hammer, B.K., & Bassler, B.L. (2003). Quorum sensing controls biofilm formation in *Vibrio cholerae*. *Mol. Microbiol.* 50: 101-114.

Harrison, L.M., Rallabhandi, P., Michalski, J., Zhou, X., Steyert, S.R., Vogel, S.N., & Kaper, J.B. (2008). *Vibrio cholerae* flagellins induce Toll-like receptor 5-mediated interleukin-8 production through mitogen-activated protein kinase and NF-κB activation. *Infect. Immun.* 76: 5524-5534.

Hase, C.C. (2001). Analysis of the role of flagellar activity in virulence gene expression in *Vibrio cholerae*. *Microbiology* 147: 831-837.

Häse, C.C., & Finkelstein, R.A. (1991). Cloning and nucleotide sequence of the *Vibrio cholerae* hemagglutinin/protease (HA/protease) gene and construction of an HA/protease-negative strain. *J. Bacteriol.* 173: 3311-3317.

Häse, C.C., & Mekalanos, J.J. (1998). TcpP protein is a positive regulator of virulence gene expression in *Vibrio cholerae*. *Proc. Natl. Acad. Sci.* USA 95:730-734.

Hase, C.C., & Mekalanos, J.J. (1999). Effects of changes in membrane sodium flux on virulence gene expression in *Vibrio cholerae*. *Proc. Natl. Acad. Sci.* USA. 96: 3183-3187.

Hase, C.C., Fedorova, N.D., Galperin, M.Y., & Dibrov, P.A. (2001). Sodium ion cycle in bacterial pathogens: evidence from cross-genome comparisons. *Microbiol. Mol. Biol. Rev.* 65: 353-370.

Haugo, A.J. & Watnick, P.I. (2002). *Vibrio cholerae* CytR is a repressor of biofilm development. *Mol. Microbiol.* 45: 471-483.

Hengge, R. (2009). Principles of c-di-GMP signaling in bacteria. *Nature Rev.* 7: 263-273.

Hengge-Aronis, R. (1999). Interplay of global regulators and cell physiology in the general stress response of *Escherichia coli*. *Curr. Opinion Microbiol.* 2: 148-152.

Hengge-Aronis, R. (2002). Signal transduction and regulatory mechanisms involved in control of the Sigma S (RpoS) subunit of RNA polymerase. *Microbiol. Mol. Biol. Rev.* 66: 373-395.

Hengge-Aronis, R. (2002a). Stationary phase gene regulation: what makes an *Escherichia coli* promoter σ^S-selective? *Curr. Opinion Microbiol.* 5: 591-595.

Herrington, D.A., Hall, R.H., Losonsky, G.A., Mekalanos, J.J., Taylor, R.K., & Levine, M.M. (1988). Toxin, the toxin co-regulated pili and the toxR regulon are essential for *Vibrio cholerae* pathogenesis in humans. *J. Exp. Med.* 168: 1487-1492.

Higgins, D.A., Poimianek, M.E., Krami, C.M., Taylor, R.K., Semmelhack, M.F., & Bassler, B.L. (2007). The major *Vibrio cholerae* autoinducer and its role in virulence factor production. *Nature* 450: 883-886.

Hommais, F., Krin, E., Laurent-Winter, C., Soutourina, O., Malpertuy, A., Le Caer, J-P., Danchin, A., & Bertin, P. (2001). Large-scale monitoring of pleiotropic regulation of gene expression by the prokaryotic nucleoid-associated protein, H-NS. *Mol. Microbiol.* 40: 20-36.

Houot, L., & Watnick, P.I. (2008). A novel role for enzyme I of the *Vibrio cholerae* phosphotransferase system in regulation of growth in a biofilm. *J. Bacteriol.* 190: 311-320.

Houot, L., Chang, S., Absalon, C., & Watnick, P.I. (2010). *Vibrio cholerae* PTS control of carbohydrate transport, biofilm formation, and colonization of the germ-free mouse intestine. *Infect. Immun.* 78: 1482-1494.

Houot, L., Chang, S., Pickering, B.S., Absalon, C., & Watnick, P.I. (2010a). The phosphoenolpyruvate phosphotransferase system regulates *Vibrio cholerae* biofilm formation through multiple independent pathways. *J. Bacteriol.* 192: 3055-3067.

Hung, D.T., Shakhnovick, E.A., Pierson, E., & Mekalanos, J.J. (2005). Small-molecule inhibitor of *Vibrio cholerae* virulence and intestinal colonization. *Science* 310: 670-674.

Huq, A., Small, E.B., West, P.A., Huq, M.I., Rahman, R., & Colwell, R.R. (1983). Ecological relationships between *Vibrio cholerae* and planktonic crustacean copepods. *Appl. Environ. Microbiol.* 45:275-283.

Hyakutake, A., Homma, M., Austin, M.J., Boin, M.A., Hase, C.C., & Kawagishi, I. (2005). Only one of the five CheY homologs in *Vibrio cholerae* directly switches flagellar rotation. *J. Bacteriol.* 187: 8403-8410.

Ichinose, Y., Ehara, M., Honda, T., & Miwatani, T. (1994). The effect on enterotoxicity of protease purified from *Vibrio cholerae* O1. *FEMS Microbiol. Lett.* 115:265–271.

Islam, S., Drasar, B.S., & Bradley, D.J. (1990). Long-term persistence of toxigenic *Vibrio cholerae* 01 in the mucilaginous sheath of blue-green-algae, *Anabaena variabilis*. *J. Trop. Med. Hygiene* 93:133-139.

Jensen, M.A., Faruque, S.M., Mekalanos, J.J., & Levin, B.R. (2006). Modeling the role of bacteriophage in the control of cholera outbreaks. *Proc. Natl. Acad. Sci.* USA 103: 4652-4657.

Jobling, M.G., & Holmes, R.K. (1997). Characterization of *hapR*, a positive regulator of the *Vibrio cholerae* HA/protease gene hap, and its identification as a functional homologue of the *Vibrio harveyi luxR* gene. *Mol. Microbiol.* 26: 1023-1034.

Joelsson, A., Kan, B., & Zhu, J. (2007). Quorum sensing enhances the stress response in *Vibrio cholerae*. *Appl. Environ. Microbiol.* 73: 3742-3746.

Joelsson, A., Liu, Z., & Zhu, J. (2006). Genetic and phenotypic diversity of quorum-sensing systems in clinical and environmental isolates of *Vibrio cholerae*. *Infect. Immun.* 74: 1141-1147.

Jude, B.A., Martinez, R.M., Skorupski, K., & Taylor, R.K. (2009). Levels of the secreted *Vibrio cholerae* attachment factor GbpA are modulated by quorum-sensing-induced proteolysis. *J. Bacteriol.* 191: 6911-6917.

Kamruzzaman, M., Udden, S.M., Cameron, D.E., Calderwood, S.B., Nair, G.B., Mekalanos, J.J., & Faruque, S.M. (2010). Quorum-regulated biofilms enhance the development of conditionally viable, environmental *Vibrio cholerae*. *Proc. Natl. Acad. Sci.* USA 107: 1588-1593.

Kannan, N., Wu, J., Anand, G.S., Yooseph, S., Neuwald, A.F., Venter, J.C., & Taylor, S.S. (2007). Evolution of allostery in the cyclic nucleotide binding module. *Genome Biol.* 8: R264.

Kaper, J.B., Lockman, H., Colwell, R.R., & Joseph, S.W. (1979). Ecology, serology, and enterotoxin production of *Vibrio cholerae* In Chesapeake Bay. *Appl. Environ. Microbiol.* 37:91-103.

Kaper, J.B., Morris Jr., G., & Levine, M.M. (1995). Cholera. *Clin. Microbiol. Rev.* 8: 48-86.

Kierek, K., & Watnick, P.I. (2003). Environmental determinants of *Vibrio cholerae* biofilm development. *Appl. Environ, Microbiol.* 69: 5079-5088.

Kim, Y-K., & McCarter, L.L. (2000). Analysis of the polar flagellar gene system of *V. parahaemolyticus*. *J. Bacteriol.* 182: 3693-3704.

Klose, K.E., & Mekalanos, J.J. (1998). Differential expression of multiple flagellins in *Vibrio cholerae*. *J. Bacteriol*. 180: 303-316.t

Klose, K.E., & Mekalanos, J.J. (1998a). Distinct roles of an alternative sigma factor during both free-swimming and colonizing phases of the *Vibrio cholerae* pathogenic cycle. *Mol. Microbiol*. 28: 501-520.

Klose, K.E., Novik, V., & Mekalanos, J.J. (1998). Identification of Multiple sigma 54-dependent transcriptional activators in *Vibrio cholerae*. *J. Bacteriol*. 180: 5256-5259.

Kojima, S., Yamamoto, K., Kawagishi, I., & Homma, M. (1999). The flagellar motor of *Vibrio cholerae* is driven by a Na^+ motive force. *J. Bacteriol*. 181: 1927-1930.

Kovacikova, G., & Skorupski, K. (2001). Overlapping binding sites for the virulence gene AphA, AphB and cAMP-CRP at the *Vibrio cholerae tcpPH* promoter. *Mol. Microbiol*. 41: 393-407.

Kovacikova, G., & Skorupski, K. (2002). The alternative sigma factor sigma E plays an important role in intestinal survival and virulence in *Vibrio cholerae*. *Infect. Immun*. 70: 5355-5362.

Kovacikova, G., & Skorupski, K. (2002a). Regulation of virulence gene expression in *Vibrio cholerae* by quorum sensing: HapR functions at the *aphA* promoter. *Mol. Microbiol*. 46:1135–1147.

Krasteva, P.V., Fong, J.C.N., Shikuma, N.J., Beyhan, S., Navarro Marcos, V.A.S., Yildiz, F.H., & Sondermann, H. (2010). *Vibrio cholerae* VpsT regulates matrix production and motility by directly sensing cyclic di-GMP. *Science* 327: 866-868.

Krishnan, H.H., Ghosh, A., Paul, K., & Chowdhury, R. (2004). Effect of anaerobiosis on expression of virulence factors in *Vibrio cholerae*. *Infect. Immun*. 72: 3961-3967.

Krueger, S., Gorshkova, I., Brown, J., Hoskins, J,M .McKenney, K.H., & Schwarz, F.P.(1998). Determination of the conformations of cAMP receptor protein and its T127L, S128A mutant with and without cAMP from small angle neutron scattering measurements. J. *Biol. Chem*. 273: 20001-20006.

Lamarche, M.G., Wanner, B.L., Crepin, S., & Harel J. (2008). The phosphate regulon and bacterial virulence: a regulatory network connecting phosphate homeostasis and pathogenesis. *FEMS Microbiol. Rev*. 32: 461-473.

Lang, B., Blot, N., Bouffartigues, E., Buckle, M., Geertz, M., Gualerzi, C.O., Mavathur, R., Muskhelishvili, G., Pon, C.L., Rimsky, S., Stella, S., Madan Babu, M., & Travers, A. (2007). High-affinity DNA binding sites for H-NS provide a molecular basis for selective silencing within proteobacterial genomes. *Nucleic Acids Res*. 35: 6330-6337.

Lee, S.H., Butler, S.M., & Camilli, A. (2001). Selection for *in vivo* regulators of bacterial virulence. *Proc. Natl. Acad. Sci*. USA 98: 6889-6894.

Lee, S.H., Hava, D.L., Waldor, M.K., & Camilli, A. (1999). Regulation and temporal expression patterns of *Vibrio cholerae* virulence genes during infection. *Cell* 99: 625-634.

Lengeler, J.W., & Jahreis, K. (2009). Bacterial PEP-dependent carbohydrate: phosphotransferase systems couple sensing and global control mechanisms. *Contrib. Microbiol*. 16: 65-87.

Lenz, D.H., & Bassler, B.L.(2007). The small nucleoid protein Fis is involved in *Vibrio cholerae* quorum sensing. *Molec. Microbiol*. 63: 859-871.

Lenz, D.H., Miller, M.B., Zhu, J., Kulkarni, R.V., & Bassler, B.L. (2005). CsrA and three redundant small RNAs regulate QS in *Vibrio cholerae*. *Mol. Microbiol*. 58: 1186-1202.

Lenz, D.H., Mok, K.C., Lilley, B.N., Kulkarni, R.V., Wingreen, N.S., & Bassler, B.L. (2004). The small RNA chaperone Hfq and multiple small RNAs control QS in *Vibrio harveyi* and *Vibrio cholerae*. *Cell* 118: 69-82.

Liang, W., Pascual-Montano, Silva, A.J., & Benitez, J.A. (2007). The cyclic AMP receptor protein modulates quorum sensing, motility and multiple genes that affect intestinal colonization in *Vibrio cholerae*. *Microbiology* 153: 2964-2975.

Liang, W., Silva, A.J., & Benitez, J.A. (2007a). The cAMP Receptor Protein Modulates Colonial Morphology Phase in *Vibrio cholerae*. *Appl. Environ. Microbiol.* 73: 7482–7487.

Liang, W., Sultan, S.Z., Silva, A.J., Benitez, J.A. (2008). Cyclic AMP posttranscriptionally regulates the biosynthesis of a major bacterial autoinducer to modulate the cell density required to activate quorum sensing. *FEBS Lett.* 582: 3744-3750.

Lim, B., Beyhan, S., & Yildiz, F.H. (2007). Regulation of *Vibrio* polysaccharide synthesis and virulence factor production by CdgC, a GGDEF-EAL domain protein, in *Vibrio cholerae*. *J. Bacteriol.* 189: 717-729.

Lim, B., Beyhan, S., Meir, J., & Yildiz, F.H. (2006). Cyclic-diGMP signal transduction systems in *Vibrio cholerae*: modulation of rugosity and biofilm formation. *Molec. Microbiol.* 60: 331.

Lin W., Fullner, K.J., Clayton, R., Sexton, J.A., Rogers, M.B., Calia, K.E., Calderwood, S.B., Fraser, C., & Mekalanos, J.J. (1999). Identification of a *Vibrio cholerae* RTX toxin gene cluster that is tightly linked to the cholera toxin prophage. *Proc. Natl. Acad. Sci.* USA 96:1071-1076.

Lin, W., Kovacikova, G., & Skorupski, K. (2005). Requirements for *Vibrio cholerae* HapR Binding and Transcriptional Repression at the *hapR* promoter are distinct from those at the *aphA* promoter. *J. Bacteriol.* 187: 3013-3019.

Lin, W., Kovacikova, G., & Skorupski, K. (2007). The quorum sensing regulator HapR downregulates the expression of the virulence gene transcription factor AphA in *Vibrio cholerae* by antagonizing Lrp- and VpsR-mediated activation. *Mol. Microbiol.* 64: 953-967.

Liu, Z., Hsiao, A., Joelsson, A., & Zhu, J. (2006). The transcriptional regulator VqmA increases expression of the quorum-sensing activator HapR in *Vibrio cholerae*. *J. Bacteriol.* 188: 2446-2453.

Liu, Z., Miyashiro, T., Tsou, A., Hsiao, A., Goulian, M., & Zhu, J. (2008). Mucosal penetration primes *Vibrio cholerae* for host colonization by repressing quorum sensing. *Proc. Natl. Acad. Sci.* USA 105: 9769-9774.

Lucchini, S., Rowley, G., Goldberg, M.D., Hurd, D., Harrison, M., & Hinton, J.C.D. (2006). H-NS mediates the silencing of laterally acquired genes in bacteria. *PLoS Pathog* 2(8): e81. DOI: 10.1371/journal.ppat.0020081.

Matson, J.S., Withey, J.H., & DiRita, V.J. (2007). Regulatory networks controlling *Vibrio cholerae* virulence gene expression. *Infect. Immun.* 75: 5542-5549.

Matz, C., McDougald, D., Moreno, A.M., Yung, P.Y., Yildiz, F.H., & Kjelleberg, S. (2005). Biofilm formation and phenotypic variation enhance predation-driven persistence of *Vibrio cholerae*. *Proc. Natl. Acad. Sci.* USA 102: 16819-16824.

McCarter, L.L. (2001). Polar flagellar motility of the *Vibrionaceae*. *Microbiol. Molec. Biol. Rev.* 65: 445-462.

Mel, S.F., Fullner, K.J., Wimer-Mackin, S., Lencer, W.I., & Mekalanos, J.J. (2000). Association of protease activity in *Vibrio cholerae* vaccine strains with decrease in transcellular epithelial resistance of polarized T84 intestinal cells. *Infect. Immun.* 68:6487–6492.

Merrell, D.S., Butler, S.M., Qadri, F., Dolganov, N.A., Alam, A., Cohen, M.B., Calderwood, S.B., Schoolnik, G.K., & Camilli, A. (2002). Host-induced epidemic spread of the cholera bacterium. *Nature* 417: 642-645.

Merrell, D.S., Tischler, A.D., Lee, S.H., & Camilli, A. (2000). *Vibrio cholerae* requires *rpoS* for efficient intestinal colonization. *Infect. Immun.* 68: 6691-6696.

Miller, M.B., Skorupski, K., Lenz, D.H., Taylor, R.K., & Bassler, B.L. (2002). Parallel quorum sensing systems converge to regulate virulence in *Vibrio cholerae. Cell* 110: 303-314.

Miller, V.L., & Mekalanos, J.J. (1985). Genetic analysis of the cholera toxin-positive regulatory gene *toxR. J. Bacteriol.* 163: 580-585.

Miller, V.L., DiRita, V.J., & Mekalanos, J.J. (1989). Identification of *toxS*, a regulatory gene whose product enhances *toxR*-mediated activation of the cholera toxin promoter. *J. Bacteriol.* 171:1288-1293.

Morris Jr., J.G. Sztein, M.B., Rice, E.B., Nataro, J.P., Losonsky, J.A., Panigrahi, P., Tacket, C.O., & Johnson, J.A. (1966). *V. cholerae* O1 can assume a chlorine-resistant rugose survival form that is virulent for humans. *J. Infect. Dis.* 174: 1364-1368.

Mwansa, J.C., Mwaba, J., Lukwesa, C., Bhuiyan, N.A., Ansaruzzaman, M., Ramamurthy, T., Alam, M., & Nair, G.B. (2007). Multiple antibiotic-resistant *Vibrio cholerae* O1 biotype El Tor strains emerge during cholera outbreaks in Zambia. *Epidemiol. Infect.* 135: 847-853.

Nagamune, K., Yamamoto, K., Naka, A., Matsuyama, J., Miwatani, T., & Honda, T. (1996). In vitro proteolytic processing and activation of the recombinant precursor of E1 Tor cytolysin/hemolysin (Pro-HlyA) of *Vibrio cholerae* by soluble hemagglutinin/protease of *V. cholerae*, trypsin, and other proteases. *Infect. Immun.* 64:4655–4658

Navarre, W.W., Porwollik, S., Wang, Y., McClelland, M., Rosen, H., Libby, S.J., & Fang, F.C. (2006). Selective silencing of foreign DNA with low GC content by the H-NS protein in *Salmonella. Science* 313: 236-238.

Nelson, E.J., Nelson, D.S., Salam, M.A., & Sack, D.A. (2011). Antibiotics for both moderate and severe cholera. *N. Engl. J. Med.* 364: 5-7.

Nielsen, A.T., Dolganov, N.A., Otto, G., Miller, M.C., Wu, C.Y., & Schoolnik G.K. (2006). *PLoS Pathog* 2(10): e109. doi:10.1371/journal.ppat.0020109.

Nogueira, T., & Springer, M. (2000). Post-transcriptional control by global regulators of gene expression in bacteria. *Current opinion in Microbiology* 3: 154-158.

Nye, M.B., & Taylor, R.K. (2003). *Vibrio cholerae* H-NS domain structure and function with respect to transcriptional repression of ToxR regulon genes reveals differences among H-NS family members. *Mol. Microbiol.* 50: 427-444.

Nye, M.B., Pfau, J.S., Skorupski, K., & Taylor, R.K. (2000). *Vibrio cholerae* H-NS silences virulence gene expression at multiple steps in the ToxR regulatory cascade. *J. Bacteriol.* 182: 4295-4303.

Ogasawara, H., Yamada, K., Kori, A., Yamamoto, K., & Ishihama, A. (2010). Regulation of the *Escherichia coli csgD* promoter: interplay between five transcription factors. *Microbiology* 156: 2470-2483.

Ogawa, N., Tzseng, C-M., Fraley, C.D.E., & Kornberg, A. (2000). Inorganic polyphosphate in *Vibrio cholerae*: genetics, biochemical, and physiological features. *J. Bacteriol.* 182: 6687-6693.

Okeke, I.N., Aboderin, O.A., Byarugaba, D.K., Ojo, K.K., & Opiuntan J.A. (2007). Growing problem of multidrug-resistant enteric pathogens in Africa. *Emerg. Infect. Dis.* 13: 1640-1646.

Oshima, T., Ishikawa, S., Kurokawa, K., Aiba, H., & Ogasawara, N. (2006). *Escherichia coli* histone-like protein H-NS preferentially binds to horizontally acquired DNA in association with RNA polymerase. *DNA Res.* 13: 141-153.

Osuna, R., Lienau, D., Hughes, K.T., & Johnson, R.C. (1995). Sequence, regulation, and functions of *fis* in *Salmonella typhimurium*. *J. Bacteriol.* 177: 2021-2032.

Owen-Hughes, T.A., Pavitt, G.D., Santos, D.S., Sidebotham, J.M., Hulton, C.S.J., Hinton, J.C.D., & Higgins, F. (1992). The chromatin-associated protein H-NS interacts with curved DNA to influence DNA topology and gene expression. *Cell* 71: 255-265.

Porter, M.E.,& Dorman, C.J. (1997). Positive regulation of *Shigella flexneri* virulence genes by integration host factor. *J. Bacteriol.* 179: 6537-6550.

Pratt, J.T., Ismail, A.M., & Camilli, A. (2010). PhoB regulates environmental and virulence gene expression in *Vibrio cholerae. Mol. Microbiol.* 77: 1595-1605.

Pratt, J.T., McDonough, E., & Camilli, A. (2009). PhoB regulates motility, biofilm, and cyclic di-GMP in *Vibrio cholerae. J. Bacteriol.* 191: 6632-6642.

Pratt, J.T., Tamayo, R., Tischler, A.D., & Camilli, A. (2007). PilZ domain proteins bind cyclic diguanylate and regulate diverse processes in *Vibrio cholerae. J. Biol. Chem.* 282: 12860-12870.

Prouty, M.G., Correa, N.E., & Klose, K.E. (2001). The novel sigma 54- and sigma 28-dependent flagellar gene transcription hierarchy of *Vibrio cholerae. Mol. Microbiol.* 39: 1595-1609.

Queiroz, M.H., Madrid, C., Paytubi, S., Balsalobre, C., & Juarez, A. (2011). Integration host factor alleviates H-NS silencing of the *Salmonella ente*rica serovar Typhimurium master regulator of SP11, *hilA*. 2011. *Microbiology* 157: 2504-2514.

Rasmussen, L., White, L., Pathak, A., Ayala, J.C., Wang, H., Wu, J-H., Benitez, J.A., & Silva, A.J. (2011). A high throughput screening assay for inhibitors of bacterial motility identifies a novel inhibitor of the Na^+-driven flagellar motor and virulence gene expression in *Vibrio cholerae. Antimicrob. Agents Chemother.* 55: 4134-4143.

Rice, E.W., Johnson, C.J., Clark, R.M., Fox, K.R., Reasoner, D.J., Dunnigan, M.E., Panigrahi, P., Johnson, J.A., & Morris, Jr., J.G. (1992). Chlorine and survival of "rugose" Vibrio cholerae. *Lancet* 340: 740.

Robert, A., Silva, A.J., Benitez, J.A., Rodriguez, B.L., Fando, R., Campos, J., Sengupta, D.K., Boesman-Finkelstein, M., & Finkelstein, R.A. (1996). Tagging a *Vibrio cholerae* El Tor candidate vaccine strain by disruption of its hemagglutinin/protease gene using a novel reporter enzyme: *Clostridium thermocellum* endoglucanase A. *Vaccine* 14: 1517-1522.

Roychowdhury, A., Pan, A., Dutta, D., Mukhopadhyay, A.K., Ramamurthy, T., Nandy, R.K., Bhattacharya, S.K., Bhattacharya, M.K. (2008). Emergence of tetracycline-resistant *Vibrio cholerae* O1serotype Inaba, in Kolkata, India. *Japan J. Infect. Dis. 61: 128-129.*

Rui, H., Ritchie, J,M. Bronson, R.T., Mekalanos, J.J., Zhang, Y., & Waldor, M.K. (2010). Reactogenicity of live-attenuated *Vibrio cholerae* vaccines is dependent on flagellins. *Proc. Natl. Acad. Sci.* USA 107: 4359-4364.

Rutherford, S.T., van Kessel, J.C., Shao, Y., Bassler, B.L. (2001). AphA and LuxR/HapR reciprocally control quorum sensing in vibrios. *Genes & Develop.* 25: 397-408.

Schoolnik, G.K., & Yildiz, F.H. (2000). The complete genome sequence of *Vibrio cholerae*: a tale of two chromosomes and two lifestyles. *Genome Biology* 1: reviews 1016.1-1016.3.

Shakhnovich, E.A., Hung, D,T, Pierson, E., Lee, K., & Mekalanos, J.J. (2007a). Virstatin inhibits dimerization of the transcriptional activator ToxT. *Proc. Natl. acad. Sci.* USA 104: 2372-2377.

Shakhnovick, E.A., Sturtevant, D., & Mekalanos, J.J. (2007). Molecular mechanisms of virstatin resistance by non-O1/non-O139 strains of *Vibrio cholerae. Mol. Microbiol.* 66: 1331-1341.

Shi, Y., Wang, S., Krueger, S., & Schwarz, F.P. (1999). Effect of mutations at the monomer-monomer interface of cAMP receptor protein on specific DNA binding. *J. Biol. Chem.* 274: 6946-6956.

Silva, A.J., & Benitez, J.A. (2004). Transcriptional regulation of *Vibrio cholerae* hemagglutinin/protease by the cyclic AMP receptor protein and RpoS. *J. Bacteriol.* 186: 6374-6382.

Silva, A.J., Leitch, G.J., Camilli, A. & Benitez, J.A. (2006). Contribution of hemagglutinin/protease and motility to the pathogenesis of El Tor biotype cholera. *Infect. Immun.* 74: 2072-2079.

Silva, A.J., Pham, K., & Benitez, J.A. (2003). Hemaglutinnin/protease expression and mucin gel penetration in El Tor biotype *Vibrio cholerae. Microbiology* 149: 1883-1891.

Silva, A.J., Sultan, S.Z., Liang, W., & Benitez, J.A. (2008). Role of the histone-like nucleoid structuring protein (H-NS) in the regulation of RpoS and RpoS-dependent genes in *Vibrio cholerae. J. Bacteriol.* 190: 7335–7345.

Simm, R., Morr, M., Kader, A., Nimtz, M., & Romling, U. (2004). GGDEF and EAL domains inversely regulate cyclic di-GMP levels and transition from sessility to motility. *Mol. Microbiol.* 53: 1123-1134.

Skorupski, K., & Taylor, R.K. (1997). Cyclic AMP and its receptor protein negatively regulate the coordinate expression of cholera toxin and toxin co-regulated pilus in *Vibrio cholerae. Proc. Natl. Acad. Sci.* USA 94, 265-270.

Spurio, R., Falconi, M., Brandi, A., Pon, C.L., & Gualerzi, C.O. (1997). The oligomeric structure of the nucleoid protein H-NS is necessary for recognition of intrinsically curved DNA and for DNA binding. *EMBO J.* 16: 1795-1805.

Stonehouse, E.A., Hulbert, R.R., Nye, M.B., Skorupski, K., & Taylor, R.K. (2011). H-NS binding and repression of the *ctx* promoter in *Vibrio cholerae. J. Bacteriol.* 193: 979-988.

Stonehouse, E.A., Kovacikova, G., Taylor, R.K., & Skorupski, K. (2008). Integration host factor positively regulates virulence gene expression in *Vibrio cholerae. J. Bacteriol.* 190: 4736-4748.

Stülke, J., & Hillen, W. (1999). Carbon catabolite repression in bacteria. *Curr. Opinion. Microbiol.* 2: 195-201.

Sudarsan, N., Lee, E.R,, Weinberg, Z., Moy, R.H., Kim, J.N., Link, K.H., & Breaker, R.R. (2008). Riboswitches in eubacteria sense the second messenger cyclic di-GMP. *Science* 321: 422-413.

Sudarsan, N., Lee, E.R., Weinberg, Z., Moy, R.H., Kim, J.M., Link, K.H., & Breaker, R.R. (2008). Riboswitches in eubacteria sense the second messenger cyclic di-GMP. *Science* 321: 411-413,

Sultan, S.Z., Silva, A.J., & Benitez, J.A. (2010). The PhoB regulatory system modulates biofilm formation and stress response in El Tor biotype *Vibrio cholerae. FEMS Microbiol. Lett.* 302: 22-31.

Svenningsen, S.L., Waters, C.M., & Bassler, B.L. (2008). A negative feedback loop involving small RNAs accelerates *Vibrio cholerae*'s transition out of quorum sensing mode. *Genes & Develop.* 22: 226-238.

Syed K.A., Beyhan, S., Correa, N., Queen, J., Liu, J., Peng, F., Satchell, K.J.F., Yildiz, F.H., & Klose, K.E. (2009). The *Vibrio cholerae* flagellar regulatory hierarchy controls expression of virulence factors. *J. Bacteriol.* 191: 6555-6570.

Tamayo, R., Patimalla, B., & Camilli, A. (2010). Growth in a biofilm induces a hyperinfective phenotype in *Vibrio cholerae. Infect. Immun.* 78: 3560-3569.

Tamayo, R., Pratt, J.T., & Camilli, A. (2007). Roles of cyclic diguanylate in the regulation of bacterial pathogenesis. *Ann. Rev. Microbiol.* 61: 131-148.

Tendeng, C., Badaut, C., Krin, E., Gounon, P., Ngo, S., Danchin, A., Rimsky, S., & Bertin, P. (2000). Isolation and Characterization of *vicH*, encoding a new pleiotropic regulator in *Vibrio cholerae. J. Bacteriol.* 182: 2026-2032.

Tischler, A.T., & Camilli, A. (2004). Cyclic diguanylate (c-di-GMP) regulates *Vibrio cholerae* biofilm formation. *Mol. Microbiol.* 53: 857-869.

Trucksis, M., Galen, J.E., Michalski, Fasano, A., & Kaper, J.B. (1993). Accessory cholera enterotoxin (Ace), the third toxin of a *Vibrio cholerae* virulence cassette. *Proc Natl Acad Sci* USA 90:5267–5271

Typas, A., Becker, G., & Hengge, R. (2007). The molecular basis of selective promoter activation by the σ^S subunit of RNA polymerase. *Mol. Microbiol.* 63: 1296-1306.

Ueguchi, C., & Mizuno, T. (1993). The *Escherichia coli* nucleoid protein H-NS functions directly as a transcriptional repressor. *EMBO J.* 12: 1039-1046.

Urakawa, H., & Rivera, I.N.G. (2006). Aquatic Environment. In: The Biology of *Vibrios* (Thompson, F.L., B. Austin and J. Swings (Eds.). ASM Press, Washington, D.C.

Van Ulsen, P., Hillebrant, M., Zulianello, L., van de Putte, P., & Goosen, N. (1996). Integration host factor alleviates the H-NS-mediated repression of the early promoter of bacteriophage Mu. *Mol. Microbiol.* 3: 567-578.

Vicente, M., Chater, K.F., & De Lorenzo, V. (1999). Bacterial transcription factors involved in global regulation. *Mol. Microbiol.* 33: 8-17.

Von Kruger, W.M., Humphreys, S., & Ketley, J.M. (1999). A role for the PhoBR regulatory system homologue in the *Vibrio cholerae* phosphate limitation response and intestinal colonization. *Microbiology* 145: 2463-2475.

Von Kruger, W.M., Lery, L.M., Soares, M.R., de Neves-Manta, F.S., Batista e Silva, B.C., Neves-Ferreira, A.G., Perales, J., & Bisch, P.M. (2006). The phosphate-starvation response in *Vibrio cholerae* O1 and *phoB* mutant under proteomic analysis: disclosing functions involved in adaptation, survival and virulence. Proteomics 6: 1495-1511.

Wai, S.N., Mizunoe, Y., Takade, A., Kawabata, S.I., & Yoshida, S.I. (1998). *Vibrio cholerae* O1 strain TSI-4 produces the exopolysaccharide materials that determine colony morphology, stress resistance, and biofilm formation. *Appl. Environ. Microbiol.* 64: 3648-3655.

Waldor, M.K. (2006). Disarming pathogens - a new approach for antibiotic development. *N. Eng. J. Med.* 354: 296-297.

Waldor, M.K., & Mekalanos, J.J. (1996). Lysogenic conversion by a filamentous phage encoding cholera toxin. *Science* 272:1910-1914.

Walker, R.L., & Owen, R.L. (1990). Intestinal barriers to bacteria and their toxins. *Ann. Rev. Medicine* 41: 393-400.

Wang, H., Wu, J-H., Ayala, J.C., Benitez, J.A., & Silva A.J. (2011). Interplay between cyclic diguanylate, HapR and the general stress response regulator (RpoS) in the regulation of *Vibrio cholerae* hemagglutinin (HA)/protease. *J. Bacteriol.* In Press.

Wang, S., Shi, Y., Gorshkova, I., & Schwarz, F.P. (2000). RNA polymerase-cNMP-ligated cAMP receptor protein (CRP) mutant interactions in the enhancement of transcription by CRP mutants. *J. Biol. Chem.* 275: 33457-33463.

Waters, C.M., Lu, W., Rabinowitz, J.D., & Bassler, B.L. (2008). Quorum sensing controls biofilm formation in *Vibrio cholerae* through modulation of cyclic di-GMP levels and repression of *vpsT*. *J. Bacteriol.* 190: 2527-2536.

Watnick, P.I., & Kolter, R. (1999). Steps in the development of a *Vibrio cholerae* El Tor biofilm. *Mol. Microbiol.* 34: 586-595.

White, P.B. (1938). The rugose variant of *Vibrios*. *J. Pathol. Bacteriol.* 46:1-6.

Wu, Z., Milton, D., Nybon, P., Sjo, A., & Magnusson, K.E.. (1996). *Vibrio cholerae* hemagglutinin/protease (HA/protease) causes morphological changes in cultured epithelial cells and perturbs their paracellular barrier function. *Microbial Pathog.* 21: 111-123.

Wu, Z., Nybom, P., & Magnusson, K.E. (2000). Distinct effects of *Vibrio cholerae* hemagglutinin/protease on the structure and localization of the tight junction-associated proteins occludin and ZO-1. *Cell. Microbiol.* 2: 11-17.

Xicohtencalt-Cortes, J., Lyons, S., Chaparro, A.P., Hernandez, D.R., Saldana, Z., Ledesma, M.A., Rondon, M.A., Gewirtz, A.T., Klose, K.E., & Giron, J.A. (2006). Identification of proinflammatory flagellin proteins in supernatants of *Vibrio cholerae* O1 by proteomic analysis. *Mol. Cell. Proteomics* 5: 12.

Xu, H-S., Roberts, N., Singleton, F.L., Attwell, R.W., Grimes, D.J., & Colwell, R.R. (1982). Survival and viability of non-culturable *Escherichia coli* and *Vibrio cholerae* in the estuaries and marine environment. *Microbiol Ecol.* 8: 313-323.

Yildiz, F.H., & Schoolnik, G.K. (1998). Role of *rpoS* in stress survival and virulence of *Vibrio cholerae*. *J. Bacteriol.* 180: 773-784.

Yildiz, F.H., & Schoolnik, G.K. (1999). *Vibrio cholerae* O1 El Tor: identification of a gene cluster required for the rugose colony type, exopolysaccharide production, chlorine resistance, and biofilm formation. *Proc. Natl. Acad. Sci.* USA 96: 4028-4033.

Yildiz, F.H., Dolganov, N.A., & Schoolnik, G.K. (2001). VpsR, a member of the response regulators of the two-component regulatory systems, is required for expression of *vps* biosynthesis genes and EPS (ETr)-associated phenotypes in *Vibrio cholerae* O1 El Tor. *J. Bacteriol.* 183:1716-1726.

Yildiz, F.H., Liu, X.S., Heydorn, A., & Schoolnik, G.K. (2004). Molecular analysis of rugosity in a *Vibrio cholerae* O1 El Tor phase variant. *Mol. Microbiol.* 53: 497-515.

Yu, R. R., & DiRita, V.J. (2002). Regulation of gene expression in *Vibrio cholerae* by *toxT* involves both antirepression and RNA polymerase stimulation. *Mol. Microbiol.* 43: 119-134.

Zhu, J., & Mekalanos, J.J. (2003). Quorum sensing-dependent biofilms enhance colonization in *Vibrio cholerae*. *Developmental Cell* 5:647-656.

Zhu, J., Miller, M.B., Vance, R.E., Dziejman, M., Bassler, B.L., Mekalanos, J.J. (2002). Quorum-sensing regulators control virulence gene expression in *Vibrio cholerae*. *Proc. Natl. Acad. Sci.* USA 99: 3129-3134.

Part 3

Cholera Toxin and Antagonists

7

The Cholera Toxin as a Biotechnological Tool

Noelia Olivera, Maia Cédola and Ricardo M Gómez
Instituto de Biotecnología y Biología Molecular, CONICET La Plata
Argentina

1. Introduction

It was as early as 1886 when Robert Koch proposed that the symptoms caused by *Vibrio cholerae* were initiated by a "poison" produced by the pathogen. However, it was not until 1959 that this postulate could be demonstrated by reproducing the disease in an animal model [De, 1959]. Today, cholera toxin (CT) is known to exhibit toxic effects in human cells and produces dehydrating diarrhea in humans. It is produced almost exclusively by few serogroups of *V. cholera*, however, sometimes may be naturally produced by other organisms, as the opportunistic pathogen *V. mimicus* [Nishibuchi and Seidler, 1983; Spira and Fedorka-Cray, 1984].

CT has important immunological properties and for that reason it has been extensively used as a systemic and mucosal adjuvant because it enhances the immunogenicity of most antigens fused or co-administered with the toxin [Sanchez and Holmgren, 2008].

The aim of this chapter will be to describe the biotechnological utilities of CT, with special attention to its adjuvant effect as well as its application in the treatment of autoimmune diseases through its ability to generate oral tolerance.

2. Structure

CT belongs to the family of AB_5-type toxins, since it is composed of two subunits in a 1:5 ratio. The A subunit (CTA), of 28 kDa, is a heterodimer associated non-covalently to a homopentamer formed by the subunits B (CTB) of 56 kDa [Merritt et al., 1994; Vanden Broeck et al., 2007]. CTA is responsible for the biological activity and CTB binds to the cell membrane receptor [Holmgren et al., 1973; Lonnroth and Holmgren, 1973] (Fig. 1.).

CTA comprises 240 amino acids, and the 11.6 kDa B subunit monomers each have 103 amino acids. CTA is synthesized as a single polypeptide chain and is post-translationally modified through the action of a *V. cholerae* protease at position R192 [Mekalanos et al., 1979]. The cleavage of this amino acid, found in an exposed loop that extends from C187 to C199 residues, generates two fragments named CTA1 and CTA2, which remain linked by a disulfide bridge [Lencer and Tsai, 2003; Tsai et al., 2001]. The toxic activity (enzymatic ADP-ribosylating) activity of CTA resides in CTA1, whereas CTA2 serves to insert CTA into the CTB pentamer [Sanchez and Holmgren, 2011]. The C-terminal hydrophobic region including residues 162-192 of CTA1, plays a key role in toxicity. It triggers the ER-associated degradation (ERAD) mechanism (see section 3) and facilitates interaction with the cytosolic ADP-ribosylation factors (ARFs) that serve as allosteric activators of CTA1 [Teter et al., 2006].

The remarkable stability of pentameric CTB is attributed to non-covalent interactions including 130 hydrogen bonds, 20 salt bridges, as well as tight packing of subunits via hydrophobic and pentamer-pentamer interactions. Consequently, the CTB pentamer is held together and remains as a complex unless boiled or monomerized by acidification at pH below 3 [Sanchez and Holmgren, 2008].

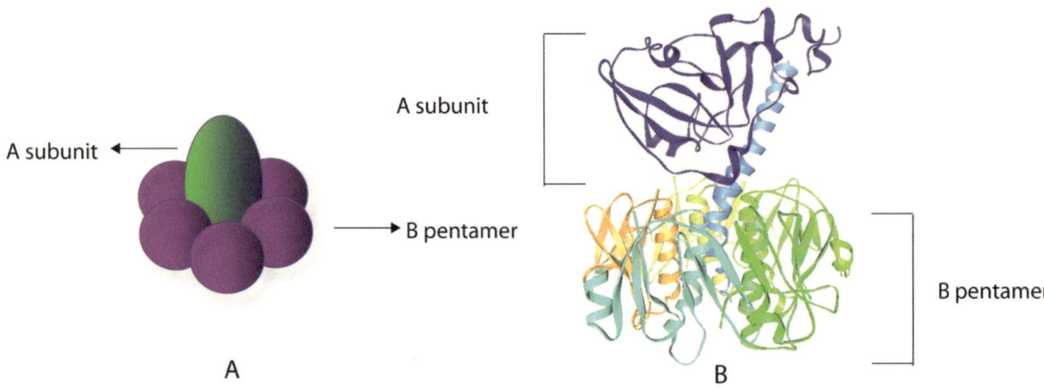

Fig. 1. Cholera toxin structure. A) Schematic model of cholera toxin. A subunit contains the toxic activity while B subunits bind to cells. B) Model based on X-ray crystallography analysis. Each subunit is represented by a different color. Adapted from Zhang et al 2005.

3. Binding and mechanism of action

CT is secreted through the outer membrane of *V. cholerae* and its toxic action begins when its B subunit binds to the high-affinity monoganglioside GM1 receptor. GM1 is a glycolipid commonly found in caveolae, organized membrane structures enriched in glycolipids, cholesterol and caveolin, involved in endocytosis and transcytosis, cellular transport and signal transduction [Shin and Abraham, 2001]. These membrane structures are present in various cell types, including immune cells [Thomas et al., 2004]. Each B subunit monomer has a binding site for GM1, however, the CTB pentamer has a much higher binding affinity for the receptor due to the important role played by a single amino acid from an adjacent B subunit that enhances this action [Merritt et al., 1994]. After binding to the receptor, CT enters human intestinal cells through endocytosis and is transported from early endosomes to the Golgi. Endocytosis of CT may follow one of three pathways: (i) lipid raft/caveolae mediated endocytic pathway, (ii) clathrin mediated endocytic pathway, or (iii) noncaveolar clathrin-independent pathway [Chinnapen et al., 2007]. GM1 is the vehicle for retrograde transport of the CT holotoxin from the plasma membrane to the ER [Fujinaga et al., 2003]. In the ER, the disulfide bond that links CTA1 and CTA2 to CTB is reduced and a protein disulfide isomerase mediates the dissociation of CTA1 from CTA2/CTB. CTA1 moves from the ER to the cytosol by the ERAD dislocation mechanism, wich recognizes misfolded proteins in the ER and exports them to the cytosol for degradation by the 26S proteasome [Massey et al., 2009]. Once inside the host cells, CTA1 catalyzes the transfer of an ADP-ribose unit from NAD^+ oxidizing agent to an arginine residue of Gs protein. This covalent modification leads to the loss of GTPase activity of the Gs protein, which remains attached to GTP, keeping the adenylate cyclase (AC) enzyme active that will produce increasing amounts of cAMP. Over 100 times the normal concentration of cAMP, the intestinal mucosa cells open a Cl^- channels in the cytoplasmic membrane, resulting in an influx of ions and water to the gut lumen that causes the characteristic acute diarrhea of cholera [Spangler, 1992]. As little as 5 µg of purified CT administered orally is sufficient to induce significant diarrhea in human volunteers while ingestion of 25 µg of CT elicits a full 20 litres cholera purge [Levine et al., 1983].

4. Immune properties

Adjuvants are substances that have the ability to enhance the immune response when co-administered with poor immunogenic molecules. CT is a bacterial immunogen with a great function as an adjuvant to a variety of antigens when given by systemic and mucosal route whether these are linked to or simply mixed with the toxin, generating a long-term immune response (Elson 1989; Vajdy and Lycke 1992).

These properties may be explained by three main characteristics of the molecule. First, CT is remarkably stable to proteases, bile salts and other compounds in the intestine. Secondly, its high affinity to GM1 ganglioside receptor, which is present on most mammalian cells including the M cells covering the Peyers patches, as well as all antigen-presenting cells (APC), facilitates the uptake and presentation of the toxin to the gut mucosal immune system. Finally, CT has strong inherent adjuvant and immunomodulating activities that depend both on its cell binding capability and its enzymatic ADP-ribosylating function (Sanchez and Holmgren 2008).

Pioneer studies carried out in 1972 showed that CT delivered by the intravenous route with a foreign antigen behaved as an adjuvant [Northrup and Fauci, 1972], a fact confirmed later by several groups using a number of unrelated antigens of little immunogenicity [Bianchi et al., 1990; Elson and Ealding, 1984]. Additional studies revealed that upon co-administration of CT and antigen through parenteral, mucosal, and transcutaneous routes resulted in substantial enhancement of mucosal immunoglobulin A (IgA) and serum IgG responses to the co-administered antigen [Chen and Strober, 1990; Drew et al., 1992; Reuman et al., 1991]. In addition to enhancing humoral immune responses, CT also augmented cellular immune responses to co-administered antigens enhancing induction of $CD4^+$ T helper (Th) and class I-restricted cytolitic T lymphocyte responses [Nurkkala et al.; Simmons et al., 1999]. In most cases, CT induced a Th2 bias response [Lavelle et al., 2004; Okahashi et al., 1996]. However, other studies have reported Th1 [Sasaki et al., 2003; Taniguchi et al., 2008] or mixed Th1/Th2 responses following oral, sublingual and intranasal immunization with antigens in the presence of CT [Cuburu et al., 2007; Fecek et al., 2010]. More importantly, subsequent studies showed that CT elicited a long-term memory response and thus was detectable long after the initial immune response [Soenawan et al., 2004; Vajdy and Lycke, 1992].

CT also acts as mucosal adjuvant against a variety of pathogens. Examples include, tetanus toxoid [Jackson et al., 1993], *Helicobacter felis* [Jiang et al., 2003], *Schistosoma japonicum* [Kohama et al., 2010], *Helicobacter pylori* [Raghavan et al., 2002], and *Sendai virus* [Liang et al., 1988]. There are many other examples where it was shown that CT has significant potential for use as adjuvant for mucosally administered antigens [Clapp et al., 2010; Jhon Carlos Castaño Osorio, 2002].

5. Mechanism of adjuvant activity

The mechanism of adjuvanticity of CT is still unclear but is has been related to: (i) the induction of increased permeability of the intestinal epithelium leading to enhanced uptake of co-administered antigens; (ii) the induction of enhanced antigen presentation by various APC; (iii) the promotion of isotype differentiation in B cells leading to increased IgA formation; and (iv) exhibition of complex stimulatory as well as inhibitory effects on T cell proliferation and cytokine production. Among these many effects, those leading to enhanced antigen presentation by various APC are probably of the greatest importance [Sanchez and Holmgren, 2011].

As mentioned before, the polarity of the immune response generated by CT is a matter of debate. Some studies indicate that CT primes naïve T cells *in vitro* and drives them towards a Th2 phenotype, with production of interleukins IL-4 (a cytokine needed for B cell differentiation), IL-5, IL-6 and IL-10, but little IFN-γ (a cytokine needed to evoke Th1 responses) and suppression of IL-12 production by dendritic cells (DC) [Braun et al., 1999; Klimpel et al., 1995; Wilson et al., 1991]. Moreover, after immunization of animals with CT co-administered antigens, IL-4 levels were significantly elevated in gut-associated tissues and in spleen, while the levels of IFN-γ either decreased or remained static [Akhiani et al., 1997; Marinaro et al., 1995]. These results are supported by evidence of increased secretory IgA, serum IgA and IgE levels [Adel-Patient et al., 2005; Bourguin et al., 1991], and higher titers of IgG1 than IgG2a [Glenn et al., 1998; Lycke et al., 1990].

In contrast, others have reported that CT induces a mixed Th1/Th2 type of immune response with the production of IFN-γ and IL-4 [Fromantin et al., 2001; Imaoka et al., 1998]. In addition, it has been shown that CT induces strong Th17-type responses after intranasal delivery [Datta et al.; Lee et al., 2009].

Furthermore, CT markedly increased antigen-presentation by DC, macrophages, and B cells [Bromander et al., 1991; George-Chandy et al., 2001]. Also, CT upregulates the expression of MHC/HLA-DR molecules, CD80/B7.1 and CD86/B7.2 co-stimulatory molecules, as well as chemokine receptors CCR7 and CXCR4, on both murine and human DC, among other APC [Cong et al., 1997; Gagliardi et al., 2000]. Importantly, CT also induced the secretion of IL-1β from both DC and macrophages. IL-1β not only induces the maturation of DC, but also acts as an efficient mucosal adjuvant when co-administered with protein antigens and might mediate a significant part of the adjuvant activity of CT [Staats and Ennis, 1999]. Treatment with CT has been demonstrated to induce maturation and mobilization of DC [Lavelle et al., 2003]. Also, CT interferes with the differentiation of monocytes into DC, giving rise to a distinct population (Ma-DC), which displays an activated macrophage-like phenotype, induces a strong allogeneic and antigen specific response, and promotes the polarization of naïve $CD4^+$ T lymphocytes toward a Th2 profile [Raghavan et al., 2010]. In additon, CT enhanced IL-6 secretion by peritoneal mast cell [Leal-Berumen et al., 1996] and production of IL-1β, IL-6, and IL-10 together with inhibition of IL-12, TNF-α, and nitric oxid in macrophages [Cong et al., 2001], depleted the $CD8^+$ intraepithelial lymphocyte population [Flach et al., 2005], and induced isotype differentiation of B cells acting synergistically with IL-4 [Salmond et al., 2002]. Recent studies show that CT enhances STAT3 gene expression

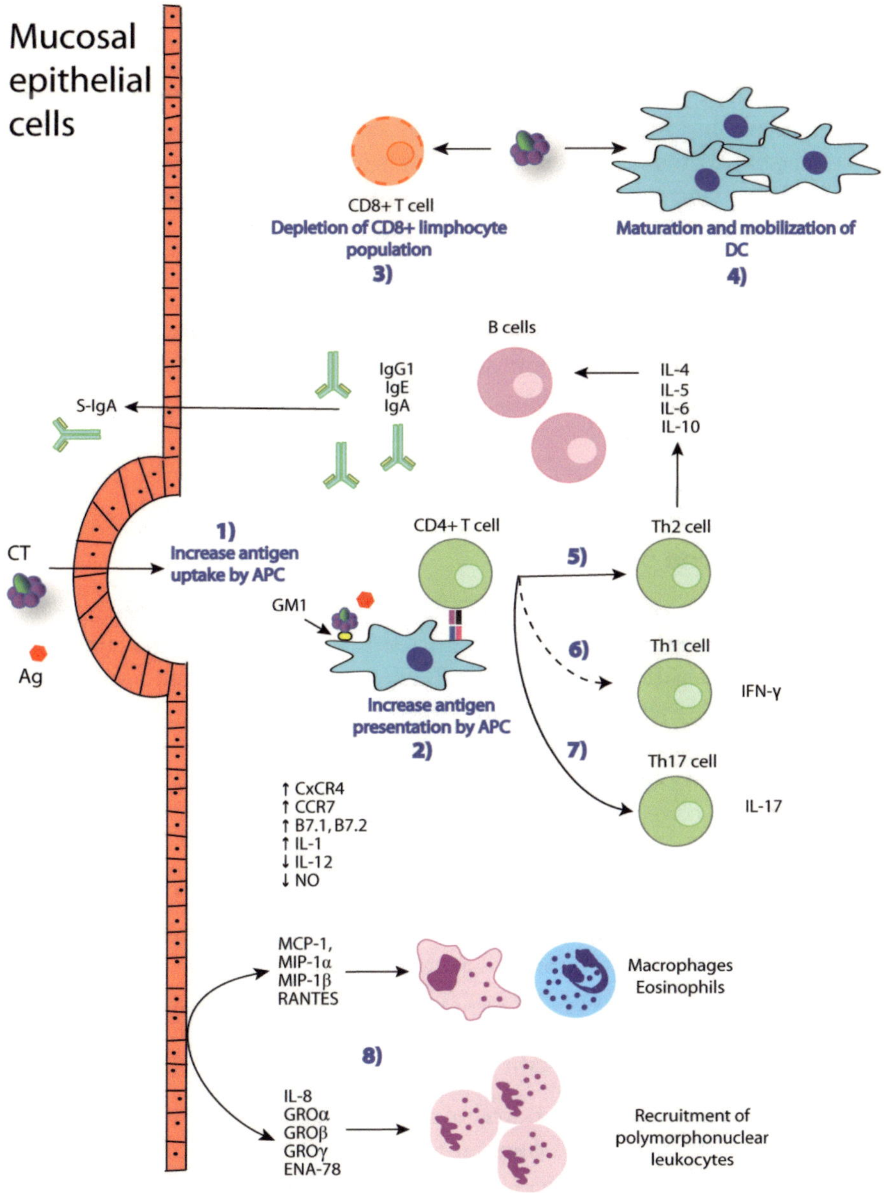

Fig. 2. Proposed mechanism of action by CT as a mucosal adjuvant. CT induces increased permeability of the intestinal epithelium leading to 1) enhanced uptake of co-administered antigens and 2) enhanced antigen-presentation by various APC. 3) It causes the depletion of $CD8^{+}$ lymphocyte population that may produce inhibitory cytokines, and 4) induces maturation and mobilization of DC. In addition, 5) CT promotes a strong Th2 dominant response to bystander antigens, and can either 6) induce or inhibit a Th1 response. Moreover, 7) CT induces strong Th17-type responses. Furthermore, 8) mucosal epithelial cells contribute to the adjuvant activity of CT by secreting a number of chemokines and acting on polymorphonuclear leukocytes, macrophages, eosinophils and T cells.

in murine B cells, and may critically modulate immune responses in both a pro-inflammatory and anti-inflammatory direction, depending on the circumstances and the types of cells involved Sjoblom-Hallen et al., (2010).

It has been suggested that mucosal epithelial cells may also play a role in adjuvanticity. Human epithelial cells express and secrete high levels of the chemoattractant cytokines IL-8, GROα, GROβ, GROγ, and ENA-78 in response to stimulation with TNF-α, IL-1β, or infection with enteroinvasive microorganisms. These chemokines attract and activate polymorphonuclear leukocytes. Activated epithelial cells also secret MCP-1, MIP-1β, MIP-1α, and RANTES, which variably act on monocytes/macrophages, eosinophils, and subpopulations of T-cells [Freytag and Clements, 2005]. One possibility is that CT interacts with epithelial cells triggering expression of one or more immunomodulatory factors that recruite APC and immune effector cells or activate those cells, or both [Lopes et al., 2000; Soriani et al., 2002].

A proposed mechanism of action of CT as adjuvant is shown in Fig. 2.

6. Genetic modifications of CT

The inherent enterotoxicity of CT has limited its widespread use as a vaccine component and adjuvant. In dogs, protection due to CT occurred only with doses that caused transient, sometimes severe, diarrhea [Pierce et al., 1982]. Moreover, murine models demonstrated that intranasal sensitization with CT as adjuvant led to increased lung inflammation with a massive recruitment of macrophages as well as accumulation in the olfactory nerves, epithelium and the olfactory bulbs of mice after binding to GM1 gangliosides [Fischer et al., 2005]. These limitations have led to mucosal strategies involving nontoxic mutants and purified B subunits.

Although early reports showed that mutants without the ADP-ribosyltransferase activity lack their adjuvant properties [Lycke et al., 1992], later studies showed that non-toxic mutants retained their adjuvant and immunogenic properties [Douce et al., 1997; Yamamoto et al., 1997] without central nervous system (CNS) toxicity [Hagiwara et al., 2006]. This suggests that the ADP-ribosyltransferase activity is not essential for its immunogenic properties, though it contributes to the adjuvant effect.

In a different approach, the CTA1 fragment linked to a synthetic analogue of *Staphylococcus aureus* protein A, the D fragment with affinity for APC, [Agren et al., 1997], proved to be non-toxic [Eriksson et al., 2004]. The fusion protein CTA1-DD binds specifically to immunoglobulins on the surface of antigen-presenting B cells through the DD polypeptide, and induces the ADP ribosylation by CTA1. Although this produces a good immune response when administered intranasally, it has been shown not to work as well after oral administration. This limitation was overcome by fusing CTA1-DD with immunostimulating complexes, such as ISCOMs (lipophilic immune stimulating complexes), producing both Th1/Th2 responses at systemic and mucosal levels [Andersen et al., 2007]. A recent report showed that CTA1 potently enhances a GeneGun-delivered DNA prime for human and simian immunodeficiency viruses antigens boost in macaques and mice [Bagley et al., 2011].

7. Immunological and adjuvant properties of CTB

Several studies using different conditions and routes of administration have described that CTB has several immunomodulatory properties opening many perspectives for future therapeutic and biotechnological applications. In this regard, intranasal immunization of women with CTB resulted in the production of long-lasting IgG and IgA anti-CTB in serum, nasal and vaginal secretions in a dose-dependent manner [Bergquist et al., 1997].

However, its capacity as mucosal adjuvant has proven to be much less than that of the toxin when given together with non-coupled antigens by the oral route [Sanchez and Holmgren, 2008]. Recombinant CTB has been successfully used as a mucosal adjuvant in vaccines for human use such as the cholera vaccine itself [Quiding et al., 1991], and the vaccine against enterotoxigenic *E. coli* that causes diarrhea [Peltola et al., 1991; Qadri et al., 2000]. Analogously, CTB proved to be good adjuvant for a *Streptococcus pneumoniae* cellular vaccine [Malley et al., 2004] and a severe acute respiratory syndrome-associated coronavirus vaccine [Qu et al., 2005] when administered intranasally in mice.

Given the potential of CTB as a regulator of the immune response, this subunit has been produced in various biological systems such as *Vibrio cholerae* [Sanchez and Holmgren, 1989], *Escherichia coli* [Arimitsu et al., 2009], *Bacillus brevis* [Goto et al., 2000], *Lactobacillus paracasei* and *plantarum* [Slos et al., 1998], in the yeasts *Hansenula polymorpha* [Song et al., 2004] and *Saccharomyces cerevisiae* [Mohsen and Rezae, 2005], and in silkworm [Gong et al., 2005]. In addition, CTB has been expressed successfully in tomato [Jani et al., 2002], lettuce [Young-Sook Kim, 2006], rice [Oszvald et al., 2008], tobacco [Hein et al., 1996], carrots [Kim et al., 2009], banana [Renuga et al., 2010] and potato transgenic plants, [Arakawa et al., 1997] where ubiquitin fusion enhances CTB expression [Mishra et al., 2006]. CTB may induce systemic immune responses in mice after gavage of the animals with the transgenic vegetal [Jiang et al., 2007]. The advantage of this approach is that plants present a low-cost agricultural-based effective production system. Different formulations, such as encapsulation in liposomes or microspheres with antigens [Seo et al., 2002] or combined with vesicles or liposomes containing antigens [Harokopakis et al., 1998; Lian et al., 1999] were also successfully tested.

CTB is a useful carrier protein for induction of mucosal IgA antibodies against chemically coupled antigens. In this regard, mice immunized intraduodenally with the horseradish peroxidase (HRP) covalently coupled to CTB showed a 33–120 fold higher level of IgA anti-HRP in intestinal washes as well as increased levels of serum IgG anti-HRP [McKenzie and Halsey, 1984]. In addition, CTB chemically conjugated to the protein I/II of *Streptococcus mutans* when administered in mice by oral [Russell and Wu, 1991], intranasal [Wu and Russell, 1998], and intragastric routes [Wu and Russell, 1993] results in the production of antistreptococcal IgG and IgA in serum and mucosa, as well as the presence of large numbers of antibody-secreting cells in salivary glands, mesenteric lymph nodes, and spleens. Similar results were found with CTB conjugated to human gamma globulin (HGG) and the recombinant *Neisseria gonorrhoeae* transferrin binding proteins, TbpA and TbpB. Vaginal and intranasal immunizations with CTB-HGG resulted in high levels of anti-HGG antibodies [Johansson et al., 1998], while rCTB-TbpA and rCTB-TbpB administered intranasally induced antibody responses in the serum and genital tract [Price et al., 2005]. Moreover, CTB was chemically conjugated to type III capsular polysaccharide from

Streptococcus group B [Shen et al., 2000] or to protein-polysaccharide conjugates [Bergquist et al., 1995] and in both cases, after subcutaneous administration, high levels of specific antibodies were detected. In addition to generating humoral response, simian immunodeficiency virus (SIV) virus-like particles (VLP) chemically conjugated to CTB showed higher levels of cytokine IFN-γ-producing splenocytes and cytotoxic-T-lymphocyte activities of immune cells than VLPs plus CTB, indicating a generation of a Th1 response in mice by CTB-VLP [Kang et al., 2003]. Finally, CTB chemically conjugated to the *Plasmodium vivax* ookinete surface protein, Pvs25, proved to be a potent transmission-blocking antigen in both intranasal and subcutaneal routes in mice [Miyata et al., 2010], and to protect against pharyngeal colonization by group A *streptococcus* when conjugated to the widely shared C repeat region of M6 protein [Bessen and Fischetti, 1990].

	Antigen	Route	CTB administration	Reference
Proteins	Nucleoprotein of Influenza A virus	in	co-administered	[Guo et al., 2010]
	Hepatitis B virus surface antigen	in	co-administered	[Isaka et al., 2001]
	MSP4 5 malaria protein	Oral	co-administered	[Wang et al., 2003]
	OVA	im	co-administered	[Rolland-Turner et al., 2004]
	HIV-1 gp41	sl	chemically coupled	[Hervouet et al., 2010]
	Epitopes from *Schistosoma mansoni* glutathione-S-transferase	in	genetically fused	[Lebens et al., 2003]
Polysacharide	Group B Streptococcus Type III Capsular Polysaccharide	in, oral, rectal, and vaginal	chemically coupled/co-administered	[Shen et al., 2000]
	Lipopolysaccharide from *V. cholerae* O1, serotype Inaba	sc	chemically coupled	[Gupta et al., 1998]
	Pseudomonas aeruginosa polysaccharide	Oral	co-administered	[Abraham and Robinson, 1991]
Micro-organisms	Measles virus	in, ig	co-administered	[Muller et al., 1995]
	Influenza virus	in	co-administered	[Yang et al.]
	Pneumocystis carinii	in	co-administered	[Pascale et al., 1999]

Table 1. Antigens towards which CT has adjuvant activity. in: intranasal, im: intramuscular, sl: sublingual, sc: subcutaneous, ig: intragastric.

Another way of using CTB as an adjuvant is in genetic constructions based on the toxin and heterologous antigens. In general, these hybrid molecules are composed of antigens fused to the amino [Laloi et al., 1996; Song et al., 2004] or carboxyl [Kim et al., 2004; Wang et al., 2010] terminus of CTB, being GM1-binding much more efficient in the latter case [Liljeqvist et al., 1997], but also protein epitopes have been introduced at internal positions in CTB

[Dertzbaugh and Elson, 1993]. Some examples of genetic incorporation of epitopes to CTB include triple glutamic acid decarboxylase [Gong et al., 2009], dodecapeptide repeat of the serine-rich *Entamoeba histolytica* protein [Zhang et al., 1995] and human insulin B-chain [Sadeghi et al., 2002]. There are many studies showing the induction of immune responses through immunization of mice with CTB fused to soluble antigens expressed both in bacteria [Larsson et al., 2004; Lee et al., 2003; Sun et al., 1999; Tsuji et al., 2003] and in transgenic plants [Jani et al., 2004; Matsumoto et al., 2009]. In all cases there was generation of IgG and IgA antigen-specific antibodies and, in some cases, protection. Some examples of the adjuvant action of CTB are shown in Table 1.

One of the strategies for using CTB as an adjuvant genetically fused to antigens has been described by Arêas *et al.* and is based on the expression vector called pAEctxB (Fig. 3.). In the generation of the vector, the gene ctxB was modified to ensure that the codons were those most frequently used by *E. coli, L. casei* and *S. typhimurium* [Areas et al., 2002]. The genetically engineered ORF was then cloned into the expression vector pAE [Ramos et al., 2004] and includes two consecutive restriction sites Mlu*I* and Hind*III*. The resulting vector allows expression, under the control of a T7 promoter, of proteins fused to the C-terminus of CTB with 6 histidine residues at the N terminus, which facilitate protein purification by immobilized metal ion affinity chromatography.

The pAE-ctxB plasmid was used to clone the pneumococcal surface adhesin A (PspA) [Areas et al., 2004], the *Leptospira interrogans* protein LipL32 [Habarta et al., 2010], the fatty-acid binding protein from *Schistosoma mansoni* S14 [Henrique Roman Ramos, 2010], and the *Bordetella pertussis* type III secretion system effector protein Bsp22 (Olivera et al., unpublished results). Intradermal immunization with CTB-PspA induced high titers of anti-PspA IgG and partially protected mice after challenge with *S. pneumonia* [Areas et al., 2005]. Moreover, intranasal immunization with CTB-PsaA protected mice against colonization with *S. pneumoniae* without alteration of the natural oral or nasopharyngeal microbiota of mice [Pimenta et al., 2006]. CTB-Sm14 itself was not able to reduce *Schistosoma mansoni* worm burden on intranasally immunized BALB/c mice, but reduced the hepatic granulomas around trapped eggs. CTB-LipL32 generated higher specific titers in mice immunized without external adjuvant than co-administration of CTB with LipL32, supporting CTB-LipL32 as a promising antigen for use in the control and study of leptospirosis.

8. CTB for mucosal immunotherapy

Mucosal administration by the oral, sublingual or nasal routes of many antigens can induce peripheral tolerance. Mucosal-induced tolerance has been recognized for a long time as a promising approach to prevent or treat allergic or autoimmune disorders and is characterized by a decreased immune response to systemic immunization with the same antigen [Sun et al., 2009; Sun et al., 1994]. In this regard, promising results have been obtained with auto-antigen coupled to CTB in order to induce oral tolerance. Although not known the mechanism by which CTB conjugated to antigens has the ability to potentiate the induction of oral tolerance, it is believed that in addition to the processes already mentioned before for CT, it may result in selected DC subsets with increased ability to induce different types of TGF-β-expressing suppressor T cells including $CD4^+$ $CD25^+$ Tr cells [Holmgren et al., 2005] and a direct depletion of effector T cells since CTB induces CD4+ and CD8+ T cell apoptosis [Christelle Basset, 2010].

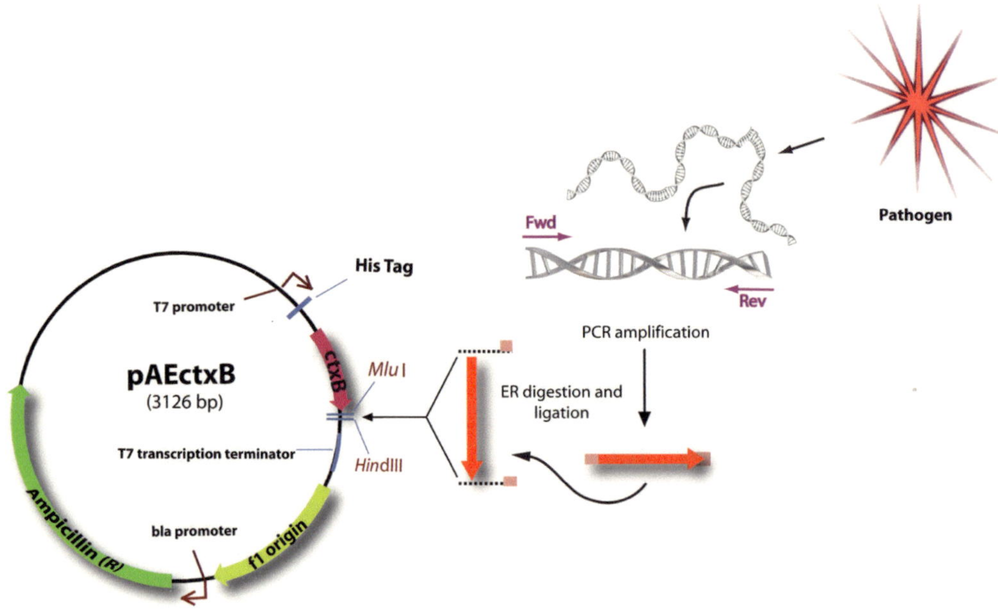

Fig. 3. Cloning strategy into pAEctxB plasmid

Oral delivery of CTB conjugated to myelin basic protein protected mice [Sun et al., 1996; Yuki et al., 2001] and rats [Sun et al., 2000b] against the development of experimental autoimmune encephalomyelitis. It was proposed that the inhibitory effect was a result of both the induction of TGF-β-producing Tr cells and down-regulation of IFNγ, IL-12, TNFα, MCP-1 and RANTES in the CNS [Wang et al., 2009].

Oral administration of a CTB-insulin conjugate prevented diabetes in non-obese diabetic (NOD) mice [Arakawa et al., 1998; Bergerot et al., 1997; Gong et al., 2007; Petersen et al., 2003; Ploix et al., 1999], which was associated with a reduction in IFNγ production and Tr cell migration into pancreatic islets [Aspord et al., 2002; Sobel et al., 1998]. On the other hand, oral administration of CTB-proinsulin fusion protein showed an increased expression of IL-4 and IL-10 in the pancreas of NOD-treated mice, suggesting that Th2 lymphocyte-mediated oral tolerance is a likely mechanism for the prevention of pancreatic insulitis [Ruhlman et al., 2007].

Oral delivery of CTB conjugated to a 60 kDa heat-shock protein derived peptide prevented mucosal induced uveitis in rats, an effect that was associated with enhanced IL-10 and TGF-β, and reduced IL-12 and IFN-γ production [Phipps et al., 2003]. Furthermore, a I/II phase clinical trial of the same peptide conjugated to CTB administered orally to 8 patients allowed the withdrawal of all immunosuppressive drugs in 5 of the 8 patients without a relapse of uveitis [Stanford et al., 2004].

In addition, oral administration of CTB in mice inhibits the induction of trinitrobenzene sulfonic acid-induced colitis and reverses such colitis after it has been established. This inhibition is associated with suppression of IL-12 and IFN-γ production [Boirivant et al., 2001; Coccia et al., 2005]. In a recent clinical trial, 40% of patients with active Crohn's disease responded to treatment with CTB [Stal et al., 2010].

CTB conjugates were also effective in the induction of tolerance to type II collagen, leading to a suppression of chondritis in a model of autoimmune ear disease [Kim et al., 2001]. Oral administration of allogeneic antigen linked to CTB induced immunological tolerance against allograft rejection [Sun et al., 2000a]. Finally, transconjunctival immunotherapy using CTB could suppress clinical effects for experimental allergic conjunctivitis in guinea pigs [Oikawa et al., 2011].

9. Conclusion

CT has been studied for over 40 years. Both CT and its non-toxic derivatives or its B subunit, have shown to be excellent mucosal adjuvants. The possibility to use them as biotechnological tools in the development of new vaccines is being intensively studied in the present. In recent years, the prospect to use CTB fused to different protein antigens became relevant because these proteins can be expressed in high levels in a soluble form and directly purified in their active form, requiring only one fermentation step. In addition, several reports have shown that CTB can generate oral tolerance to different conjugated antigens, opening ways for the treatment of autoimmune diseases. Hopefully, future studies will focus on the use of CTB in such important issues.

10. Acknowledgements

This work was supported by grants from Agencia Nacional de Promoción Científica y Tecnológica (ANPCyT) PICT 07-00642 and PICT 07-00028 (RMG).

11. References

Abraham E, Robinson A. 1991. Oral immunization with bacterial polysaccharide and adjuvant enhances antigen-specific pulmonary secretory antibody response and resistance to pneumonia. Vaccine 9(10):757-764.

Adel-Patient K, Bernard H, Ah-Leung S, Creminon C, Wal JM. 2005. Peanut- and cow's milk-specific IgE, Th2 cells and local anaphylactic reaction are induced in Balb/c mice orally sensitized with cholera toxin. Allergy 60(5):658-664.

Agren LC, Ekman L, Lowenadler B, Lycke NY. 1997. Genetically engineered nontoxic vaccine adjuvant that combines B cell targeting with immunomodulation by cholera toxin A1 subunit. J Immunol 158(8):3936-3946.

Akhiani AA, Nilsson LA, Ouchterlony O. 1997. Intranasal administration of Schistosoma mansoni adult worm antigen in combination with cholera toxin induces a Th2 cell response. Parasite Immunol 19(4):183-190.

Andersen CS, Dietrich J, Agger EM, Lycke NY, Lovgren K, Andersen P. 2007. The combined CTA1-DD/ISCOMs vector is an effective intranasal adjuvant for boosting prior Mycobacterium bovis BCG immunity to Mycobacterium tuberculosis. Infect Immun 75(1):408-416.

Arakawa T, Chong DK, Merritt JL, Langridge WH. 1997. Expression of cholera toxin B subunit oligomers in transgenic potato plants. Transgenic Res 6(6):403-413.

Arakawa T, Yu J, Chong DK, Hough J, Engen PC, Langridge WH. 1998. A plant-based cholera toxin B subunit-insulin fusion protein protects against the development of autoimmune diabetes. Nat Biotechnol 16(10):934-938.

Areas AP, Oliveira ML, Miyaji EN, Leite LC, Aires KA, Dias WO, Ho PL. 2004. Expression and characterization of cholera toxin B-pneumococcal surface adhesin A fusion protein in Escherichia coli: ability of CTB-PsaA to induce humoral immune response in mice. Biochem Biophys Res Commun 321(1):192-196.

Areas AP, Oliveira ML, Miyaji EN, Leite LC, Ho PL. 2005. Intradermal immunization of mice with cholera toxin B-pneumococcal surface protein A fusion protein is protective against intraperitoneal challenge with Streptococcus pneumoniae. Infect Immun 73(6):3810-3813.

Areas AP, Oliveira ML, Ramos CR, Sbrogio-Almeida ME, Raw I, Ho PL. 2002. Synthesis of cholera toxin B subunit gene: cloning and expression of a functional 6XHis-tagged protein in Escherichia coli. Protein Expr Purif 25(3):481-487.

Arimitsu H, Tsukamoto K, Ochi S, Sasaki K, Kato M, Taniguchi K, Oguma K, Tsuji T. 2009. Lincomycin-induced over-expression of mature recombinant cholera toxin B subunit and the holotoxin in Escherichia coli. Protein Expr Purif 67(2):96-103.

Aspord C, Czerkinsky C, Durand A, Stefanutti A, Thivolet C. 2002. alpha4 integrins and L-selectin differently orchestrate T-cell activity during diabetes prevention following oral administration of CTB-insulin. J Autoimmun 19(4):223-232.

Bagley KC, Lewis GK, Fouts TR. 2011. Adjuvant activity of the catalytic A1 domain of cholera toxin for retroviral antigens delivered by GeneGun. Clin Vaccine Immunol 18(6):922-930.

Bergerot I, Ploix C, Petersen J, Moulin V, Rask C, Fabien N, Lindblad M, Mayer A, Czerkinsky C, Holmgren J, Thivolet C. 1997. A cholera toxoid-insulin conjugate as an oral vaccine against spontaneous autoimmune diabetes. Proc Natl Acad Sci U S A 94(9):4610-4614.

Bergquist C, Johansson EL, Lagergard T, Holmgren J, Rudin A. 1997. Intranasal vaccination of humans with recombinant cholera toxin B subunit induces systemic and local antibody responses in the upper respiratory tract and the vagina. Infect Immun 65(7):2676-2684.

Bergquist C, Lagergard T, Lindblad M, Holmgren J. 1995. Local and systemic antibody responses to dextran-cholera toxin B subunit conjugates. Infect Immun 63(5):2021-2025.

Bessen D, Fischetti VA. 1990. Synthetic peptide vaccine against mucosal colonization by group A streptococci. I. Protection against a heterologous M serotype with shared C repeat region epitopes. J Immunol 145(4):1251-1256.

Bianchi AT, Zwart RJ, Van der Heijden PJ. 1990. Induction of an enteric Ig-response against ovalbumin and stimulation of the response by cholera toxin and its B-subunit in mice. Reg Immunol 3(3):131-138.

Boirivant M, Fuss IJ, Ferroni L, De Pascale M, Strober W. 2001. Oral administration of recombinant cholera toxin subunit B inhibits IL-12-mediated murine experimental (trinitrobenzene sulfonic acid) colitis. J Immunol 166(5):3522-3532.

Bourguin I, Chardes T, Mevelec MN, Woodman JP, Bout D. 1991. Amplification of the secretory IgA response to Toxoplasma gondii using cholera toxin. FEMS Microbiol Lett 65(3):265-271.

Braun MC, He J, Wu CY, Kelsall BL. 1999. Cholera toxin suppresses interleukin (IL)-12 production and IL-12 receptor beta1 and beta2 chain expression. J Exp Med 189(3):541-552.

Bromander A, Holmgren J, Lycke N. 1991. Cholera toxin stimulates IL-1 production and enhances antigen presentation by macrophages in vitro. J Immunol 146(9):2908-2914.

Clapp B, Golden S, Maddaloni M, Staats HF, Pascual DW. 2010. Adenovirus F protein as a delivery vehicle for botulinum B. BMC Immunol 11:36.

Coccia EM, Remoli ME, Di Giacinto C, Del Zotto B, Giacomini E, Monteleone G, Boirivant M. 2005. Cholera toxin subunit B inhibits IL-12 and IFN-{gamma} production and signaling in experimental colitis and Crohn's disease. Gut 54(11):1558-1564.

Cong Y, Oliver AO, Elson CO. 2001. Effects of cholera toxin on macrophage production of co-stimulatory cytokines. Eur J Immunol 31(1):64-71.

Cong Y, Weaver CT, Elson CO. 1997. The mucosal adjuvanticity of cholera toxin involves enhancement of costimulatory activity by selective up-regulation of B7.2 expression. J Immunol 159(11):5301-5308.

Cuburu N, Kweon MN, Song JH, Hervouet C, Luci C, Sun JB, Hofman P, Holmgren J, Anjuere F, Czerkinsky C. 2007. Sublingual immunization induces broad-based systemic and mucosal immune responses in mice. Vaccine 25(51):8598-8610.

Chen KS, Strober W. 1990. Cholera holotoxin and its B subunit enhance Peyer's patch B cell responses induced by orally administered influenza virus: disproportionate cholera toxin enhancement of the IgA B cell response. Eur J Immunol 20(2):433-436.

Chinnapen DJ, Chinnapen H, Saslowsky D, Lencer WI. 2007. Rafting with cholera toxin: endocytosis and trafficking from plasma membrane to ER. FEMS Microbiol Lett 266(2):129-137.

Christelle Basset FT, Cyrille Di Martino, John Holton, John D. Clements and Evelyne Kohli. 2010. Cholera-Like Enterotoxins and Regulatory T cells. Toxins 2:1774-1795.

Datta SK, Sabet M, Nguyen KP, Valdez PA, Gonzalez-Navajas JM, Islam S, Mihajlov I, Fierer J, Insel PA, Webster NJ, Guiney DG, Raz E. Mucosal adjuvant activity of cholera toxin requires Th17 cells and protects against inhalation anthrax. Proc Natl Acad Sci U S A 107(23):10638-10643.

De SN. 1959. Enterotoxicity of bacteria-free culture-filtrate of Vibrio cholerae. Nature 183(4674):1533-1534.

Dertzbaugh MT, Elson CO. 1993. Reduction in oral immunogenicity of cholera toxin B subunit by N-terminal peptide addition. Infect Immun 61(2):384-390.

Douce G, Fontana M, Pizza M, Rappuoli R, Dougan G. 1997. Intranasal immunogenicity and adjuvanticity of site-directed mutant derivatives of cholera toxin. Infect Immun 65(7):2821-2828.

Drew MD, Estrada-Correa A, Underdown BJ, McDermott MR. 1992. Vaccination by cholera toxin conjugated to a herpes simplex virus type 2 glycoprotein D peptide. J Gen Virol 73 (Pt 9):2357-2366.

Elson CO, Ealding W. 1984. Cholera toxin feeding did not induce oral tolerance in mice and abrogated oral tolerance to an unrelated protein antigen. J Immunol 133(6):2892-2897.

Eriksson AM, Schon KM, Lycke NY. 2004. The cholera toxin-derived CTA1-DD vaccine adjuvant administered intranasally does not cause inflammation or accumulate in the nervous tissues. J Immunol 173(5):3310-3319.

Fecek RJ, Marcondes Rezende M, Busch R, Hassing I, Pieters R, Cuff CF. 2010. Enteric reovirus infection stimulates peanut-specific IgG2a responses in a mouse food allergy model. Immunobiology 215(12):941-948.

Fischer R, McGhee JR, Vu HL, Atkinson TP, Jackson RJ, Tome D, Boyaka PN. 2005. Oral and nasal sensitization promote distinct immune responses and lung reactivity in a mouse model of peanut allergy. Am J Pathol 167(6):1621-1630.

Flach CF, Lange S, Jennische E, Lonnroth I, Holmgren J. 2005. Cholera toxin induces a transient depletion of CD8+ intraepithelial lymphocytes in the rat small intestine as detected by microarray and immunohistochemistry. Infect Immun 73(9):5595-5602.

Freytag LC, Clements JD. 2005. Mucosal adjuvants. Vaccine 23(15):1804-1813.

Fromantin C, Jamot B, Cohen J, Piroth L, Pothier P, Kohli E. 2001. Rotavirus 2/6 virus-like particles administered intranasally in mice, with or without the mucosal adjuvants cholera toxin and Escherichia coli heat-labile toxin, induce a Th1/Th2-like immune response. J Virol 75(22):11010-11016.

Fujinaga Y, Wolf AA, Rodighiero C, Wheeler H, Tsai B, Allen L, Jobling MG, Rapoport T, Holmes RK, Lencer WI. 2003. Gangliosides that associate with lipid rafts mediate transport of cholera and related toxins from the plasma membrane to endoplasmic reticulm. Mol Biol Cell 14(12):4783-4793.

Gagliardi MC, Sallusto F, Marinaro M, Langenkamp A, Lanzavecchia A, De Magistris MT. 2000. Cholera toxin induces maturation of human dendritic cells and licences them for Th2 priming. Eur J Immunol 30(8):2394-2403.

George-Chandy A, Eriksson K, Lebens M, Nordstrom I, Schon E, Holmgren J. 2001. Cholera toxin B subunit as a carrier molecule promotes antigen presentation and increases CD40 and CD86 expression on antigen-presenting cells. Infect Immun 69(9):5716-5725.

Glenn GM, Scharton-Kersten T, Vassell R, Mallett CP, Hale TL, Alving CR. 1998. Transcutaneous immunization with cholera toxin protects mice against lethal mucosal toxin challenge. J Immunol 161(7):3211-3214.

Gong Z, Jin Y, Zhang Y. 2007. Suppression of diabetes in non-obese diabetic (NOD) mice by oral administration of a cholera toxin B subunit-insulin B chain fusion protein vaccine produced in silkworm. Vaccine 25(8):1444-1451.

Gong Z, Long X, Pan L, Le Y, Liu Q, Wang S, Guo J, Xiao B, Zhou M, Mei D. 2009. Cloning, expression, purification and characterization of the cholera toxin B subunit and triple glutamic acid decarboxylase epitopes fusion protein in Escherichia coli. Protein Expr Purif 66(2):191-197.

Gong ZH, Jin HQ, Jin YF, Zhang YZ. 2005. Expression of cholera toxin B subunit and assembly as functional oligomers in silkworm. J Biochem Mol Biol 38(6):717-724.

Goto N, Maeyama J, Yasuda Y, Isaka M, Matano K, Kozuka S, Taniguchi T, Miura Y, Ohkuma K, Tochikubo K. 2000. Safety evaluation of recombinant cholera toxin B subunit produced by Bacillus brevis as a mucosal adjuvant. Vaccine 18(20):2164-2171.

Guo L, Zheng M, Ding Y, Li D, Yang Z, Wang H, Chen Q, Sui Z, Fang F, Chen Z. 2010. Protection against multiple influenza A virus subtypes by intranasal administration of recombinant nucleoprotein. Arch Virol 155(11):1765-1775.

Gupta RK, Taylor DN, Bryla DA, Robbins JB, Szu SC. 1998. Phase 1 evaluation of Vibrio cholerae O1, serotype Inaba, polysaccharide-cholera toxin conjugates in adult volunteers. Infect Immun 66(7):3095-3099.

Habarta A, Abreu PA, Olivera N, Hauk P, Cedola MT, Ferrer MF, Ho PL, Gomez RM. 2010. Increased immunogenicity to LipL32 of Leptospira interrogans when expressed as a fusion protein with the cholera toxin B subunit. Curr Microbiol 62(2):526-531.

Hagiwara Y, Kawamura YI, Kataoka K, Rahima B, Jackson RJ, Komase K, Dohi T, Boyaka PN, Takeda Y, Kiyono H, McGhee JR, Fujihashi K. 2006. A second generation of double mutant cholera toxin adjuvants: enhanced immunity without intracellular trafficking. J Immunol 177(5):3045-3054.

Harokopakis E, Hajishengallis G, Michalek SM. 1998. Effectiveness of liposomes possessing surface-linked recombinant B subunit of cholera toxin as an oral antigen delivery system. Infect Immun 66(9):4299-4304.

Hein MB, Yeo TC, Wang F, Sturtevant A. 1996. Expression of cholera toxin subunits in plants. Ann N Y Acad Sci 792:50-56.

Henrique Roman Ramos PAM, Celso Raul Romero Ramos, Ana Paula de Mattos Arêas, Toshie Kawano and Paulo Lee Ho. 2010. A Genetic Fusion between Sm14 and CTB does not Reduce Schistosoma mansoni Worm Burden on Intranasally Immunized BALB/c Mice. J Vaccin Vaccinat 1(3):doi: 10.4172/2157-7560.1000111.

Hervouet C, Luci C, Cuburu N, Cremel M, Bekri S, Vimeux L, Maranon C, Czerkinsky C, Hosmalin A, Anjuere F. 2010. Sublingual immunization with an HIV subunit vaccine induces antibodies and cytotoxic T cells in the mouse female genital tract. Vaccine 28(34):5582-5590.

Holmgren J, Adamsson J, Anjuere F, Clemens J, Czerkinsky C, Eriksson K, Flach CF, George-Chandy A, Harandi AM, Lebens M, Lehner T, Lindblad M, Nygren E, Raghavan S, Sanchez J, Stanford M, Sun JB, Svennerholm AM, Tengvall S. 2005. Mucosal adjuvants and anti-infection and anti-immunopathology vaccines based on cholera toxin, cholera toxin B subunit and CpG DNA. Immunol Lett 97(2):181-188.

Holmgren J, Lonnroth I, Svennerholm L. 1973. Tissue receptor for cholera exotoxin: postulated structure from studies with GM1 ganglioside and related glycolipids. Infect Immun 8(2):208-214.

Imaoka K, Miller CJ, Kubota M, McChesney MB, Lohman B, Yamamoto M, Fujihashi K, Someya K, Honda M, McGhee JR, Kiyono H. 1998. Nasal immunization of nonhuman primates with simian immunodeficiency virus p55gag and cholera toxin adjuvant induces Th1/Th2 help for virus-specific immune responses in reproductive tissues. J Immunol 161(11):5952-5958.

Isaka M, Yasuda Y, Mizokami M, Kozuka S, Taniguchi T, Matano K, Maeyama J, Mizuno K, Morokuma K, Ohkuma K, Goto N, Tochikubo K. 2001. Mucosal immunization against hepatitis B virus by intranasal co-administration of recombinant hepatitis B surface antigen and recombinant cholera toxin B subunit as an adjuvant. Vaccine 19(11-12):1460-1466.

Jackson RJ, Fujihashi K, Xu-Amano J, Kiyono H, Elson CO, McGhee JR. 1993. Optimizing oral vaccines: induction of systemic and mucosal B-cell and antibody responses to tetanus toxoid by use of cholera toxin as an adjuvant. Infect Immun 61(10):4272-4279.

Jani D, Meena LS, Rizwan-ul-Haq QM, Singh Y, Sharma AK, Tyagi AK. 2002. Expression of cholera toxin B subunit in transgenic tomato plants. Transgenic Res 11(5):447-454.

Jani D, Singh NK, Bhattacharya S, Meena LS, Singh Y, Upadhyay SN, Sharma AK, Tyagi AK. 2004. Studies on the immunogenic potential of plant-expressed cholera toxin B subunit. Plant Cell Rep 22(7):471-477.

Jhon Carlos Castaño Osorio JSP. 2002. Inmunización intranasal de ratones con la proteína Sag2 de Toxoplasma gondii asociada con la toxina colérica. Rev Cubana Invest Biomed 1:35-45.

Jiang W, Baker HJ, Smith BF. 2003. Mucosal immunization with helicobacter, CpG DNA, and cholera toxin is protective. Infect Immun 71(1):40-46.

Jiang XL, He ZM, Peng ZQ, Qi Y, Chen Q, Yu SY. 2007. Cholera toxin B protein in transgenic tomato fruit induces systemic immune response in mice. Transgenic Res 16(2):169-175.

Johansson EL, Rask C, Fredriksson M, Eriksson K, Czerkinsky C, Holmgren J. 1998. Antibodies and antibody-secreting cells in the female genital tract after vaginal or intranasal immunization with cholera toxin B subunit or conjugates. Infect Immun 66(2):514-520.

Kang SM, Yao Q, Guo L, Compans RW. 2003. Mucosal immunization with virus-like particles of simian immunodeficiency virus conjugated with cholera toxin subunit B. J Virol 77(18):9823-9830.

Kim N, Cheng KC, Kwon SS, Mora R, Barbieri M, Yoo TJ. 2001. Oral administration of collagen conjugated with cholera toxin induces tolerance to type II collagen and suppresses chondritis in an animal model of autoimmune ear disease. Ann Otol Rhinol Laryngol 110(7 Pt 1):646-654.

Kim TG, Gruber A, Langridge WH. 2004. HIV-1 gp120 V3 cholera toxin B subunit fusion gene expression in transgenic potato. Protein Expr Purif 37(1):196-202.

Kim YS, Kim MY, Kim TG, Yang MS. 2009. Expression and assembly of cholera toxin B subunit (CTB) in transgenic carrot (Daucus carota L.). Mol Biotechnol 41(1):8-14.

Klimpel GR, Asuncion M, Haithcoat J, Niesel DW. 1995. Cholera toxin and Salmonella typhimurium induce different cytokine profiles in the gastrointestinal tract. Infect Immun 63(3):1134-1137.

Kohama H, Harakuni T, Kikuchi M, Nara T, Takemura Y, Miyata T, Sato Y, Hirayama K, Arakawa T. 2010. Intranasal administration of Schistosoma japonicum paramyosin induced robust long-lasting systemic and local antibody as well as delayed-type hypersensitivity responses, but failed to confer protection in a mouse infection model. Jpn J Infect Dis 63(3):166-172.

Laloi P, Munro CL, Jones KR, Macrina FL. 1996. Immunologic characteristics of a Streptococcus mutans glucosyltransferase B sucrose-binding site peptide-cholera toxin B-subunit chimeric protein. Infect Immun 64(1):28-36.

Larsson C, Holmgren J, Lindahl G, Bergquist C. 2004. Intranasal immunization of mice with group B streptococcal protein rib and cholera toxin B subunit confers protection against lethal infection. Infect Immun 72(2):1184-1187.

Lavelle EC, Jarnicki A, McNeela E, Armstrong ME, Higgins SC, Leavy O, Mills KH. 2004. Effects of cholera toxin on innate and adaptive immunity and its application as an immunomodulatory agent. J Leukoc Biol 75(5):756-763.

Lavelle EC, McNeela E, Armstrong ME, Leavy O, Higgins SC, Mills KH. 2003. Cholera toxin promotes the induction of regulatory T cells specific for bystander antigens by modulating dendritic cell activation. J Immunol 171(5):2384-2392.

Leal-Berumen I, Snider DP, Barajas-Lopez C, Marshall JS. 1996. Cholera toxin increases IL-6 synthesis and decreases TNF-alpha production by rat peritoneal mast cells. J Immunol 156(1):316-321.

Lebens M, Sun JB, Sadeghi H, Backstrom M, Olsson I, Mielcarek N, Li BL, Capron A, Czerkinsky C, Holmgren J. 2003. A mucosally administered recombinant fusion protein vaccine against schistosomiasis protecting against immunopathology and infection. Vaccine 21(5-6):514-520.

Lee JB, Jang JE, Song MK, Chang J. 2009. Intranasal delivery of cholera toxin induces th17-dominated T-cell response to bystander antigens. PLoS One 4(4):e5190.

Lee SF, Halperin SA, Salloum DF, MacMillan A, Morris A. 2003. Mucosal immunization with a genetically engineered pertussis toxin S1 fragment-cholera toxin subunit B chimeric protein. Infect Immun 71(4):2272-2275.

Lencer WI, Tsai B. 2003. The intracellular voyage of cholera toxin: going retro. Trends Biochem Sci 28(12):639-645.

Levine MM, Kaper JB, Black RE, Clements ML. 1983. New knowledge on pathogenesis of bacterial enteric infections as applied to vaccine development. Microbiol Rev 47(4):510-550.

Lian T, Bui T, Ho RJ. 1999. Formulation of HIV-envelope protein with lipid vesicles expressing ganglioside GM1 associated to cholera toxin B enhances mucosal immune responses. Vaccine 18(7-8):604-611.

Liang XP, Lamm ME, Nedrud JG. 1988. Oral administration of cholera toxin-Sendai virus conjugate potentiates gut and respiratory immunity against Sendai virus. J Immunol 141(5):1495-1501.

Liljeqvist S, Stahl S, Andreoni C, Binz H, Uhlen M, Murby M. 1997. Fusions to the cholera toxin B subunit: influence on pentamerization and GM1 binding. J Immunol Methods 210(2):125-135.

Lonnroth I, Holmgren J. 1973. Subunit structure of cholera toxin. J Gen Microbiol 76(2):417-427.

Lopes LM, Maroof A, Dougan G, Chain BM. 2000. Inhibition of T-cell response by Escherichia coli heat-labile enterotoxin-treated epithelial cells. Infect Immun 68(12):6891-6895.

Lycke N, Severinson E, Strober W. 1990. Cholera toxin acts synergistically with IL-4 to promote IgG1 switch differentiation. J Immunol 145(10):3316-3324.

Lycke N, Tsuji T, Holmgren J. 1992. The adjuvant effect of Vibrio cholerae and Escherichia coli heat-labile enterotoxins is linked to their ADP-ribosyltransferase activity. Eur J Immunol 22(9):2277-2281.

Malley R, Morse SC, Leite LC, Areas AP, Ho PL, Kubrusly FS, Almeida IC, Anderson P. 2004. Multiserotype protection of mice against pneumococcal colonization of the nasopharynx and middle ear by killed nonencapsulated cells given intranasally with a nontoxic adjuvant. Infect Immun 72(7):4290-4292.

Marinaro M, Staats HF, Hiroi T, Jackson RJ, Coste M, Boyaka PN, Okahashi N, Yamamoto M, Kiyono H, Bluethmann H, Fujihashi K, McGhee JR. 1995. Mucosal adjuvant effect of cholera toxin in mice results from induction of T helper 2 (Th2) cells and IL-4. J Immunol 155(10):4621-4629.

Massey S, Banerjee T, Pande AH, Taylor M, Tatulian SA, Teter K. 2009. Stabilization of the tertiary structure of the cholera toxin A1 subunit inhibits toxin dislocation and cellular intoxication. J Mol Biol 393(5):1083-1096.

Matsumoto Y, Suzuki S, Nozoye T, Yamakawa T, Takashima Y, Arakawa T, Tsuji N, Takaiwa F, Hayashi Y. 2009. Oral immunogenicity and protective efficacy in mice of transgenic rice plants producing a vaccine candidate antigen (As16) of Ascaris suum fused with cholera toxin B subunit. Transgenic Res 18(2):185-192.

McKenzie SJ, Halsey JF. 1984. Cholera toxin B subunit as a carrier protein to stimulate a mucosal immune response. J Immunol 133(4):1818-1824.

Mekalanos JJ, Collier RJ, Romig WR. 1979. Enzymic activity of cholera toxin. II. Relationships to proteolytic processing, disulfide bond reduction, and subunit composition. J Biol Chem 254(13):5855-5861.

Merritt EA, Sarfaty S, van den Akker F, L'Hoir C, Martial JA, Hol WG. 1994. Crystal structure of cholera toxin B-pentamer bound to receptor GM1 pentasaccharide. Protein Sci 3(2):166-175.

Mishra S, Yadav DK, Tuli R. 2006. Ubiquitin fusion enhances cholera toxin B subunit expression in transgenic plants and the plant-expressed protein binds GM1 receptors more efficiently. J Biotechnol 127(1):95-108.

Miyata T, Harakuni T, Tsuboi T, Sattabongkot J, Kohama H, Tachibana M, Matsuzaki G, Torii M, Arakawa T. 2010. Plasmodium vivax ookinete surface protein Pvs25 linked to cholera toxin B subunit induces potent transmission-blocking immunity by intranasal as well as subcutaneous immunization. Infect Immun 78(9):3773-3782.

Mohsen Arzanlou AR, Nader Shahrokhi, Ahmad Zavaran Hossini, Yoko Yasuda, Kunio Tochikubo, Rezaee MA. 2005. Expression of cholera toxin B subunit in Saccharomyces cerevisiae. Annals of Microbiology(2):145-150.

Muller CP, Beauverger P, Schneider F, Jung G, Brons NH. 1995. Cholera toxin B stimulates systemic neutralizing antibodies after intranasal co-immunization with measles virus. J Gen Virol 76 (Pt 6):1371-1380.

Nishibuchi M, Seidler RJ. 1983. Medium-dependent production of extracellular enterotoxins by non-O-1 Vibrio cholerae, Vibrio mimicus, and Vibrio fluvialis. Appl Environ Microbiol 45(1):228-231.

Northrup RS, Fauci AS. 1972. Adjuvant effect of cholera enterotoxin on the immune response of the mouse to sheep red blood cells. J Infect Dis 125(6):672-673.

Nurkkala M, Wassen L, Nordstrom I, Gustavsson I, Slavica L, Josefsson A, Eriksson K. Conjugation of HPV16 E7 to cholera toxin enhances the HPV-specific T-cell recall responses to pulsed dendritic cells in vitro in women with cervical dysplasia. Vaccine 28(36):5828-5836.

Oikawa A, Shoji J, Inada N, Sawa M. 2011. Transconjunctival immunotherapy using cholera toxin B to treat experimental allergic conjunctivitis in a mouse model. Jpn J Ophthalmol 55(5):534-540.

Okahashi N, Yamamoto M, Vancott JL, Chatfield SN, Roberts M, Bluethmann H, Hiroi T, Kiyono H, McGhee JR. 1996. Oral immunization of interleukin-4 (IL-4) knockout mice with a recombinant Salmonella strain or cholera toxin reveals that CD4+ Th2 cells producing IL-6 and IL-10 are associated with mucosal immunoglobulin A responses. Infect Immun 64(5):1516-1525.

Oszvald M, Kang TJ, Tomoskozi S, Jenes B, Kim TG, Cha YS, Tamas L, Yang MS. 2008. Expression of cholera toxin B subunit in transgenic rice endosperm. Mol Biotechnol 40(3):261-268.

Pascale JM, Shaw MM, Durant PJ, Amador AA, Bartlett MS, Smith JW, Gregory RL, McLaughlin GL. 1999. Intranasal immunization confers protection against murine Pneumocystis carinii lung infection. Infect Immun 67(2):805-809.

Peltola H, Siitonen A, Kyronseppa H, Simula I, Mattila L, Oksanen P, Kataja MJ, Cadoz M. 1991. Prevention of travellers' diarrhoea by oral B-subunit/whole-cell cholera vaccine. Lancet 338(8778):1285-1289.

Petersen JS, Bregenholt S, Apostolopolous V, Homann D, Wolfe T, Hughes A, De Jongh K, Wang M, Dyrberg T, Von Herrath MG. 2003. Coupling of oral human or porcine insulin to the B subunit of cholera toxin (CTB) overcomes critical antigenic differences for prevention of type I diabetes. Clin Exp Immunol 134(1):38-45.

Phipps PA, Stanford MR, Sun JB, Xiao BG, Holmgren J, Shinnick T, Hasan A, Mizushima Y, Lehner T. 2003. Prevention of mucosally induced uveitis with a HSP60-derived peptide linked to cholera toxin B subunit. Eur J Immunol 33(1):224-232.

Pierce NF, Cray WC, Jr., Sacci JB, Jr. 1982. Oral immunization of dogs with purified cholera toxin, crude cholera toxin, or B subunit: evidence for synergistic protection by antitoxic and antibacterial mechanisms. Infect Immun 37(2):687-694.

Pimenta FC, Miyaji EN, Areas AP, Oliveira ML, de Andrade AL, Ho PL, Hollingshead SK, Leite LC. 2006. Intranasal immunization with the cholera toxin B subunit-pneumococcal surface antigen A fusion protein induces protection against colonization with Streptococcus pneumoniae and has negligible impact on the nasopharyngeal and oral microbiota of mice. Infect Immun 74(8):4939-4944.

Ploix C, Bergerot I, Durand A, Czerkinsky C, Holmgren J, Thivolet C. 1999. Oral administration of cholera toxin B-insulin conjugates protects NOD mice from autoimmune diabetes by inducing CD4+ regulatory T-cells. Diabetes 48(11):2150-2156.

Price GA, Russell MW, Cornelissen CN. 2005. Intranasal administration of recombinant Neisseria gonorrhoeae transferrin binding proteins A and B conjugated to the cholera toxin B subunit induces systemic and vaginal antibodies in mice. Infect Immun 73(7):3945-3953.

Qadri F, Wenneras C, Ahmed F, Asaduzzaman M, Saha D, Albert MJ, Sack RB, Svennerholm A. 2000. Safety and immunogenicity of an oral, inactivated enterotoxigenic Escherichia coli plus cholera toxin B subunit vaccine in Bangladeshi adults and children. Vaccine 18(24):2704-2712.

Qu D, Zheng B, Yao X, Guan Y, Yuan ZH, Zhong NS, Lu LW, Xie JP, Wen YM. 2005. Intranasal immunization with inactivated SARS-CoV (SARS-associated coronavirus) induced local and serum antibodies in mice. Vaccine 23(7):924-931.

Quiding M, Nordstrom I, Kilander A, Andersson G, Hanson LA, Holmgren J, Czerkinsky C. 1991. Intestinal immune responses in humans. Oral cholera vaccination induces strong intestinal antibody responses and interferon-gamma production and evokes local immunological memory. J Clin Invest 88(1):143-148.

Raghavan S, Ostberg AK, Flach CF, Ekman A, Blomquist M, Czerkinsky C, Holmgren J. 2010. Sublingual immunization protects against Helicobacter pylori infection and induces T and B cell responses in the stomach. Infect Immun 78(10):4251-4260.

Raghavan S, Svennerholm AM, Holmgren J. 2002. Effects of oral vaccination and immunomodulation by cholera toxin on experimental Helicobacter pylori infection, reinfection, and gastritis. Infect Immun 70(8):4621-4627.

Ramos CR, Abreu PA, Nascimento AL, Ho PL. 2004. A high-copy T7 Escherichia coli expression vector for the production of recombinant proteins with a minimal N-terminal His-tagged fusion peptide. Braz J Med Biol Res 37(8):1103-1109.

Renuga G, Saravanan* R, Babu Thandapani A, Arumugam KR. 2010. Expression of Cholera toxin B subunit in Banana callus culture. JPharm Sci & Res 2:26-33.

Reuman PD, Keely SP, Schiff GM. 1991. Similar subclass antibody responses after intranasal immunization with UV-inactivated RSV mixed with cholera toxin or live RSV. J Med Virol 35(3):192-197.

Rolland-Turner M, Farre G, Muller D, Rouet N, Boue F. 2004. Immunological tools for the assessment of both humoral and cellular immune responses in Foxes (Vulpes vulpes) using ovalbumin and cholera toxin B as an antigenic model. Vaccine 22(31-32):4163-4172.

Ruhlman T, Ahangari R, Devine A, Samsam M, Daniell H. 2007. Expression of cholera toxin B-proinsulin fusion protein in lettuce and tobacco chloroplasts--oral administration protects against development of insulitis in non-obese diabetic mice. Plant Biotechnol J 5(4):495-510.

Russell MW, Wu HY. 1991. Distribution, persistence, and recall of serum and salivary antibody responses to peroral immunization with protein antigen I/II of Streptococcus mutans coupled to the cholera toxin B subunit. Infect Immun 59(11):4061-4070.

Sadeghi H, Bregenholt S, Wegmann D, Petersen JS, Holmgren J, Lebens M. 2002. Genetic fusion of human insulin B-chain to the B-subunit of cholera toxin enhances in vitro antigen presentation and induction of bystander suppression in vivo. Immunology 106(2):237-245.

Salmond RJ, Luross JA, Williams NA. 2002. Immune modulation by the cholera-like enterotoxins. Expert Rev Mol Med 4(21):1-16.

Sanchez J, Holmgren J. 1989. Recombinant system for overexpression of cholera toxin B subunit in Vibrio cholerae as a basis for vaccine development. Proc Natl Acad Sci U S A 86(2):481-485.

Sanchez J, Holmgren J. 2008. Cholera toxin structure, gene regulation and pathophysiological and immunological aspects. Cell Mol Life Sci 65(9):1347-1360.

Sanchez J, Holmgren J. 2011. Cholera toxin - a foe & a friend. Indian J Med Res 133(2):153-163.

Sasaki K, Kato M, Takahashi T, Ochi S, Ichinose Y, Shiraki K, Asano Y, Iwanaga M, Tsuji T. 2003. Live varicella vaccine polarizes the mucosal adjuvant action of cholera toxin or its B subunit on specific Th1-type helper T cells with a single nasal coadministration in mice. J Med Virol 70(2):329-335.

Seo JY, Seong SY, Ahn BY, Kwon IC, Chung H, Jeong SY. 2002. Cross-protective immunity of mice induced by oral immunization with pneumococcal surface adhesin a encapsulated in microspheres. Infect Immun 70(3):1143-1149.

Shen X, Lagergard T, Yang Y, Lindblad M, Fredriksson M, Holmgren J. 2000. Systemic and mucosal immune responses in mice after mucosal immunization with group B streptococcus type III capsular polysaccharide-cholera toxin B subunit conjugate vaccine. Infect Immun 68(10):5749-5755.

Shin JS, Abraham SN. 2001. Cell biology. Caveolae--not just craters in the cellular landscape. Science 293(5534):1447-1448.

Simmons CP, Mastroeni P, Fowler R, Ghaem-maghami M, Lycke N, Pizza M, Rappuoli R, Dougan G. 1999. MHC class I-restricted cytotoxic lymphocyte responses induced by enterotoxin-based mucosal adjuvants. J Immunol 163(12):6502-6510.

Sjoblom-Hallen A, Marklund U, Nerstedt A, Schon K, Ekman L, Bergqvist P, Lowenadler B, (2010) Lycke NY. Gene expression profiling identifies STAT3 as a novel pathway for immunomodulation by cholera toxin adjuvant. Mucosal Immunol 3(4):374-386.

Slos P, Dutot P, Reymund J, Kleinpeter P, Prozzi D, Kieny MP, Delcour J, Mercenier A, Hols P. 1998. Production of cholera toxin B subunit in Lactobacillus. FEMS Microbiol Lett 169(1):29-36.

Sobel DO, Yankelevich B, Goyal D, Nelson D, Mazumder A. 1998. The B-subunit of cholera toxin induces immunoregulatory cells and prevents diabetes in the NOD mouse. Diabetes 47(2):186-191.

Soenawan E, Srivastava I, Gupta S, Kan E, Janani R, Kazzaz J, Singh M, Shreedhar V, Vajdy M. 2004. Maintenance of long-term immunological memory by low avidity IgM-secreting cells in bone marrow after mucosal immunizations with cholera toxin adjuvant. Vaccine 22(11-12):1553-1563.

Song H, Zhou L, Fang W, Li Y, Wang X, Fang H, Li X, Wu M, Qiu B. 2004. High-level expression of codon optimized foot-and-mouth disease virus complex epitopes and cholera toxin B subunit chimera in Hansenula polymorpha. Biochem Biophys Res Commun 315(1):235-239.

Soriani M, Bailey L, Hirst TR. 2002. Contribution of the ADP-ribosylating and receptor-binding properties of cholera-like enterotoxins in modulating cytokine secretion by human intestinal epithelial cells. Microbiology 148(Pt 3):667-676.

Spangler BD. 1992. Structure and function of cholera toxin and the related Escherichia coli heat-labile enterotoxin. Microbiol Rev 56(4):622-647.

Spira WM, Fedorka-Cray PJ. 1984. Purification of enterotoxins from Vibrio mimicus that appear to be identical to cholera toxin. Infect Immun 45(3):679-684.

Staats HF, Ennis FA, Jr. 1999. IL-1 is an effective adjuvant for mucosal and systemic immune responses when coadministered with protein immunogens. J Immunol 162(10):6141-6147.

Stal P, Befrits R, Ronnblom A, Danielsson A, Suhr O, Stahlberg D, Brinkberg Lapidus A, Lofberg R. 2010. Clinical trial: the safety and short-term efficacy of recombinant cholera toxin B subunit in the treatment of active Crohn's disease. Aliment Pharmacol Ther 31(3):387-395.

Stanford M, Whittall T, Bergmeier LA, Lindblad M, Lundin S, Shinnick T, Mizushima Y, Holmgren J, Lehner T. 2004. Oral tolerization with peptide 336-351 linked to cholera toxin B subunit in preventing relapses of uveitis in Behcet's disease. Clin Exp Immunol 137(1):201-208.

Sun JB, Czerkinsky C, Holmgren J. 2009. Mucosally induced immunological tolerance, regulatory T cells and the adjuvant effect by cholera toxin B subunit. Scand J Immunol 71(1):1-11.

Sun JB, Holmgren J, Czerkinsky C. 1994. Cholera toxin B subunit: an efficient transmucosal carrier-delivery system for induction of peripheral immunological tolerance. Proc Natl Acad Sci U S A 91(23):10795-10799.

Sun JB, Li BL, Czerkinsky C, Holmgren J. 2000a. Enhanced immunological tolerance against allograft rejection by oral administration of allogeneic antigen linked to cholera toxin B subunit. Clin Immunol 97(2):130-139.

Sun JB, Mielcarek N, Lakew M, Grzych JM, Capron A, Holmgren J, Czerkinsky C. 1999. Intranasal administration of a Schistosoma mansoni glutathione S-transferase-cholera toxoid conjugate vaccine evokes antiparasitic and antipathological immunity in mice. J Immunol 163(2):1045-1052.

Sun JB, Rask C, Olsson T, Holmgren J, Czerkinsky C. 1996. Treatment of experimental autoimmune encephalomyelitis by feeding myelin basic protein conjugated to cholera toxin B subunit. Proc Natl Acad Sci U S A 93(14):7196-7201.

Sun JB, Xiao BG, Lindblad M, Li BL, Link H, Czerkinsky C, Holmgren J. 2000b. Oral administration of cholera toxin B subunit conjugated to myelin basic protein protects against experimental autoimmune encephalomyelitis by inducing transforming growth factor-beta-secreting cells and suppressing chemokine expression. Int Immunol 12(10):1449-1457.

Taniguchi T, Harada T, Hayashi T, Tanikawa T, Kurohane K, Miyake M, Imai Y. 2008. Elevated production of Legionella-specific immunoglobulin A in A/J mice is accompanied by T-helper 1-type polarization. Immunol Lett 121(2):123-126.

Teter K, Jobling MG, Sentz D, Holmes RK. 2006. The cholera toxin A1(3) subdomain is essential for interaction with ADP-ribosylation factor 6 and full toxic activity but is not required for translocation from the endoplasmic reticulum to the cytosol. Infect Immun 74(4):2259-2267.

Thomas S, Preda-Pais A, Casares S, Brumeanu TD. 2004. Analysis of lipid rafts in T cells. Mol Immunol 41(4):399-409.

Tsai B, Rodighiero C, Lencer WI, Rapoport TA. 2001. Protein disulfide isomerase acts as a redox-dependent chaperone to unfold cholera toxin. Cell 104(6):937-948.

Tsuji N, Suzuki K, Kasuga-Aoki H, Isobe T, Arakawa T, Matsumoto Y. 2003. Mice intranasally immunized with a recombinant 16-kilodalton antigen from roundworm Ascaris parasites are protected against larval migration of Ascaris suum. Infect Immun 71(9):5314-5323.

Vajdy M, Lycke NY. 1992. Cholera toxin adjuvant promotes long-term immunological memory in the gut mucosa to unrelated immunogens after oral immunization. Immunology 75(3):488-492.

Vanden Broeck D, Horvath C, De Wolf MJ. 2007. Vibrio cholerae: cholera toxin. Int J Biochem Cell Biol 39(10):1771-1775.

Wang BN, Yang Y, Kuang Y, Cao K, Li MY, Li WY. 2010. [Construction eukaryotic plasmids of the ureI and ctB-ureI and profile its' expression in cell]. Xi Bao Yu Fen Zi Mian Yi Xue Za Zhi 26(8):764-766.

Wang J, Lu ZH, Gabius HJ, Rohowsky-Kochan C, Ledeen RW, Wu G. 2009. Cross-linking of GM1 ganglioside by galectin-1 mediates regulatory T cell activity involving TRPC5 channel activation: possible role in suppressing experimental autoimmune encephalomyelitis. J Immunol 182(7):4036-4045.

Wang L, Kedzierski L, Wesselingh SL, Coppel RL. 2003. Oral immunization with a recombinant malaria protein induces conformational antibodies and protects mice against lethal malaria. Infect Immun 71(5):2356-2364.

Wilson AD, Bailey M, Williams NA, Stokes CR. 1991. The in vitro production of cytokines by mucosal lymphocytes immunized by oral administration of keyhole limpet hemocyanin using cholera toxin as an adjuvant. Eur J Immunol 21(10):2333-2339.

Wu HY, Russell MW. 1993. Induction of mucosal immunity by intranasal application of a streptococcal surface protein antigen with the cholera toxin B subunit. Infect Immun 61(1):314-322.

Wu HY, Russell MW. 1998. Induction of mucosal and systemic immune responses by intranasal immunization using recombinant cholera toxin B subunit as an adjuvant. Vaccine 16(2-3):286-292.

Yamamoto S, Takeda Y, Yamamoto M, Kurazono H, Imaoka K, Fujihashi K, Noda M, Kiyono H, McGhee JR. 1997. Mutants in the ADP-ribosyltransferase cleft of cholera toxin lack diarrheagenicity but retain adjuvanticity. J Exp Med 185(7):1203-1210.

Yang P, Tang C, Luo D, Zhan Z, Xing L, Duan Y, Jia W, Peng D, Liu X, Wang X. Cross-clade protection against HPAI H5N1 influenza virus challenge in BALB/c mice intranasally administered adjuvant-combined influenza vaccine. Vet Microbiol 146(1-2):17-23.

Young-Sook Kim B-GK, Tae-Geum Kim, Tae-Jin Kang, Moon-Sik Yang. 2006. Expression of a cholera toxin B subunit in transgenic lettuce (Lactuca sativa L.) using Agrobacterium-mediated transformation system. Plant Cell Tiss Organ Cult 87:203-210.

Yuki Y, Byun Y, Fujita M, Izutani W, Suzuki T, Udaka S, Fujihashi K, McGhee JR, Kiyono H. 2001. Production of a recombinant hybrid molecule of cholera toxin-B-subunit and proteolipid-protein-peptide for the treatment of experimental encephalomyelitis. Biotechnol Bioeng 74(1):62-69.

Zhang T, Li E, Stanley SL, Jr. 1995. Oral immunization with the dodecapeptide repeat of the serine-rich Entamoeba histolytica protein (SREHP) fused to the cholera toxin B subunit induces a mucosal and systemic anti-SREHP antibody response. Infect Immun 63(4):1349-1355.

8

Brefeldin A and Exo1 Completely Releave the Block of Cholera Toxin Action by a Dipeptide Metalloendoprotease Substrate

Davy Vanden Broeck and Marc J.S. De Wolf
International Centre for Reproductive Health, Ghent University, Ghent, Belgium

1. Introduction

Cholera toxin (CT), the enterotoxin secreted by *Vibrio cholerae* classical as well as *El Tor* biotypes, is the major causative agent of the acute diarrheal disease of humans. CT and the *Escherichia coli* heat labile enterotoxin (LT),are structurally and immunologically highly homologous,seeing that they belong to the same enterotoxin family (de Haan and Hirst, 2004; Spangler, 1992; Vanden Broeck et al., 2007). Both are oligomeric proteins of the A-B type. CT is composed of one A or activating subunit (CT-A Mr 27,400), which consists of two distinct polypeptide chains CT-A_1 (Mr 22,000) and CT-A_2 (Mr 5,400), linked by a single disulfide bridge, and 5 identical B subunits (Mr 11,600) arranged in a ring like configuration (CT-B).

The subunits are arranged in such a manner that CT-A occupies the central channel of the CT-B pentamer extending well above the plane of the pentameric ring (Sixma et al., 1991; Zhang et al., 1995). The CT-A_2peptide goes through the pore in the doughnut-like structure of the CT-B pentamer, and protrudes on the side, which binds cell surface receptors with its COOH-terminal KDEL sequence exposed. CT elicits a secretory response from intestinal epithelia by binding to the apical cell membrane through interaction between CT-B and the monosialoganglioside $GM_{1,}$ followed by entry of polypeptide A_1 into the cell, where it is able to stimulate the basolateral adenylatecyclase by catalyzing the ADP-ribosylation of Arg201 of the $G_{s\alpha}$ subunit of the stimulatory GTP-binding regulatory protein (de Haan and Hirst, 2004; Spangler, 1992; Vanden Broeck et al., 2007a; Sixma et al., 1991).

There is a distinct lag period between toxin binding and the activation of adenylatecyclase, during which the toxin must be internalized and processed.At the end of this lag period small amounts of CT-A_1 appear in the cells parallel to activation of the cyclase(Kassis et al., 1982).

Early morphologic studies showed that CT is preferentially clustered into non-coated membrane invaginations characteristic of caveolae and enters several cell types via smooth, non clathrin coated vesicles (Lencer et al., 1999).

Studies using cholesterol perturbing agents and chimeric toxins have shown that GM_1-mediated association with detergent-resistant membrane fractions (DRMS) or lipid rafts is required for toxic entry of CT (Orlandi and Fishman, 1998; Wolf et al., 1998, 2002).

Although CT is currently used as a marker for endocytosis without utilising clathrin-coated pits,it appears to be endocytosed simultaneously through both clathrin -dependent and-independent routes (Orlandi and Fishman, 1998; Nichols et al., 2001; Shogomori and Futerman, 2001; Torgersen et al., 2001; Vanden Broeck et al., 2007b).

In a recent study using fluorescence microscopy (Massol et al., 2004)it has been shown that apart from clathrin-, caveolin-endocytic pathways, CT also enters cells via a pathway that is regulated by the small GTPase Arf6 and possibly a fourth pathway that is dynamin and Arf6-independent. However, after blocking all three known endocytic payhways simultaneously by over expression of negative dominant mutants of dynamin and Arf6, fluorescent CT in the Golgi and ER became undetectable, although CT induced toxicity was hardly affected (Massol et al., 2004).These findings illustrate the difficulty in correlating morphologic data with the functional entry of a potent toxin such as CT.

Consistent with the multiple ports of entry into the cell, CT can be found in early and recycling endosomes (Tran et al., 1987; Nichols, 2002)and in caveolin-1 containing endocytic intermediates (Nichols, 2002),which have been proposed to be responsible for the functional transport of CT. For CT to be toxic it must be transported through the Golgi to the ER. Brefeldin A (BFA), a fungal metabolite that disrupts the structural and functional integrity of the Golgi apparatus (Klausner et al., 1992),renders cells resistant to CT cytotoxicity and blocks intracellular formation of CT-A_1(Orlandi et al., 1993; Nambiar et al., 1993; Lencer et al., 1993).

Movement into the Golgi can also be inhibited by blockage of COPI- and COPII- mediated vesicular transport, and this affects toxin function further implicating trafficking through the Golgi apparatus as a necessary step in toxin action (Richards et al., 2002; Majoul et al., 1998).

On reaching the ER, the reduced form of the lumenal chaperone protein disulfideisomerase binds to the A_1 chain, dissociates it from the B subunit and unfolds it(Tsai et al., 2001; Tsai and Rapoport, 2002; Fujinaga et al., 2003). Subsequent oxidation of PDI by the ER lumenal ERO1, the A_1 chain is released (Tsai and Rapoport, 2002)and is translocated to the cytosol probably via the Sec61 channel, identifying the rough ER as the compartment from which translocation occurs (Schmitz et al., 2000). It has been suggested that the rapid refolding (Tsai and Rapoport, 2002)may render the A_1 chain resistant to poly ubiquitination and provide the driving force for retro translocation to the cytosol (Rodighiero et al., 2002).

We previously reported that the metalloendoprotease substrate N-benzoyloxycarbonyl-Gly-Phe-NH_2(Cbz-Gly-Phe-NH_2) completely blocked the response of different celltypes in culture to CT. The effect was reversible, dose-and time-dependent. The dipeptide had no effect on the binding of CT to the cell surface and did not decrease its internalization but appeared to affect a later step in toxin action (De Wolf, 2000).

In this study we further investigated the mechanism by which Cbz-Gly-Phe-NH_2 blocks CT action.

2. Materials and methods

2.1.Materials

Highly purified CT was obtained from List Biological Laboratories (Campbell, Ca.). CT was radiolabeled with ^{125}I using the Iodo-gen method as described by Fraker and Speck (1978).

Unreacted ^{125}I-Na was removed using gel filtration on a Sephadex G-50 mini-column using the centrifugation procedure of Tuszynski et al. (1980).Cbz-Gly-Phe-NH_2, brefeldinA, 3-isobutylmethylxanthine, iodixanol (Optiprep™), 1,9-dideoxyforskolin, nocodazole and 2-deoxy-D-glucose were from Sigma. 2-(4-Fluorobenzoylamino)-benzoic acid methylester (Exo1) was from Calbiochem.1,3-Cyclohexane-bis(methylamine) (CBM) was purchased from Acros Organics. Na^{125}I was obtained from MP Biochemicals& Reagents (formerly ICN).

2.2.Cell culture

Vero cells originally obtained from Flow Laboratories were cultured in Medium 199 with Earle's salts supplemented with 5% fetal calf serum (FCS).Human intestinal epithelial T84 cells (obtained from ATCC) were propagated in a 1:1 mixture of Ham's F12 medium and Dulbecco's modified Eagle's medium with 2.5mM L-glutamine and 5% fetal bovine serum.Madin-Darby canine kidney (MDCK) cells (obtained from ATCC) were grown in Eagle's Minimum Essential Medium with 2mM L-glutamine and Earle's BSS adjusted to contain 1.5g/l sodium bicarbonate, 0.1mM non-essential amino acids, and 1.0mM sodium pyruvate with 10% fetal bovine serum. Growth medium was changed twice a week and cells were passed weekly (at confluency) using a 0.05% (w/v) trypsin solution (Gibco). Cells were counted in a hemocytometer.

2.3 Preparation of membranes from post nuclear supernatant of a Vero cell homogenate

Vero cells were grown to confluency in 175cm^2 culture flasks and maintained in culture for at least 14 days before harvesting. Cells were washed once with serum free medium to remove serum and harvested by short trypsinisation with a 0.05% trysin, EDTA solution in HBSS (Gibco). After 1 min the trypsinisation solution was removed by aspiration and the culture flasks were put at 37°C until the cells detached from the bottom. Cells needed for one gradient centrifugation experiment (5 culture flasks for each time interval) were collected in an Eppendorf tube, washed twice and suspended in 2ml of serum-free medium buffered with 25mM HEPES containing 0.1% BSA and chilled. Cells were then labeled with ^{125}I-CT (10^{6}cpm /2 ml≈ 10nM) in the same medium containing 0.01 % bovine serum albumin for 30 min at 4°C to allow binding without endocytosis. Subsequently, cells were washed and harvested immediately (t=0) or washed and incubated for 10,30,60 or 120 min in serum-free medium at 37°C and harvested.Cells were pelleted by low speed centrifugation. The pellets were resuspended in 50mM tris-HCl pH 7.4 containing 250mM sucrose (Tris-sucrose) buffer and homogenized on ice with 4 x 4 strokes of a Potter Elvejhem homogenizer (position 9). The homogenates were spun at 3,000 x g for 10 min to pellet unbroken cells, cell debris and nuclei to yield the PNS. Membranes from PNS were obtained by centrifugation of the PNS at 100,000 x g for 1 h at 4°C. The membrane pellet was resuspended in Tris-sucrose buffer.

2.4 Gradient centrifugation

Subcellular fractionation was always performed on freshly prepared post nuclear membranes or PNS from cells labeled with ^{125}I-CT. Membrane pellets prepared from PNS (post nuclear membranes),resuspended in 3 ml of homogenization buffer (50mM Tris-HCl, pH 7.4 containing 0.25M sucrose) or equal volumes of PNS,werelayered on top of two layers of respectively 4 ml of 25% iodixanol and 4 ml of 50% iodixanol each in isoosmotic homogenization buffer in a 11.5 ml centrifugation tube (Sorvall). The tubes were centrifuged in a (Sorvall TV-850) vertical rotor at 35,000 rpm for 18 h at 4°C using a Kontron centrifuge Centricon T2060. Fractions of 0.3 ml were collected from the bottom of the gradient using a device with a perforation needle and a density gradient fractionator. A 15 µl portion of each gradient fraction was used to determine its refractive index (η) as measured by an Abbe refractometer. From the refractive indices the densities of individual gradient fractions were calculated using the equation $\varsigma=3.4911\eta-3.6664$ as reported by Graham et al. (1994). Fractions were further analyzed for protein by the method of Bradford (1976) and for the trans-Golgi marker UDP-galactosyltransferase(Verdon and Berger, 1983) as well as the classical subcellular organelle markers rotenone-insensitive NADPH cytochrome creductase, alkaline phosphatase, acid phosphatase and cytochromecoxidase as described before (De Wolf et al., 1985).

2.5 Assay of cellular cyclic AMP content

Monolayer cultures of cells were washed twice with Earle's balanced salt solution without Ca^{2+} and Mg^{2+} and treated with 0.05% (w/v) trypsin solution containing 0.02% EDTA in HBSS. After 1 min the trypsin solution was removed and 10-15 min later cells were suspended in culture medium. Cells were collected by centrifugation at 750 rpm for 5 min and resuspended in 1 ml serum-free medium containing 25mM Hepes, 0.01% (w/v) bovine serum albumin and 1mM 3-isobutyl-1-methylxanthine. 1 ml aliquots of cell suspension (10^5 cells/ml were divided over Eppendorf tubes and incubated with CT (1µg/ml) and the required effectors were added at the indicated times as described in the legend of figures. Afterwards, cell suspensions were put on ice, centrifuged for 6 min at 1000 rpm and resuspended in 0.1 ml 0.5M sodium acetate buffer (pH 6.2). The suspensions were boiled for 10 min and then sonicated for 30 s. After centrifugation for 10 min at 10000 rpm, 20 µl of cell extract was taken for cyclic AMP (cAMP) assay. cAMP was assayed using a cAMP assay kit (Pharmacia Amersham) based on a competitive protein-binding method. Results for cAMP represent the mean of values from duplicate samples each assayed in triplicate.

2.6 Generation of CT-A_1 and analysis by SDS-polyacrylamide gel electrophoresis

Vero cells were grown to confluency in small (∅=3cm) petri dishes (250.10^6 cells) and maintained in culture for at least one week before use. Cells were washed once with serum-free medium buffered with 25mM Hepes and incubated with and without Cbz-Gly-Phe-NH_2(3mM) for 30 min at 37°C.The medium was replaced with ice-cold serum-free medium/Hepes (total volume=3 ml) containing ^{125}I-CT (10^6cpm/ml;≈1nM CT) and 0.01% BSA and the cells were further incubated at 4°C for 30 min.The cells were then washed with ice-cold serum-free medium/Hepes and incubated at 37°C for 60 min by replacing the medium with warm serum-free medium-/Hepes. With each medium change, Cbz-Gly-Phe-NH_2(3mM) wasadded as required. The cell incubations were either stopped immediately or after the addition of BFA (1µg/ml), further incubated for 30 min at 37°C and then stopped. Incubations were stopped by adding 1 ml of ice-cold N-ethylmaleimide (NEM) (1mM) in phosphate-buffer saline to prevent any further reduction of CT (Kassis et al., 1982), scraped in PBS, and pelleted by low speed centrifugation. The cells were lysed and solubilised by addition of a small volume of 0.125M Tris/HCl (pH 8.0), 2mM phenyl-methyl sulfonylfluoride and 1 % SDS. After 10 min at 37°C the solubilised material was adjusted to 20% glycerol and 0.02% bromphenol blue and applied to the gels. The amount of CT-A_1 generated was determined by SDS-PAGE.

Each sample (≈10,000 cpm) was separated on 16% tris-glycine gel (Novex pre-cast gels). After the gels were run and stained with coomassie blue, protein bands corresponding to CT-A_1 were cut from the gel, which was subsequently dissolved in lumasolveand, after addition of lipoluma (Lumac, LSC), counted in a liquid scintillation counter. CT reduced with dithiothreitol and dialysed against 10mM tris/HCl pH 7.4 containing 10mM NEM, to remove the excess of reducing agent, was adjusted to 1% SDS, 20% glycerol and 0.02% bromphenol blue, warmed at 37°C for 10 min and run on each slab gel.

3. Results

3.1 Effect of Cbz-Gly-Phe-NH_2 on the intracellular retrograde transport of CT

In order to assess whether the metalloendoprotease substrate Cbz-Gly-Phe-NH_2 perturbs the uptake and intracellular trafficking of CT, we performed subcellular fractionation experiments on post-nuclear membranes of Vero cells with prebound^{125}I-CT.

The distribution profiles of marker enzymes after isopycnic gradient centrifugation of these membranes, using self-generating gradients of iodixanol, showed a reasonable separation of Golgi fractions (as represented by UDP-galactosyltransferase) from the ER fractions (rotenone-insensitive NADPH cytochrome c reductase) and plasma membranes (alkaline phosphatase) (Fig.1,C). Membrane proteins were distributed all over the gradient (profile not shown).

At the outset,^{125}I-CT was allowed to bind to Vero cells in suspension for 30 min at 4°C, minimizing endocytosis.Cells were washed and homogenized immediately (t=0) or they were washed and re-cultured for an additional 10 min (t=10); 30 min (t=30); 60 min (t=60) and 120 min (t=120) at 37°C prior to preparation of membranes from PNS. It was noticed that during re-culture, radioactivity was progressively released into the culture medium (after 10 h more than 60%, mostly (80%) as non-precipitable material).However, when the re-culture time was 120 min this amount was less than 10%.

As shown in Fig.1 panels A and C, the radioactivity profile at zero time corresponded to that of alkaline phosphatase, a cell-surface membrane marker. Upon increasing the re-culture time,ra-dioactivity shifted to higher densities. After 30 min most of the radioactivity equilibrated at densities (1.127g/ml) corresponding to Golgi-derived membranes, as evidenced by the distribution of the Golgi marker UDP-galactosyltransferase.At still later time points (60–120min),^{125}I-CT further moved to higher densities corresponding to those of membranes from the rough ER, which is in agreement with the generally accepted retrograde transport of the toxin to the ER. The distribution profiles of marker enzymes were not affected upon increasing the re-culture time (data not shown).

As shown in Fig.1,B, pre-treatment of Vero cells with Cbz-Gly-Phe-NH_2 (3mM) for 30 min at 37° C, before binding and internalization of ^{125}I-CT, markedly affected the distribution profiles of radioactivity upon increasing re-culture times. Whereas the internalization,in agreement with our previous results (Schmitz et al., 2000), was not affected, further transport of the toxin appeared to be strongly perturbed. After re-culture the toxin still moved to densities corresponding to those of Golgi-derived membranes, but at an apparently lower rate, and further transport to the ER appeared to be blocked. Pre-exposure of cells to Cbz-Gly-Phe-NH_2 (3mM) did not significantly affect the distribution profiles of marker enzymes. Only the Golgi marker equilibrated at a somewhat higher density

(1.132g/ml versus 1.127g/ml) but clearly did not shift to densities corresponding to the ER, as was the case after pretreatment of cells with BFA (data not shown).

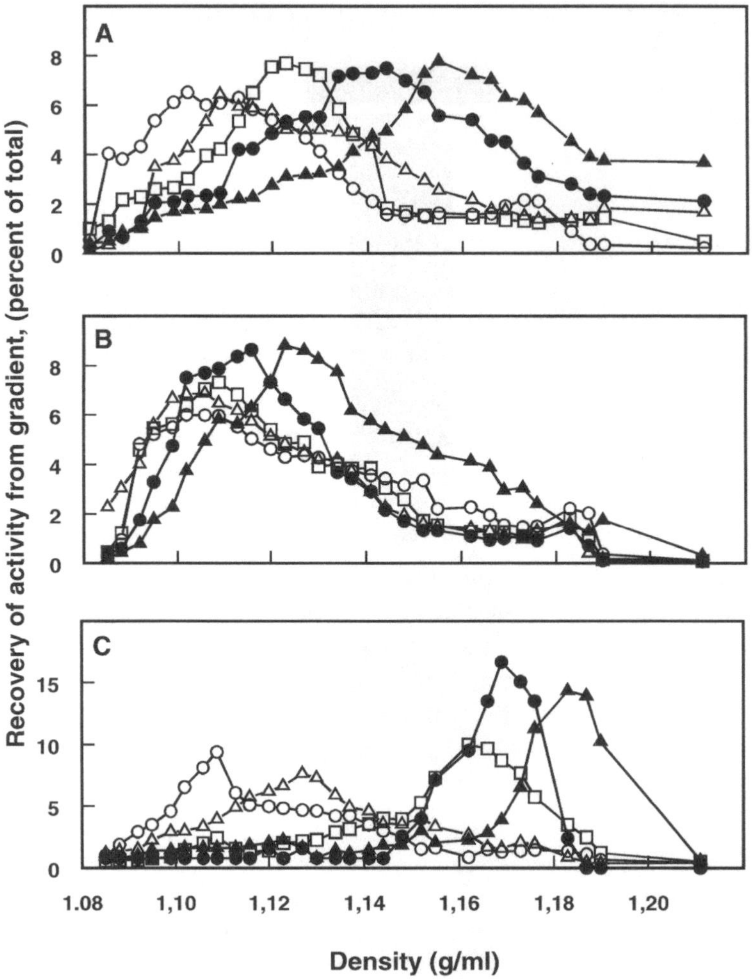

Fig. 1. Subcellular fractionation of post-nuclear membranes from Vero cells prelabeled with ^{125}I-CT.Vero cells prelabeled with ^{125}I-CT at low temperature to block endocytosis were, after washing, incubated at 37°C for 0 time (○), 15 min (△), 30 min (□), 60 min (●) or 120 min (▲) and post-nuclear membranes were prepared and centrifuged through a self-generating gradient of iodixanol as described under Materials and Methods. A. Subcellular distribution profiles of membrane-bound ^{125}I-CT after increasing re-culture periods.B. Subcellular distribution profiles of membrane-bound ^{125}I-CT after pretreatment of Vero cells with Cbz-Gly-Phe-NH_2 and different re-culture periods. Vero cells in suspension were pretreated with Cbz-Gly-Phe-NH_2 (3mM) for 30 min at 37°C. The cells were chilled and after binding of ^{125}I-CT at 4°C, washed and re-cultured for different periods of time in the presence of Cbz-Gly-Phe-NH_2 (3mM) at 37°C.C. Distribution profiles of subcellular marker enzymes at zero time (no-reculture),(○) Alkaline phosphatase, (△) UDP- galactosyltransferase, (●) NADPH - cytochrome creductase, (□) Acid phosphatase, (▲) cytcoxidase. The distribution profiles are representative for three similar experiments.

3.2 Effect of drugs perturbing the Golgi structure on theCbz-Gly-Phe-NH_2-mediated inhibition of CT action

From the density gradient centrifugation experiments it is clear that the metalloendoprotease substrate Cbz-Gly-Phe-NH_2 affects the intracellular transport of CT and that in its presence the toxin appears to be trapped in an intracellular compartment, which cofractionated with a marker of the Golgi apparatus.In order to find out whether in the presence of Cbz-Gly-Phe-NH_2 the toxin travels beyond the trans-Golgi network (TGN) and reaches the cisternae of the Golgi complex, we explored whether drugs that are able to redistibute Golgi membranes and its content into the ER also caused a reversal of Cbz-Gly-Phe-NH_2-mediated inhibition of CT action.

As shown in Fig.2,A,C and in agreement with previous results (De Wolf, 2000),prior incubation of Vero cells and T84 cells with Cbz-Gly-Phe-NH_2 or with BFA for 30 min at 37°C resulted in respectively a complete or strong inhibition of CT action in a dose-dependent way.

However, when these cells were preincubated with Cbz-Gly-Phe-NH_2 (3mM) for 30 min at 37 °C and then incubated in the presence of CT (1µg/ml) for an additional 60 min time period, a time at which CT - as evidenced by the gradient centrifugation experiments - becomes trapped in a compartment where it is unable to reach the cytosol and raise intracellular cAMP levels, subsequent addition of BFA completely reversed the Cbz-Gly-Phe-NH_2-mediated inhibition of CT action in a dose-dependent way(EC_{50}≈0.5µg/ml) (Fig.2,B,D).

The concentrations at which reversal of the inhibition occurred, corresponded to the concentrations needed for inhibition of CT action and induction of the redistribution of Golgi membranes into the ER (Fig.2,A,C) (Doms et al., 1989; Lippincott-Schwartz et al., 1989).

We next determined the effect of 2-(4-fluoro-benzoylamino)-benzoic acid methylester (Exo1), a novel chemical inhibitor of the exocytotic pathway (Feng et al., 2003).Like BFA, Exo1 induces the release of ADP-ribosylation factor (ARF)1 from Golgi membranes, inducing/generating/stimulating a rapid collapse of the Golgi into the endoplasmic reticulum in different cell types. However, unlike BFA this drug has less effect on the organization of the trans-Golgi network (Feng et al., 2003). As shown in Fig.2,A,C,E, prior exposure to Exo1 blocked the CT induced cAMP accumulation in all cell types tested. The effect was dose-dependent with an IC_{50} value of ≈0.35µM. This value is almost two orders of magnitude lower than that reported for its inhibitory effect on the anterograde movement of the viral glycoprotein VSVG from the ER to the Golgi and its stimulation of the release or ARF1 from Golgi membranes in BSC1 fibroblasts (Feng et al., 2003).

As expected, Exo1 also completely reversed the Cbz-Gly-Phe-NH_2-mediated inhibition of CT ac-tion in a similar dose-dependent way (Fig.2,B,-D,F).

We previously showed (De Wolf, 2000)that there are some similarities in the inhibitory effects of Cbz-Gly-Phe-NH_2 and BFA on CT action. However, Madin-Darby canine kidney epithelial (MDCK) cells, of which the Golgi structure is BFA resistant (Hunziker et al., 1991)and as a consequence are insensitive to the inhibitory effect of BFA on CT action, were sensitive to the inhibitory effect of Cbz-Gly-Phe-NH_2.In agreement with our previous results (De Wolf, 2000),prior exposure of these cells toCbz-Gly-Phe-NH_2(Fig.2,E) completely suppressed (IC_{50}=0.5mM) CT action. Therefore, it was of interest to determine whether BFA is also able to reverse the inhibitory effect of Cbz-Gly-Phe-NH_2 on CT action in MDCK cells.

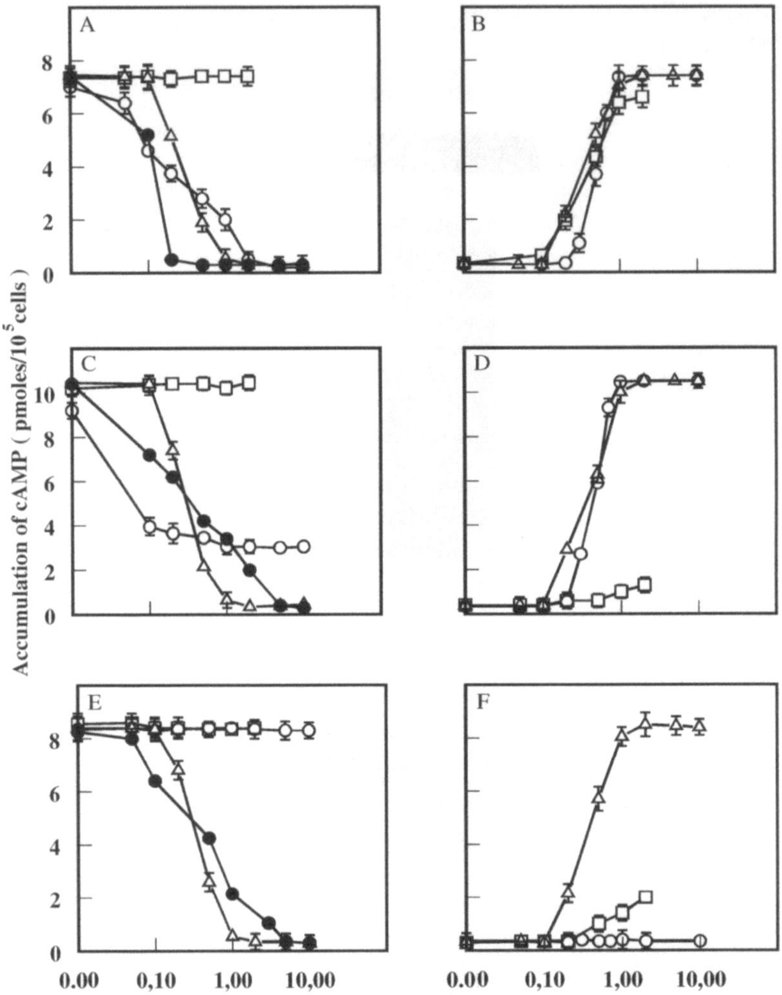

Fig. 2. Inhibition of CT action by different concentrations of BFA, Exo1 and nocodazole and their effect on the Cbz-Gly-Phe-NH_2 - mediated inhibition of CT action in several cell types. A, Vero cells; C, T84 human intestinal epithelial cells and E, MDCK cells in suspension were preincubated at 37°C for 30 min in the presence of the indicated amounts of BFA (○), Exo1 (△), nocodazole (□) or Cbz-Gly-Phe-NH_2 (●). After the addition of CT (1μg/ml) cells were further incubated for 90 min at 37°C and the cAMP accumulation measured. B, Vero cells; D, T84 human, intestinal epithelial cells and F, MDCK cells were preincubated with Cbz-Gly-Phe-NH_2 (3mM) for 30 min at 37°C. Following the addition of CT (1μg/ml) cells were further incubated for 60 min at 37°C. Finally, the indicated amounts of BFA (○),Exo1 (△) and nocodazole (□)were added and the cells incubated for an additional 30 min at 37°C and cAMP measured. Values are the means ±SD of triplicate assays from one of three similar experiments. Error bars are indicated when they were more than 5% of the mean.

As shown in Fig.2,E,F, BFA did neither prevent CT induced cAMP accumulation nor reverse the inhibitory effect of Cbz-Gly-Phe-NH_2 on CT action in MDCK cells. In contrast, Exo1, which is able to prevent CT action in these cells, was also able to reverse the inhibition by Cbz-Gly-Phe-NH_2 in a similar dose-dependent way (Fig.2,-E,F).

This is in line with the proposal (Feng et al., 2003)that although Exo1 and BFA are exerting similar effects they probably have different protein targets. Whereas BFA blocks GDP to GTP exchange on ARF1 and therefore reduces the concentration of ARF1-GTP on Golgi membranes, it is believed that Exo1 also reduces the concentration of ARF1-GTP on Golgi membranes by accelerating the hydrolysis of GTP bound to ARF1 by an activation of ARF1-GAP activity(Feng et al., 2003).

By causing the release of ARF1 and COPI from membranes, BFA and Exo1 directly interfere with the Golgi-ER retrograde trafficking machinery and this likely perturbs normal recycling from the Golgi to the ER. Therefore it was of interest to see whether a treatment of cells, which affects the Golgi structure without directly interfering with the retrograde transport, also caused a reversal of the inhibition of the CT action by Cbz-Gly-Phe-NH_2.

A constant influx of membrane from the ER is required to maintain the Golgi structure. Microtubule disruption prevents this influx by blocking the peripherial pre-Golgi intermediates from tracking into the Golgi region (Cole et al., 1996; Storrie et al., 1998). The microtubule depolymerizing agent nocodazole, which blocks the forward traffic into the Golgi complex without a corresponding effect on recycling, leads to the fragmentation of the Golgi complex and redistribution of its material to the site of perturbation (Cole et al., 1996).

Whereas prior exposure of cells to nocodazole did not affect CT action (Fig.2,A,C,E), it was able to reverse the Cbz-Gly-Phe-NH_2-mediated inhibition of CT action in a dose-dependent way. Maximal reversal was observed at a concentration of 0.5μg/ml. The effect was most pronounced in Vero cells (Fig.2,B), whereas in T84 and MDCK cells the effect was minimal. Increasing the concentration of nocodazole above 2μg/ml impairedthe effect because of strongly reduced cell viability.

3.3 Time dependence of the BFA-, Exo1-and nocodazole-induced reversal of the inhibitory effect of Cbz-Gly-Phe-NH_2on CTaction in Vero cells

As depicted in Fig.3 BFA (2μg/ml), Exo1 (2μM) and nocodazole (1μg/ml) caused a rapid increase in the cAMP concentration after CT had accumulated in an intracellular compartment in the presence of Cbz-Gly-Phe-NH_2 (3mM). Already within 1 min after the addition of each drug a significant increase in cAMP accumulation could be observed and after a 5 to 10 min time period the cAMP concentration reached its maximal value. This time course is similar to that observed for the redistribution of Golgi membranes into the ER (Lippincott-Schwartz et al., 1989; Feng et al., 2003; Sciaky et al., 1997)and indicates that once CT has reached the Golgi, the BFA-, Exo1-or nocodazole-induced redistribution of Golgi membranes and content into the ER is followed by a very fast activation of the adenylyl cyclase.Thisimplies that within approximately one minute a fraction of the toxin reaches the ER, becomes activated by reduction, translocates into the cytosol and gains access to its substrate the $G_{S\alpha}$subunit of G_S, which finally activates the cyclase after mono-ADP ribosylation.

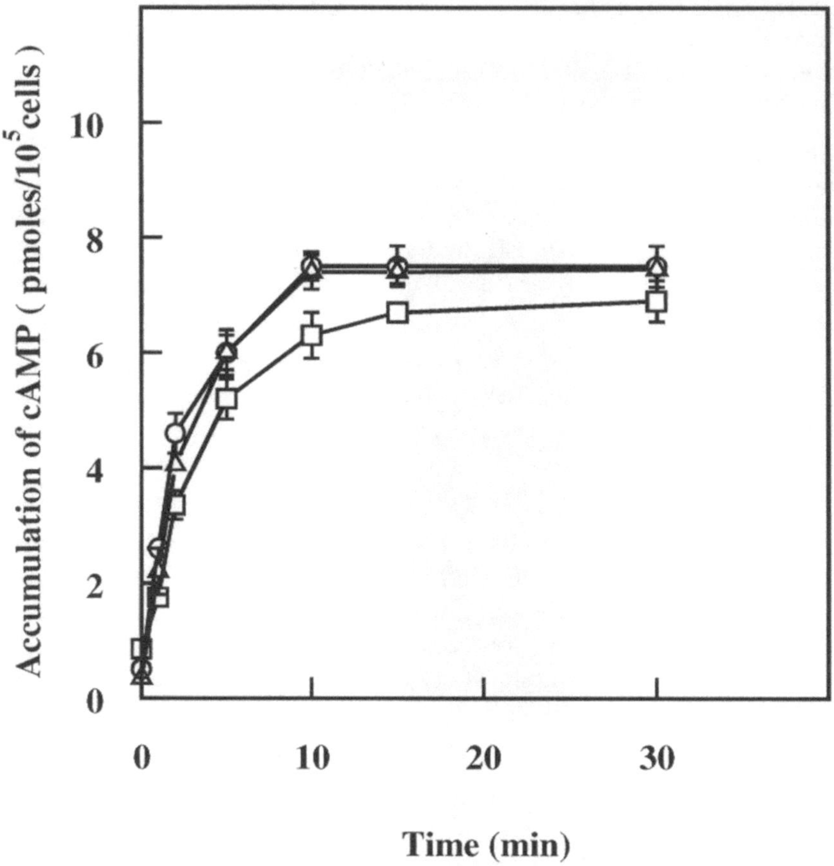

Fig. 3. Time dependence of the BFA-, Exo1- and nocodazole-induced reversal of the inhibitory effect of Cbz-Gly-Phe-NH_2 on the CT-induced accumulation of cAMP in Vero cells. Vero cells in suspension were preincubated with Cbz-Gly-Phe-NH_2 (3mM) for 30 min at 37°C. After the addition of CT (1μg/ml) cells were further incubated for 60 min at 37°C. Subsequently, BFA (2μg/ml) (○), Exo1 (2μM) (△) and nocodazole (1μg/ml) (□) were added and the cells incubated for the indicated times followed by a determination of cAMP. Data points are the means of triplicate assays from one of at least three similar experiments.

Therefore we assume that, at least in the presence of Cbz-Gly-Phe-NH_2,CT also becomes activated at the level of the Golgi apparatus, and that in the ER the A_1 fragment is rapidly translocated into the cytosol. A generation of CT-A_1 at the level of the Golgi complex is in line with our previous observation (De Wolf, 2000)that in the presence of Cbz-Gly-Phe-NH_2 (3mM), CT-A_1 can still be formed. Furthermore, in this study we found that upon direct quantitation of the amount of CT-A_1 generated, the BFA-induced redistribution of Golgi membranes into the ER did not increase the fraction of CT-A that became reduced in cells pretreated with Cbz-Gly-Phe-NH_2 (3mM) (data not shown).

Likewise, the BFA-induced reversal of the inhibitory effect ofCbz-Gly-Phe-NH_2on the CT action was hardly affected by the addition of agents that are able to change the redox potential of the ER and affect the unfolding of CT and the generation of CT-A_1 fragment

(Tsai and Rapoport, 2002). As shown in Table I, incubation of cells with 5mM dithiothreitol (DTT), a reducing agent known to permeate into the ER of intact cells (Braakman et al., 1992)or the oxidant diamide (0.5mM),did almost not influence the BFA-induced reversal of the inhibitory effect ofCbz-Gly-Phe-NH_2. Also, the membrane-permeant sulfhydryl blocker NEM, which at a concentration of 10μM has been shown to completely inhibit the reduction of CT to CT-A_1 by intact CaCo-2 cells (Orlandi, 1997),had only a minor effect on the BFA-induced restoration of CT toxicity in the presence of Cbz-Gly-Phe-NH_2 (Table I).

Treatment	Accumulation of cAMP
	pmoles/10^5 cells
Control	7.5 ± 0.3
DTT (5mM)	6.7 ± 0.3
Diamide (0.5mM)	7.5 ± 0.3
NEM (0.01mM)	7.4 ± 0.2
NEM (0.1mM)	5.8 ± 0.2
2-deoxy-D-glucose (50mM) + 0.02 % sodium azide	2.0 ± 0.2
Nocodazole (2μM)	7.4 ± 0.3
1,3-cyclohexanebis(methylamine) (2mM)	7.5 ± 0.2
All treatments no BFA added	0.4 ± 0.2

Table 1. Effect of several treatments on the BFA-induced reversal of the inhibitory effect of Cbz-Gly-Phe-NH_2 on CT cytotoxicity. Vero cells in suspension were preincubated for 30 min at 37°C with Cbz-Gly-Phe-NH_2 (3mM). After addition of CT (1μg/ml) cells were further incubated for 60 min at 37°C. The indicated amounts of agents were added and the cells incubated for 15 min at 37°C. Finally, BFA (1μg/ml) wad added and the incubation continued for 30 min at 37°C.

3.4 Kinetics of CT transport in the presence of Cbz-Gly-Phe-NH_2 to a compartment that redistributes into the ER upon addition of BFA

The rapidBFA-induced reversal of the inhibition of CT action by Cbz-Gly-Phe-NH_2 allowed us to estimate the time it takes for CT to reach, in the presence of Cbz-Gly-Phe-NH_2,a compartment that redistributes into the ER following the addition of BFA.

In these experiments, cells (Vero,T84 and MDCK) were preincubated with Cbz-Gly-Phe-NH_2 (3mM) for 30 min at 37°C. CT (1μg/ml) was added and the cells further incubated for the indicated times. Finally, BFA (5μg/ml) was added and the incubation continued for 90 min and cAMP accumulation measured.

As shown in Fig.4, in the presence of Cbz-Gly-Phe-NH_2 substantial amounts of CTreached, within approximately 5 to10 min, a compartment that redistributes into the ER following the addition of BFA.

This time period corresponds to the time needed for CT to reach the Golgi complex, as evidenced by our subcellular fractionation experiments (Fig.1) and previous immunofluorescence studies (Majoul et al., 1996) on Vero cells.

In these experiments theBFA concentration was kept high to induce rapid (within less than 5 min) redistribution of the Golgi lipids and proteins into the ER.

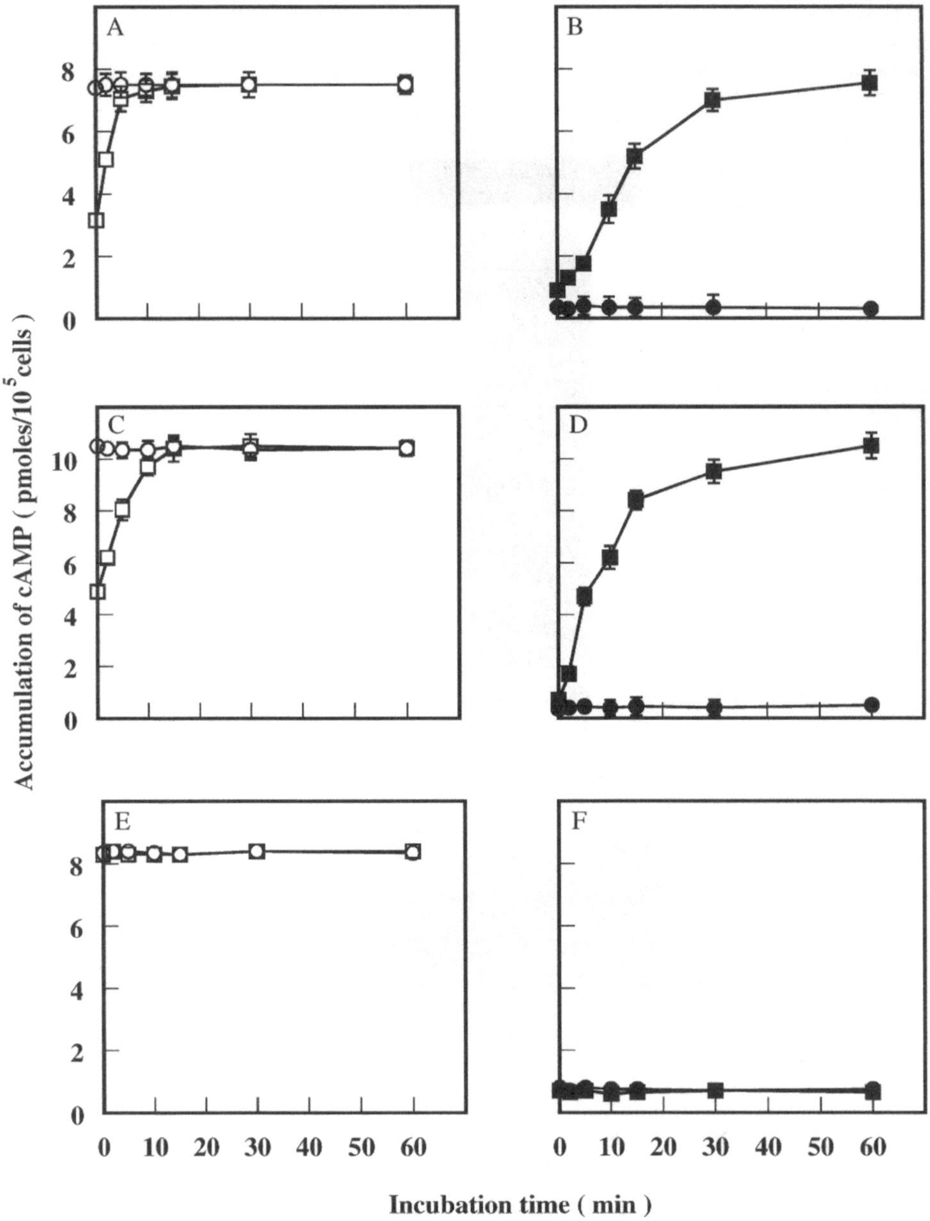

Fig. 4. Kinetics of CT transport in the presence of Cbz-Gly-Phe-NH2 to a compartment which is redistributed to the ER following the addition of BFA. Vero cells (A,B), T84 (C,D) and MDCK cells (E,F) were preincubated with (●,■) and without (○,□) Cbz-Gly-Phe-NH_2 (3mM) for 30 min at 37°C. Subsequently, CT (1μg/ml) was added and the cells incubated at 37°C for the indicated times. Finally, cells were incubated in the presence (□,■) and absence (○,●) of BFA (2μg/ml) for 90 min at 37°C and the cAMP accumulation determined. Values are the means ±SD of triplicate assays from one of three similar experiments. Error bars are indicated when they were more than 5% of the mean.

3.5 Characteristics of the BFA-and Exo1- induced reversal of the inhibition of CT action by Cbz-Gly-Phe-NH_2

It has been shown previously (Lippincott-Schwartz, 1990)that within minutes of adding BFA to most cells, the Golgi apparatus disassembles, giving rise to long, uncoated tubules that extend along microtubules fusing uniquely with the ER. Several treatments have been shown to inhibit this BFA-induced tubule formation. These included AlF_4^-, nocodazole, forskolin and some of its derivatives, reduced temperature and energy depletion (Orlandi, 1997; Majoul et al., 1996; Lippincott-Schwartz, 1990).

In order to further examine whether the BFA- and Exo1-induced reversal of the inhibition of CT action by Cbz-Gly-Phe-NH_2 is related to tubulation and disassembly of the Golgi apparatus, similar treatments affecting Golgi tubule formation were applied.

To this end, Vero cells in suspension were preincubated for 30 min at 37°C with Cbz-Gly-Phe-NH_2 (3mM). Subsequently, CT (1μg/ml) was added and the cells further incubated for 60 min at 37°C. The cells were then treated with the different reagents and finally BFA (1μg/ml) or Exo1 (2μM) wasadded and the incubation continued for 30 min at 37°C and thecAMP content determined.

3.5.1 Effect of AlF_4^-on the BFA- and Exo1- induced reversal of the inhibition of CT action by Cbz-Gly-Phe-NH_2

AlF_4^- stabilizes coatomer binding to Golgi membranes in vitro and in vivo and renders COPI highly resistant to removal by BFA, apparently by inhibition of COPI dissociation(Donaldson et al., 1991a; Finazzi et al., 1994).

The mechanism by which AlF_4^- stabilizes COPI binding is not well understood but probably in-volvestrimeric G-proteins(Donaldson et al., 1991b; Helms et al., 1998). Another possibility is that AlF_4^-locksARF1 in a GDP.AlF_4^-binding transition state together with a limiting cofactor GAP, as shown for other small GTPases,and in this way reduces the overall rate of GTP hydrolysis (Rittinger et al., 1997; Scheffzek et al., 1997).

As shown in Fig.5,A, treatment of Vero cells with 30mM NaF plus 50μM $AlCl_3$ elicted, however, only a minor inhibitory effect on the BFA induced reversal of the inhibition of CT action by Cbz-Gly-Phe-NH_2. This slight reduction of the reversal of the inhibition of CT action by Cbz-Gly-Phe-NH_2 appearedto be cell specific, since it was not observed with T84 cells (data not shown).

It has been reported that AlF_4^-blocks the ability of Exo1 to induce dissociation of membrane-bound ARF^{wt}-GTP from Golgi membranes (Feng et al., 2003). Therefore, we also determined the effect of AlF_4^-on the Exo1-induced reversal of the inhibition of CT action by Cbz-Gly-Phe-NH_2. From Fig.5,A it is clear that AlF_4^-almostcompletely blocked the ability of Exo1 to reverse the effect of Cbz-Gly-Phe-NH_2.

AlF_4^- is able to directly interact with heterotrimeric G-proteins and, as described above, with small GTP binding proteins complexed with specific GTPase activating proteins.

However, the effect of AlF_4^-on the BFA-and Exo1-induced reversal of the inhibitory action of Cbz-Gly-Phe-NH_2 wasmost likely not influenced by an increase of the cAMP level by a direct activation of G_S,since addition of $AlF_4^-$to intact cells hadonly a minor effect on the cAMP level

(Fig.5,B). This is in contrast to its effect on the adenylyl cyclase activity of membrane preparations or crude cell lysates. In addition, CT- induced mono ADP ribosylation of Gs_{α} depends on active ARF1 as a cofactor, therefore, an effect of AlF_4-at the level of ARF1 should also be considered. A previous study (Kahn, 1991), however , has demonstrated that AlF_4^- does not activate ARF1 and does not affect the CT induced mono ADP ribosylation of Gs.

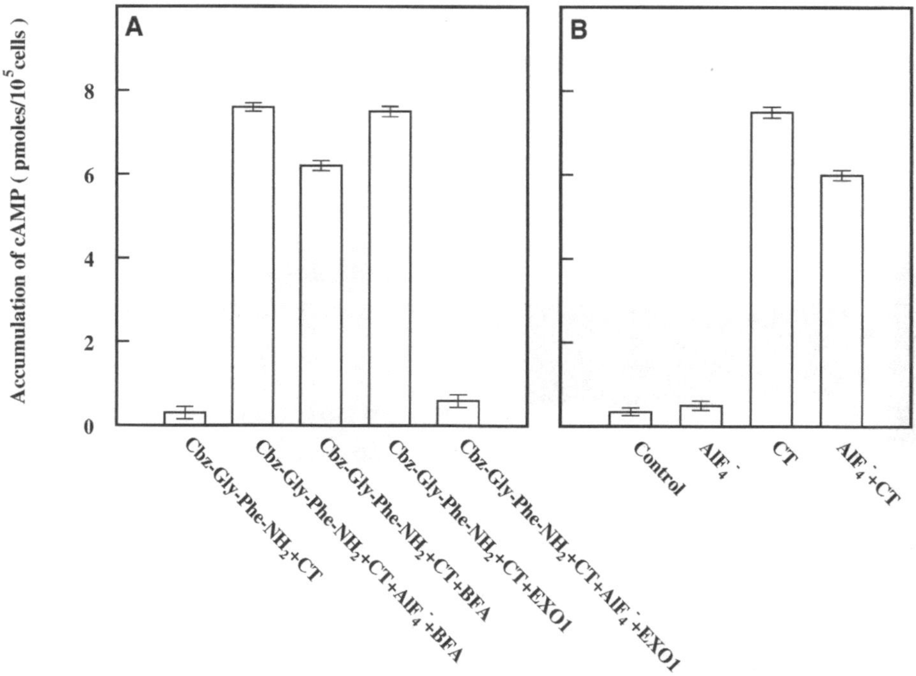

Fig. 5. Effect of AlF4 on the BFA- and Exo1-induced reversal of the inhibition of CT action by Cbz-Gly-Phe-NH2.A. Vero cells in suspension were incubated with Cbz-Gly-Phe-NH2 (3mM) for 30 min at 37°C. CT (1µg/ml) was added and the cells were incubated for an additional 60 min at 37°C. Then cells were further incubated for 15 min at 37°C with and without NaF (30mM) and AlC13 (50µM). Finally cells were treated with BFA (1 µg/ml) or Exo1 (2µM) for 30 min at 37°C and the intracellular concentration of cAMP measured. B. In parallel experiments Vero cells were preincubated with and without NaF (30mM) and AlC13 (50µM) for 15 min at 37°C and further incubated for 60 min at 37°C with or without CT (1mg/ml) and the intracellular concentration of cAMP determined. Values are the means ±SD of triplicate assays from one of three similar experiments. Error bars are indicated when they were more than 5% of the mean.

Furthermore, as shown in Fig.5,B, prior exposure of Vero cells to AlF_4^- did not enhance but rather slightly reduced the CT-induced cAMP accumulation. A similar reduction was observed in the BFA-induced reversal of the inhibition of CT action by Cbz-Gly-Phe-NH_2. Wealso looked whether1,3-cyclohexanebis-(methylamine)(CBM), a drug that interacts with COPI coatomer and inhibits coatomer binding to Golgi membranes (Hu et al., 1999), interferes with the BFA- or Exo1-induced reversal of the inhibition of CT action byCbz-Gly-Phe-NH_2. As shown in Table I, CBM (2mM) had no effect on the BFA- or Exo1-induced reversal of the inhibition of CT action by Cbz-Gly-Phe-NH_2.This dibasic compound itself did also not reverse the inhibitory effect of Cbz-Gly-Phe-NH_2 (data not shown), which is consistent with its inability to cause a redistribution of Golgi membranes into the ER (Hu et al., 1999).

In agreement with previous results (Chen et al., 2002),pre-treatment of Vero cells with CBM (2mM) did not affect the CT-induced elevation of the cAMP level (data not shown).

These experiments indicate that there is no straightforward relationship between COPI dissociation and redistribution of Golgi membranes into the ER and also argue against COPI-and KDEL-dependent functional retrograde transport of CT.

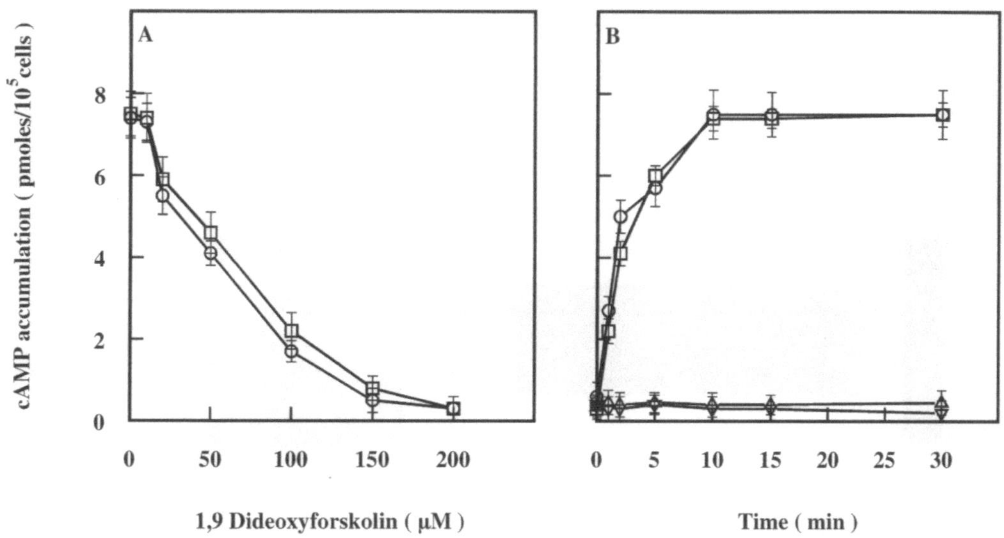

Fig. 6. Effect of 1,9-dideoxyforskolin on the BFA- or Exo1-induced reversal of the inhibition of CT action by Cbz-Gly-Phe-NH2. A. Effect of 1,9-dideoxyforskolin concentration.Vero cells in suspension were preincubated for 30 min at 37°C with Cbz-Gly-Phe-NH2 (3mM). CT (1µg/ml) was added and the cells further incubated for 60 min at 37°C. The indicated amounts of 1,9-dideoxyforskolin were added and after 15 min BFA (1 µg/ml) (O) or Exo1 (2µM) (□) were added and the cells finally incubated for an additional 30 min at 37°C and cAMP accumulation measured. B. Effect of 1,9-dideoxyforskolin on the time courses of the BFA or Exo1 induced reversal of the inhibition of CT action by Cbz-Gly-Phe-NH2.Cells were preincubated as described under A. After CT treatment cells were incubated in the presence and absence of 1,9 dideoxyforskolin (150µM) for 15 min and BFA (1µg/ml) (O,△) or Exo1 (2µM) (□,▽) were added and the cells further incubated at 37°C for the indicated times. Values are the means ±SD of triplicate assays from one of three similar experiments. Error bars are indicated when they were more than 5% of the mean.

3.5.2 Effect of 1,9-dideoxyforskolin on the BFA- and Exo1-induced reversal of the inhibition of CT action byCbz-Gly-Phe-NH_2

It has previously been shown that forskolin inhibits and reverses the effects of BFA on Golgi morphology(Lippincott-Schwartz, 1991a).Also, 1,9-dideoxyforskolin, a naturally occurring analogue of forskolin that does not activate adenylyl cyclase and reproduces many of the cAMP independent effects of forskolin(Laurenza et al., 1989),exerted a similar effect (Lippincott-Schwartz, 1991a). Therefore, it was of interest to look at the effect of 1,9-dideoxyforskolin on the BFA- and Exo1-induced reversal of the inhibition of CT action by Cbz-Gly-Phe-NH_2.

As illustrated in Fig.6,A, the forskolin analogue completely antagonized the effect of BFA or Exo1 on the Cbz-Gly-Phe-NH_2-induced inhibition of CT action in a dose-dependent (IC_{50} ≈60μM) way. The effect of 1,9-dideoxyforskolin was very fast,since after its additionno raise in cAMP level could be observed one minute after the further addition of BFA or Exo1 (Fig.6,B).

3.5.3 Effect of reduced temperature and energy depletion on the BFA-induced reversal of the inhibition of CT action byCbz-Gly-Phe-NH_2

As shownin Table I, reduction in cellular ATP levels using the metabolic inhibitors 2-deoxy-D-glucose (50mM) and sodium azide (0.02%) strongly suppressed the BFA-induced reversal of the inhibition of CT action by Cbz-Gly-Phe-NH_2. Also, lowering the temperature to below 15°C abolished (Fig.7) the BFA-induced restoration of toxicity. The inhibitory effectsof these treatments are in line with their influence on the BFA-induced disassembly of the Golgi apparatus (Lippincott-Schwartz et al., 1990).

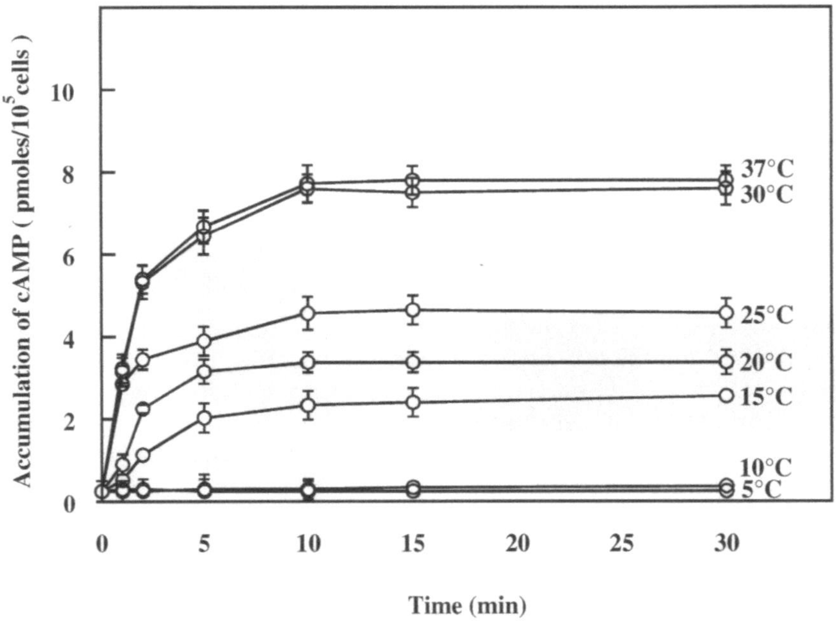

Fig. 7. Temperature dependence of the kinetics of the BFA-induced reversal of the Cbz-Gly-Phe-NH_2-mediated inhibition of CT action on Vero cells. Vero cells in suspension were preincubated with Cbz-Gly-Phe-NH_2 (3mM) for 30 min at 37°C. CT (1μg/ml) was added and the cells further incubated for 60 min at 37°C. Cells were subsequently cooled to the indicated temperatures and after the addition of BFA (5μg/ml) incubated for the indicated times and cAMP measured.Values are the means ±SD of triplicate assays from one of three similar experiments. Error bars are indicated when they were more than 5% of the mean.

4. Discussion

The metalloendoprotease substrate Cbz-Gly-Phe-NH_2, but not its inactive analogue Cbz-Gly-Gly-NH_2, renders cells completely resistant to the action of CT without apparently affecting the binding and internalization of the toxin (De Wolf, 2000).

In this study we further examined the Cbz-Gly-Phe-NH_2-induced inhibition of CT action by looking at the effect of thisdipeptide on the intracellular trafficking of the toxin by using gradient centrifugation experiments and treatment of cells with agents affecting intracellular vesicular transport.

Density gradient centrifugation experiments of post nuclear membranes or supernatants of Vero cells prelabeled with ^{125}I-CT revealed that Cbz-Gly-Phe-NH_2 does not affect the internalization of the toxin but blocks its transport to the ER. Following pretreatment of cells with Cbz-Gly-Phe-NH_2 (3mM) the toxin appears to be trapped in an intracellular compartment, which cofractionates with UDP-galactosyltransferase a marker of the Golgi apparatus.

To further explore whether in the presence of Cbz-Gly-Phe-NH_2 the toxin travels beyond the trans Golgi-network (TGN) and actually reaches cisternae of the Golgi complex, we looked whether drugs known to redistribute Golgi membranes into the ER are also able to cause a reversal of Cbz-Gly-Phe-NH_2-induced inhibition of CT action.

The idea for such an approach came from our previous experiments on the time dependence of the BFA effect on the CT-induced cAMP accumulation in Vero cells (De Wolf, 2000).In these experiments we noticed that addition of BFA 15 min after the addition of CT did not inhibit but rather enhanced the CT-induced increase in the cAMP level. As an explanation we proposed that once the toxin has reached the Golgi complex, the BFA-mediatedredistribution of Golgi membranes into the ER increases the rate of delivery of the toxin to the ER.

In this study we showed that the fungal metabolite brefeldin A (BFA) and a novel chemical inhibitor of anterograde vesicular transport Exo1 are able to completely reverse the Cbz-Gly-Phe-NH_2-induced inhibition of CT action. Both drugs have been shown to cause a rapid release of ADP-ribosylation factor (ARF)1 and COPI from Golgi membranes into the cytosol, followed by massive tubulation and collapse of the Golgi apparatus into the endoplasmic reticulum (Feng et al., 2003; Sciaky et al., 1997; Lippincott-Schwartz et al., 1991a). BFA and to a much lesser extent Exo1 also cause tubulation of the trans-Golgi network (TGN), however, no redistribution of TGN membranes into the ER occurs, instead theyfuse with early and recycling endosomes (Feng et al., 2003; Lippincott-Schwartz et al., 1991b).Therefore, our results indicated that, in the presence of Cbz-Gly-Phe-NH_2, CT is able to travel to the Golgi, however, further retrograde transport to the ER is blocked.

The modes of action of BFA and Exo1, however, appear to be different, as illustrated by the effect of AlF_4^-. Whereas AlF_4^- has only a minor or no effect (depending on the cell type) on the BFA-induced reversal of inhibition of CT action by Cbz-Gly-Phe-NH_2, it completely preventsthe reversal of inhibition by Exo1. This is consistent with earlier observations showing that, whereas AlF_4^- slows but does not prevent the BFA-induced dissociation of ARF1 from Golgi membranes (Feng et al., 2003),it completely blocks the Exo1-induced dissociation of ARF1 from these membranes (Feng et al., 2003).

This agrees with the proposal (Feng et al., 2003)that BFA and Exo1 have different targets. In contrast with BFA, Exo1 appears not to interfere with the activity of guanine nucleotide exchange factors specific for Golgi associated ARF's, but probably acts at a step downstream from the ARF1-GTP loading step, most likely by increasing the rate of GTP hydrolysis through the activation of an ARF-GAP-dependent step (Feng et al., 2003).

The difference in the mechanisms of action of BFA and Exo1 is also apparent from their divergent effects on the action of CT in MDCK cells and reversal of the Cbz-Gly-Phe-NH_2-induced inhibition of CT action in these cells. MDCK cells have a Golgi complex which is resistant to the action of BFA (Hunziker et al., 1991),but apparently,as shown in this study,not to that of Exo1. Kinetic analysis of the BFA- or Exo1-induced reversal of the inhibition of CT action by Cbz-Gly-Phe-NH_2 revealed that the redistribution of Golgi membranes into the ER is a fast process. Furthermore, sincethe toxin-induced increase in cAMP content reached 50%of its maximal levelonly two minutes after the addition of BFA or Exo1, the subsequent steps in toxin action must also be taken very rapidly. Golgi tubules are known to mediate retrograde traffic in cells treated with BFA. In BFA treated cells, Golgi tubules resembling those of untreated cells are observed, but they are formed at a more rapid rate. Moreover, the tubules fail to detach from Golgi structures. This leads to the formation of a dynamic Golgi tubule network within 5-8 min of adding the drug. When one or more of the Golgi tubules fuses with the ER, Golgi membranes redistribute rapidly (within 30 sec) in the ER, leaving no Golgi structure behind (Sciaky et al., 1997).

Since BFA and Exo1, by perturbing ARF1 function and COPI binding, directly interfere with the Golgi to ER retrograde trafficking machinery, we also investigated the effect of the microtubule depolimerizing drug nocodazole. Microtubule disruption by nocodazole is known to block the inward translocation of pre-Golgi intermediates along microtubules without significant effects on the Golgi to ER traffic (Cole et al., 1996),causing a more naturalrecyclingof Golgi components to the ER. As shown in this study,nocodazole also partially reverses the Cbz-Gly-Phe-NH_2 induced inhibition of CT action. The extent of reversal, however, appears to be cell type dependent.

We previously reported (De Wolf, 2000)that whereas Vero cells pretreated with BFA areunable to reduce CT to the CT-A_1 peptide and arecompletely resistant to CT action, treatment of the same cells with Cbz-Gly-Phe-NH_2 only partially reduced their ability to generate the CT-A_1 peptide, although they also become completely insensitive to toxin action. To account for this observation we argued that the total amount of reduced toxin may not reflect toxin that can be translocated to the cytosol, for instance, in the presence of Cbz-Gly-Phe-NH_2, reduced toxin may be trapped in a compartment where translocation to the cytosol is impossible or much less efficient. Several lines of evidence have indicated that a protein-disulfideisomerase (PDI; EC 5.34.1) mediates the reduction of CT-A (Tsai et al., 2001; Orlandi, 1997). This enzyme is found predominantly as a resident soluble protein within the lumen of the ER (Freedman et al., 1989),but has also been ascribed to the Golgi apparatus (Taylor and Varandani, 1985), the trans-Golgi network and the plasma membrane of mammalian cells (Varandani et al., 1978). Our results indicated that at least in the presence of Cbz-Gly-Phe-NH_2, CT can be reduced and thus activated at the level of the Golgi complex. Modifications of CT structure at the level of the Golgi complex have been reported previously (Bastiaens et al., 1996). In this study evidence waspresented indicating that CT-A dissociates from CT-B in the Golgi, after which CT-A is transported in oxidized form to the ER via a KDEL-dependent mechanism. Reduction of CT in an intermediate compartment before reaching the Golgi is unlikely, since in the presence of BFA, which as Cbz-Gly-Phe-NH_2 does not impair the binding and internalization of CT, no reduction of CT-A occurs. Conditions prevailing in the Golgi (lower pH, less oxidizing) may also be favourable for the reduction of CT-A. For instance, it has been shown that in vitro the PDI mediated reduction of CT-A is maximalat a pH 5.5-6.0 (Tsai et al., 2001).

Previous studies (Lippincott-Schwartz et al., 1991a)have reported that forskolin inhibits and even reverses the effects of BFA on Golgi structure. These effects arealso reproduced by 1,9-dideoxyforskolin, a naturally occurring analogue of forskolin that does not activate adenylyl cyclase(Laurenza et al., 1989). In this study we demonstrated that 1,9-dideoxyforskolin also antagonizes the effect of BFA on the Cbz-Gly-Phe-NH_2-induced inhibition of CT action in a dose-dependent way. It has been speculated that forskolin interferes with the action of BFA by (competition)/competing for the binding of BFA to its target protein, the Golgi-localized nucleotide exchange factor specific for ARF1(Lippincott-Schwartz et al., 1991a). A subsequent study (Nickel et al., 1996), however, showed that in vitro forskolin does not prevent inhibition of Golgi-catalyzed nucleotide exchange by BFA. Therefore, it was concluded that it is unlikely that forskolin and BFA bind to the same target protein. Forskolin treatment of CHO cells, however, resultsin increased levels of Cys-BFA, the major BFA conjugate secreted by CHO cells, in the medium, which led to the suggestion that the effect of forskolin on BFA-induced disassembly of the Golgi apparatus might be due to an enhanced detoxification of the drug. The present results do not favor this hypothesis, since 1,9-dideoxyforskolin also blocks the Exo1-induced reversal of the inhibition of CT action by Cbz-Gly-Phe-NH_2. In addition,the fast action of 1,9-dideoxyforskolin is difficult to reconcile with the proposed enhanced detoxification and removal of BFA. In this light it is also interesting to note that forskolin also prevents the redistribution of Golgi membranesinto the ER, induced by the Epidermal-cell differentiation inhibitor (EDIN), an exoenzyme (ADP-ribosyltransferase) produced by Staphylococcus aureus with a substrate specificity of the rho protein (Sugai et al., 1992). Therefore, it is clear that forskolin inhibits the action of structurally totally unrelated compounds, which all cause disassembly of the Golgi complex. The exact target and mechanism of action of forskolin and its derivatives in this phenomenon therefore remains to be defined.

Taken together, the results of this study are in agreement with the view that intoxication by CT requires retrograde transport of CT from the plasma membrane to the ER, involving passage through the TGN and Golgi apparatus. A direct transport from the TGN to the ER as recently proposed (Feng et al., 2004)is unlikely since Cbz-Gly-Phe-NH_2 and Exo1 completely abolish toxicity,whereastransport of the toxin to the TGN still occurs. We also demonstrated that the metalloendoprotease substrate blocks the retrograde transport of CT from the Golgi complex to the ER. Therefore,metalloendoproteases may not only play a role in vesicular transport and secretion of newly synthesized proteins as previously proposed (Lennarz and Strittmatter, 1991),but may also be involved in retrograde transport between the Golgi and the ER. Finally, we also showed that successive addition of two strong inhibitors of CT action at the appropriate time points can annihilate their inhibitory effects.

5. Acknowledgment

I thank R. Goossens for skilled technical assistance.

6. References

Bastiaens PIH, Majoul IV, Verveer PJ, Söling H-D, Jovin TM.Imaging the intracellular trafficking and state of the AB5 quaternary structure of cholera toxin.EMBO J1196; 15:4246 - 53.

Braakman I, Helenius J, Helenius A. Manipulating disulfide bond formation and protein folding in the endoplasmic reticulum. EMBO J1992; 11:1717 - 22.

Bradford MM.A rapid and sensitive method for the quantitation of microgram quantities of protein utilizing the principle of protein-dye binding. Anal Biochem. 1976; 72:248 - 54.

Chen A, Hu T, Miroyak C, Draper RK. Retrograde transport of protein toxins under conditions of COPI dysfunction.BiochimBiophysActa2002; 1589:124 - 39.

Cole NB, Sciaky N, Marotta A, Song J, Lippincott-Schwartz J. Golgi dispersal during microtubule disruption: regeneration of Golgi stacks at peripheral endoplasmic reticulum exit sites. MolBiol Cell1996; 7:631 - 50.

de Haan L, Hirst TR. Cholera toxin: a paradigm for multi-functional engagement of cellular mechanisms (Review).Mol MembrBiol. 2000; 21:77 - 92.

De Wolf MJS, Van Dessel GAF, Lagrou AR, Hilderson HJJ, Dierick WSH. Topography, purification and characterization of thyroidal NAD+ glycohydrolase.Biochem J1985; 226:415-27.

De Wolf MJS.A dipeptide metalloendoprotease substrate completely blocks the response of cells in culture to cholera toxin. J BiolChem.2000; 275:30240 - 7.

Doms RW, Russ G, Yewdell JW. Brefeldin A redistributes resident and itinerant Golgi proteins to the endoplasmic reticulum.J Cell Biol.1989; 109:61-72.

Donaldson JG, Lippincott-Schwartz J, Klausner RD.Guanine nucleotides modulate the effects of brefeldin A in semipermeable cells: regulation of the association of a 110-kD peripheral membrane protein with the Golgi apparatus. J Cell Biol.1991a; 112:579 - 88.

Donaldson JG, Kahn RA, Lippincott-Schwartz J, Klausner RD. Binding of ARF and beta-COP to Golgi membranes: possible regulation by a trimeric G protein. Science1991b; 254:1197 - 9.

Feng Y, Yu S, Lasell TKR, Jadhav AP, Macia E, Chardin P et al. Exo1: a new chemical inhibitor of the exocytic pathway. ProcNatlAcad Sci. USA2003; 100:6469 - 74.

Feng Y, Jadhav AP, Rodighiero C, Fujinaga Y, Kirchausen T, Lencer WI. Retrograde transport of cholera toxin from the plasma membrane to the endoplasmic reticulum requires the trans-Golgi network but not the Golgi apparatus in Exo2-treated cells. EMBO reports2004; 5:596-601.

Finazzi D, Cassel D, Donaldson JG, Klausner RD. Aluminum fluoride acts on the reversibility of ARF1-dependent coat protein binding to Golgi membranes.J Biol Chem.1994; 269:13325 - 30.

Fraker PJ,Speck JC.Protein and cell membrane iodinations with a sparingly soluble chloroamide, 1,3,4,6-tetrachloro-3a,6a-diphrenylglycoluril. BiochemBiophys Res Commun 1978;80:849 - 57.

Freedman RB, Bulleid NJ, Hawkins HC, Paver JL.Role of protein disulphide-isomerase in the expression of native proteins.BiochemSocSymp1989; 55:167 - 92.

Fujinaga Y, Wolf AA, Rodighiero C,Wheeler H, Tsai B, Allen L et al. Gangliosides that associate with lipid rafts mediate transport of cholera and related toxins from the plasma membrane to endoplasmic reticulum.Mol BiolCell2003; 14:4783-93.

Graham J, Ford T,Rickwood D. The preparation of subcellular organelles from mouse liver in self-generated gradients of iodixanol. Anal Biochem.1994; 220:367 - 73.

Helms JB, Helms-Brons D, Brüger B, Gkanteragas I, Eberle H, Nickel W et al. A putative heterotrimeric G protein inhibits the fusion of COPI-coated vesicles. Segregation of heterotrimeric G proteins from COPI-coated vesicles. J BiolChem 1998; 273:15203 – 8.

Hu T, Kao C-Y, Hudson RT, Chen A, Draper RK.Inhibition of secretion by 1,3-cyclohexanebis(methylamine), a dibasic compound that interferes with coatomer function.MolBiol Cell1999; 10:921 – 33.

Hunziker W, Whitney JW, Mellman I.Selective inhibition of transcytosis by brefeldin A in MDCK cells. Cell 1991;67:617 – 27.

Kahn RA. Fluoride is not an activator of the smaller (20-25 kDa) GTP-binding proteins.J BiolChem1991; 266:15595 – 7.

Kassis S, Hagmann J, Fishman PH, Chang PP. Moss J.Mechanism of action of cholera toxin on intact cells. Generation of A1 peptide and activation of adenylatecyclise.J BiolChem1982; 257:12148-52.

Klausner RD, Donaldson JG, Lippincott-Schwartz J. Brefeldin A: insights into the control of membrane traffic and organelle structure. J Cell Biol 1992;116:1071-80.

Laurenza A, Sutkowski EM, Seamon KB. Forskolin: a specific stimulator of adenylyl cyclase or a diterpene with multiple sites of action?Trends PharmacolSci 1989; 10:442 – 7.

Lencer WI, de Almeida JB, Moe S, Stow JL, Ausiello DA, Madara JL.Entry of cholera toxin into polarized human intestinal epithelial cells. Identification of an early brefeldin A sensitive event required for A1-peptide generation. J Clin Invest.1993; 92:2941-51.

Lencer WI, Hirst TR, Holmes RK.Membrane traffic and the cellular uptake of cholera toxin.BiochimBiophysActa 1999; 1450:177-90.

Lennarz WJ, Strittmatter WJ. Cellular functions of metallo-endoproteinases. BiochemBiophysActa1991; 1071:149 – 58.

Lippincott-Schwartz J, Yuan LC, Bonifacino JS, Klausner RD. Rapid redistribution of Golgi proteins into the ER in cells treated with brefeldin A: evidence for membrane cycling from Golgi to ER. Cell1989; 56:801 - 13.

Lippincott-Schwartz J, Donaldson JG, Schweizer A, Berger EG, Houri H-P, Yuan LC,Klausner RD. Microtubule-dependent retrograde transport of proteins into the ER in the presence of brefeldin A suggests an ER recycling pathway. Cell1990; 60:821 – 36.

Lippincott-Schwartz J, Glickman J, Donaldson JG, Robbins J, Kreis TE, Seamon KB et al. Forskolin inhibits and reverses the effects of brefeldin A on Golgi morphology by a cAMP-independent mechanism. J Cell Biol1991a; 112:567 – 77.

Lippincott-Schwartz J, Yuan L, Tipper C, Amherdt M, Orci L, Klausner RD. Brefeldin A's effects on endosomes, lysosomes, and the TGN suggest a general mechanism for regulating organelle structure and membrane traffic. Cell1991b; 67:601 – 16.

Majoul IV, Bastiaens PIH, Söling H-D. Transport of an external Lys-Asp-Glu-Leu (KDEL) protein from the plasma membrane to the endoplasmic reticulum: studies with cholera toxin in Vero cells. J Cell Biol.1996; 133:777 – 89.

Majoul I, Sohn K, Wieland FT, Pepperkok R, Pizza M, Hillemann J, Söling H-D. KDEL receptor (Erd2p)-mediated retrograde transport of the cholera toxin A subunit from the Golgi involves COPI, p23, and the COOH terminus of Erd2p. J Cell Biol.1998; 143:601-12.

Massol RH, Larsen JE, Fujinaga Y, Lencer WI, Kirchhausen T. Cholera toxin toxicity does not require functional Arf6- and dynamin-dependent endocytic pathways.MolBiol Cell 2004; 15:3631-41.

Nambiar M, Oda T, Chen C, Kuwazuru Y, Wu HC. Involvement of the Golgi region in the intracellular trafficking of cholera toxin. J Cell Physiol.1993; 154:222-8.

Nichols BJ, Kenworthy AK, Polishchuk RS,Lodge R, Roberts TH,Hirshberg K, Phair RD, Lippincott-Schwartz J.Rapid cycling of lipid raft markers between the cell surface and Golgi complex. J Cell Biol.2001; 153:529-41.

Nichols BJ.A distinct class of endosome mediates clathrin-independent endocytosis to the Golgi complex. Nat Cell Biol.2002; 4:374-8.

Nickel W, Helms JB, Kneusel RE, Wieland FT. Forskolin stimulates detoxification of brefeldin A. J Biol Chem. 1996; 271:15870 - 73.

Orlandi PA, Curran PK, Fishman PH. Brefeldin A blocks the response of cultured cells to cholera toxin. Implications for intracellular trafficking in toxin action. J BiolChem 1993;268:12010-16.

Orlandi PA. Protein-disulfideisomerase-mediated reduction of the A subunit of cholera toxin in a human intestinal cell line. J Biol Chem.1997; 272:4591 – 9.

Orlandi PA, Fishman PH. Filipin-dependent inhibition of cholera toxin: evidence for toxin internalization and activation through caveolae-like domains. J Cell Biol 1998;141:905-15.

Richards AA, Stang E,Pepperkok R, Parton RG.Inhibitors of COP-mediated transport and cholera toxin action inhibit simian virus 40 infection.MolBiol Cell 2002; 13:1750-64.

Rittinger K, Walker PA, Eccleston JF, Smerdon SJ, Gamblin SJ. Structure at 1.65 A of RhoA and its GTPase-activating protein in complex with a transition-state analogue.Nature1997; 389:758 – 62.

Rodighiero C, Tsai B, Rapoport TA, Lencer WI. Role of ubiquitination in retro-translocation of cholera toxin and escape of cytosolic degradation.EMBO Rep2002; 3: 1222 – 7.

Scheffzek K, Ahmadian MR, Kabsch W, Wiesmuller L, Lautwein A, Schmitz F, Wittinghofer A. The Ras-RasGAP complex: structural basis for GTPase activation and its loss in oncogenic Ras mutants. Science1997; 277:333 – 8.

Schmitz A, Herrgen H, Winkeler A, Herzog V. Cholera toxin is exported from microsomes by the Sec61p complex. J CellBiol.2000; 148:1203 – 12.

Sciaky N, Presley J, Smith C, Zaal KJM, Cole N, Moreira JE et al. Golgi tubule traffic and the effects of brefeldin A visualized in living cells. J Cell Biol.1997; 139:1137 – 55.

Shogomori H, Futerman AH.Cholera toxin is found in detergent-insoluble rafts/domains at the cell surface of hippocampal neurons but is internalized via a raft-independent mechanism. J BiolChem. 2001; 276:9182 - 8.

Sixma TK, Pronk SE, Kalk KH, Wartna ES, Van Zanten BAM, Witholt B, Hol WGJ. Crystal structure of a cholera toxin-related heat-labile enterotoxin from E. coli. Nature1991; 351:371 - 7.

Spangler BD. Structure and function of cholera toxin and the related Escherichia coli heat-labile enterotoxin.Microbiol Rev 1992; 56:622 - 47.

Storrie B, White J, Röttger S, Stelzer EHK, Suganuma T, Nilsson T. Recycling of golgi-resident glycosyltransferases through the ER reveals a novel pathway and provides an explanation for nocodazole-induced Golgi scattering. J Cell Biol. 1998; 143: 1505 – 21.

Sugai M, Chen C-H, Wu HC. Bacterial ADP-ribosyltransferase with a substrate specificity of the rho protein disassembles the Golgi apparatus in Vero cells and mimics the action of brefeldin A.ProcNatlAcadSci USA1992; 89:8903 – 7.

Taylor CA, Varandani PT. Localization of glutathione-insulin transhydrogenase (protein-disulfide interchange enzyme) in pancreas using immunocytochemistry, immunodiffusion, and enzymatic activity assay techniques. Eur J Cell Biol. 1985;39:97-102.

Torgersen ML, Skretting G, van Deurs B, Sandvig K. Internalization of cholera toxin by different endocytic mechanisms. J Cell Sci. 2001; 114:3737 - 47.

Tran D, Carpentier JL, Sawano F, Gorden P, Orci L.Ligands internalized through coated or noncoated invaginations follow a common intracellular pathway. ProcNatlAcadSci USA. 1987;84:7957-61.

Tsai B, Rodighiero C, Lencer WI, Rapoport T.Protein disulfideisomerase acts as a redox-dependent chaperone to unfold cholera toxin.Cell2001; 104:937-48.

Tsai B, Rapoport T. Unfolded cholera toxin is transferred to the ER membrane and released from protein disulfideisomerase upon oxidation by Ero1. J CellBiol.2002 ; 159:207-15.

Tuszynski GP, Knight L, Piperno JR, Walsh PN. A rapid method for removal of [125I]iodide following iodination of protein solutions. AnalBiochem. 1980; 106:118 – 22.

Vanden Broeck D, Horvath C,De Wolf MJS.Vibrio cholerae: cholera toxin. Int J Biochem Cell Biol 2007a; 39:1771-5.

Vanden Broeck D, Lagrou AR, De Wolf MJS. Distinct role for clathrin-mediated endocytosis in the uptake of cholera toxin. ActaBiochimicaPolonica 2007b; 54:757 - 67.

Varandani PT, Raveed D, Nafz MA. Insulin degradation. XXIII. Distribution of glutathione-insulin transhydrogenase in isolated rat hepatocytes as studied by immuno-ferritin and electron microscopy. BiochimBiophysActa1978; 538:343 – 53.

Verdon B, Berger EG. Methods Enzymol Anal. 1983; 3:374 - 81.

Wolf AA, Fujinaga Y,Lencer WI.Uncoupling of the cholera toxin-G(M1) ganglioside receptor complex from endocytosis, retrograde Golgi trafficking, and downstream signal transduction by depletion of membrane cholesterol. J Biol Chem.2002; 277:16249-56.

Wolf AA, Jobling MG, Wimer-Mackin S, Ferguson-Maltzman M, Madara JL, Holmes RK, Lencer WI.Ganglioside Structure Dictates Signal Transduction by Cholera Toxin and Association with Caveolae-like Membrane Domains in Polarized Epithelia. J Cell Biol.1998; 141:917-27.

Zhang R-G, Scott DL,Westbrook ML, Nance S, Spangler BD, Shipley GG. Westbrook EM.The three-dimensional crystal structure of cholera toxin. J Mol Biol.1995; 251:563- 73.

9

Structure Based Design of Cholera Toxin Antagonists

Črtomir Podlipnik[1] and Jose J. Reina[2]
[1]*Faculty of Chemistry and Chemical Technology, University of Ljubljana*
[2]*Department of Organic and IndustrialChemistry, University of Milano*
[1]*Slovenia*
[2]*Italy*

1. Introduction

Cholera is an acute enteric infection, with huge pandemic potential, caused by ingestion of food or water contaminated with the bacterium *Vibrio cholerae*, the gram negative bacteria (Sack, Sack et al. 2004). The etiologic agent responsible for cholera was identified in 1883 when Robert Koch demonstrated that comma(-shaped) bacteria, later designated as *V. cholerae*, causes cholera infection (Koch 1884). Since Koch's discovery of cholera virulent factor, different specific strain variants of *V. cholerae* have been identified. For the majority of cholera's disease outbreaks two biotypes of *V. cholerae*'sserogroup O1 are responsible: Clasical and "El Tor", as well serogroup O139 that was responsible for a large epidemic in Bangladesh and India (Ramamurthy, Garg et al. 1993). Non-O1 and non-O139 *V. cholerae* can cause mild diarrhoea but do not generate epidemics (Ramamurthy, Bag et al. 1993). Cholera transmission is closely related to inadequate environmental conditions that can be find in suburban slums where the basic infrastructure is not available, as well as in camps for internally displaced people or refugees, where minimum requirements of clean water and sanitation are not met. A typical example of such non-promising situation has induced an outbreak of Cholera after earthquake in Haiti in January 2010 (Andrews and Basu 2011). The short incubation period of two hours to five days, enhances the potentially explosive pattern of outbreaks. Intensive efforts for the identification of the basis of Cholera disease at a molecular level were done by different research groups during the 1960s, until Finkelstein and co-workers recognized a protein toxin as a major virulent factor that causes the massive fluid release in Cholera infection (Finkelstein, Atthasampunna et al. 1966). The efforts to solve a complete structure of Cholera toxin by X-ray diffraction analysis were concluded during the 1990s (Spangler 1992; Zhang, Scott et al. 1995). Up to date, 27 X-ray structures related to Cholera toxin (CT) are deposited in the Protein Databank. The structure and function of CT at the molecular level will be the subject of our review. In this work we will also show some examples of structure based design of various types of CT inhibitors; we will introduce catechin-like compounds as inhibitors of the enzymatic A unit of CT; mimics of oGM1 as inhibitors of the non-toxic pentamer of B subunits of CT (CTB); as well as multivalent inhibitors that very effectively prevent adhesion of CTB to GM1 receptors at the surface of epithelial cells. At the end, we will also describe a new strategy for developing inhibitors via targeting binding site for blood group antigens in Cholera Toxin.

2. Cholera toxin – structure and mode of action

Cholera toxin (CT) belongs to the family of AB_5 bacterial toxins, which includes CT itself and the *Escherichia coli* heat-labile toxins (LTs) LT-I and LT-II, among others. This family of bacterial toxins is named after the characteristic architecture comprising a single catalytically active component, A, and a non-toxic pentamer of B subunits (B_5) (Fig. 1a). The structure and function of AB_5 toxins have been reviewed in detail on several occasions (Bernardi, Podlipnik et al. 2006; Hol, Fan et al. 2004; Hayes, Turnbull 2011).

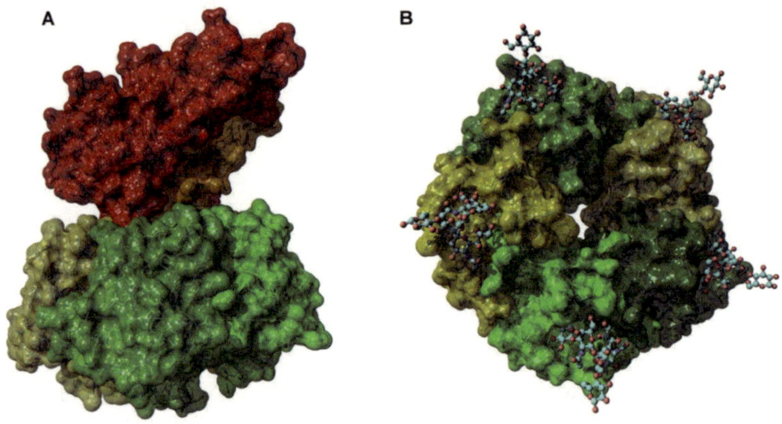

Fig. 1. (A) Holotoxin CT and (B) pentamer B complexed with oGM1.

The A subunit of CT is composed of two distinct parts A_1 and A_2. The A_1 component is responsible for the toxic enzyme activity, while the A_2 component serves as non-covalent linker of subunit A to subunit B. Each of five CT's B-subunits is composed from two α helices and two three-stranded β sheets, that form together a doughnut-shaped structure, which has a central pore into which the C-terminal of A_2 subunit extends. The B pentamer is responsible for binding CT to ganglioside GM1 on the external membrane of intestinal epithelial cells. This binding is recognized as a key event for initiation of the threatening action of CT. The interaction of the oligosaccharidic head groups of ganglioside GM1 (Galβ1-3GalNAcβ1-4(NeuAcα2-3)Galβ1-4Glcβ1-OH,oGM1) with B_5 unit of CT is depicted in Fig. 1b. It is interesting that the binding ability of the B-pentamer to cell surface receptors is retained even in absence of the A-subunit. However, the complete AB_5 holotoxin is needed for actual intoxication.

The B pentamer of CT (CTB) interacts with the soluble, monovalent oligosaccharide portion of GM1 (oGM1) with strong affinity, the binding process is weakly cooperative. The close view of the interaction based on 1.25 Å resolution structure of oGM1:CTB complex (Merritt, Sarfaty et al. 1994) is shown in Fig 2b. We may observe that branched oGM1 (Fig 3) is attached to CTB binding site with two fingers: the first one is a sialic acid "thumb" and the second one a GalB(1->3)GalNAc "forefinger" (two-fingered grip). Most of the contacts are given by the "finger" tips: in terms of buried protein surface, the terminal Gal and Neu5Ac residues contribute 39% and 43%, the rest and minor part of protein surface is buried with GalNAc. The most recent value of the dissociation constant for interaction between one oGM1 and one CTB binding site has been evaluated by Isothermal Titration Calorimetry (ITC) and it was found to be 43 nM (Turnbull, Precious et al. 2004), this is one of the strongest known protein-carbohydrate interaction. It has been also observed that all of the mono- or disaccharide fragments of oGM1 bind to CTB much more weakly; for example, the terminal galactose residue displays K_d=15 mM, which is in the case of the Gal-GalNAc forefinger improved by only a factor of two.

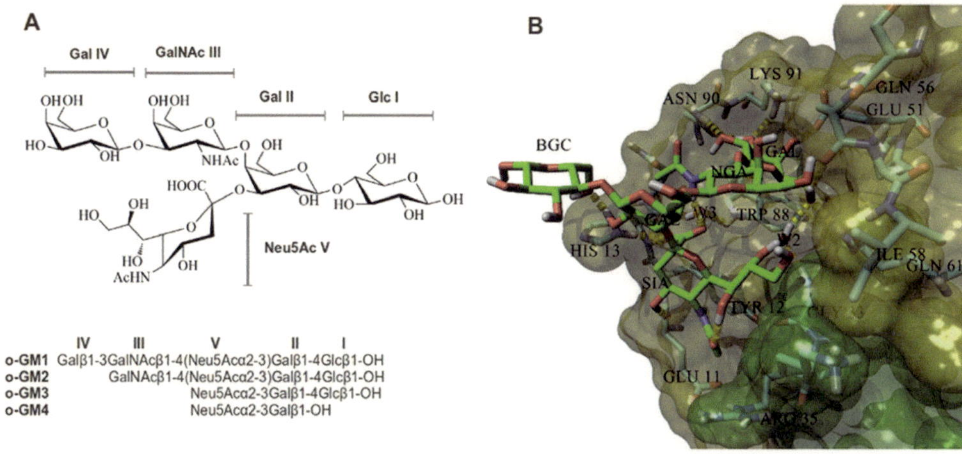

Fig. 2. (A) *Structure of ganglioside head groups. (B)* Close view of CTB:oGM1 interaction.

The other important binding determinant, Neu5Ac, binds even more weakly to the protein (K_d ≈ 200 mM). The analysis of results obtained by dissecting of the oGM1:CTB interaction by ITC has shown that high affinity and selectivity of oGM1:CTB interaction originates mainly from the conformational pre-organisation of the branched GM1 pentasaccharide rather than through the effect of cooperativity of terminal moieties galactose and sialic acid. The terminal galactose residue in the "forefinger" binds to the CTB binding site very specifically. The pyranose ring of this galactose is stacked on top of Trp88 (CH/pi interaction) and forms an extensive hydrogen bond network involving Asn90, Lys91, Glu51 and Gln61 residues from CTB_5. The terminal galactose is docked in a deep cavity that is shielded from the solvent, on the other hand the rest of the toxin's binding site is shallow and solvent exposed. The sialic acid (Neu5Ac) represents the second important moiety of GM1 required for recognition of Cholera toxin. The sugar ring of sialic acid makes hydrophobic interaction with Tyr12, whereas hydroxyl, and N-acetyl substituents form hydrogen bonds with CTB residues, while carboxyl group forms water-mediated hydrogen bond with Trp88.

The action of CT is initiated by binding of CT via the B_5 pentamer to GM1s receptors that are part of the external membrane of intestinal epithelial cells. When CT binds to the cell, the whole toxin is transferred into the cell via receptor-mediated endocytosis. The toxin is then transported to the endoplasmic reticulum (ER), where A subunit dissociates from the rest of the protein assembly. Subunit A is then split to subunits A_1 and A_2 by peptide-disulfide isomerase in the ER. Subunit A_1 is then translocated to the cytosol of the host cell, where it catalyses the covalent transfer of an ADP-ribose moiety from NAD^+ to Arg201 of the signalling protein $G_{s\alpha}$ (a component of an adenylate cyclase system). Adenylate cyclase system is normally activated by a regulatory protein G_s and GTP; however the activation is normally brief, because another regulatory protein (G_i) hydrolyses GTP. The normal situation is described in Fig 3a. Cholera toxin catalyses transfer of ADP to adenyl cyclase cycle. Ribosylated form of G_s stabilizes the GTP bound form of protein, which stays continually activated (Cassel and Pfeuffer 1978). This situation is shown in Fig 3b.

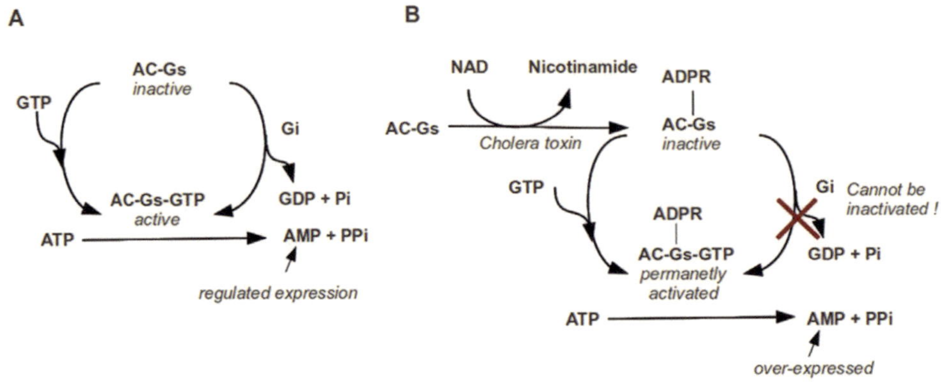

Fig. 3. Action of enzymatic unit of Cholera Toxin. (A) Normal action. (B) Permanent activation of Adenylate cyclase system.

This modification of the adenylate cyclase system results in an elevated level of AMP which causes the activation of the sodium pumps in the lumen of the cells through an AMP-dependent kinase pathway, forcing the Na^+ ions out. The electrochemical imbalance is then compensated by driving Cl^- and H_2O out of the cells. The process of Cholera Toxin action is followed by enormous loss of water from the epithelial cells into the intestinal lumen, causing water diarrhoea characteristic for cholera.

It has been shown that A_1 by itself has relatively low enzymatic activity in vitro. The interaction of A_1 with ADP-ribosylation factor (ARF) protein from human host increases the enzymatic activity of A_1. Numerous studies *in vitro* and *in vivo* have indicated the importance of tight interaction between A_1 fragment and ARF. Recent structural investigations of a CTA_1 :ARF_6-GTP complex pointed out that binding of ARF_6-GTP causes dramatic changes in the CTA_1 loop regions that open the binding site for NAD^+ (Hol, O'Neal et al. 2005).

Taking into account structural information and given mechanism of action of CT, three different strategies are possible to design a prophylactic cure against Cholera:

- Inhibition of the action of the catalytically active unit A of CT.
- Design of small molecules that act as a decoys for the toxin's GM1 binding site and thus prevent adhesion of CT to cell membranes of epithelial cells.
- Prevention of assembly of AB_5 complex that takes place in the cytosol.

In further writing, the first two strategies of the development the Cholera toxin inhibitors will be reviewed, with special attention to experience based on our recent work in this field of medicinal chemistry.

3. Natural products as Cholera toxin inhibitors

During the history, traditional healers have prepared medicaments for the treatment (prevention) of Cholera infections from various medicinal plants. The most common ways to administer such natural remedies are infusions or decoctions that are usually compositions of numerous natural products. The active substances from medicinal plants can treat Cholera via different pharmacological mechanisms; from the direct antimicrobial against *V. cholerae*, prevention of adhesion of CT to the GM1 receptors at surface of epithelial cells, to direct inhibition of ADP-ribosylation of active unit of CT. The improved understanding of the CT toxicity at the molecular level and the further set up of modern biological assays, has allowed in recent years the identification of different classes of bioactive natural products. An important class of such products are polyphenols from green and black tea, green apples, hop bract and the Chinese rhubarb rhizome. Garlic extract is another example of traditional cure against diarrhoea diseases such as cholera. Recent researches have recognized a galactan polysaccharide as a major anti-choleric component of garlic (Politi, Alvaro-Blanco et al. 2006). Some interesting natural inhibitors of CT are shown in Fig 4.

Toda *et al.* (1992) reported that polyphenol catechins (EGC, 3, ECG, 4, and EGCG, 5) isolated from green tea have protective function against infection with *V. cholerae* O1. EGCG and ECG also protect against hemolysin (another toxin from *V. cholerae* that causes red blood cell rupture) in a dose dependent manner–the more green tea catechins, the better the protection. Animal studies also showed that these catechins reduced the fluid accumulation (the primary cause of cholera fatality) from CT (Toda, Okubo et al. 1992).

Toda *et al.* (1991) have also suggested that extracts of black tea have anti-bactericidal function against *V. cholerae* O1. The major active components of black tea that could be responsible for protective activity against *V. cholerae* O1 are theaflavin-3,3'-digallate, 9 and thearubigin, 10.

Saito *et al.* (2002) have shown the anti-choleric activity of natural polyphenols extracted from immature apples. They described that the inhibitory effect of apple polyphenols extract (APE) on CT-catalyzed ADP-ribosylation of agmantine is dose-dependent and it is due to the inhibition of the enzymatic activity of the A subunit of CT. The concentration of APE at which 50% of the enzymatic activity of CT (15 μg/ml) is inhibited was approximately 8.7 μg/ml. Bioassay oriented fractionation of APE indicated that the highly polymerized catechins, also named procyanidine polymers, are the major inhibitory components of this apple extract. Other constituents like the non-catechin-type polyphenols (chlorogenic acid, phloridzin, phloretin, caffeic acid, and p-coumaric acid) and the monomeric catechins (catechin and epicatechin) have shown week inhibitory activity. The results indicate that APE disturbs the biological activity of CT *in vivo*, also but not only via inhibition of the enzymatic activity of A-subunit. An additional explanation for the *in vivo* reduction of secretory activity of APE can also be the protection of the intestine's mucosa with polymerized catechins. Procyanidins B1, 6, C2, 7 and tetracatechin, 8 representative structures from Saito study are shown in Fig. 4.

Hor *et al.* (1995) also reported *in vivo* CTA inhibitory activity of proantho-cyanidines extracted from *Guazuma ulimfolia,* a medicinal plant used in Mexico for traditional treatment of diarrhoea.

Oi *et al.* (2002) studied the bioactivity of rhubarb galloyl tannin (RG-tannin), a compound isolated from *Rhei rhizome,* against CT activities including ADP-ribosylation and fluid accumulation. This kind of heterologuos polyphenol gallate inhibits fluid accumulation in mouse and rabbit ileal loops that is induced by CT action, as well as catalytic activity of

CTA. It was also observed that RG-tannin, had no effect on the binding of CTB to the ganglioside GM1 or an endogenous ADP-ribosylation of membrane proteins. The authors prepared and tested a small library of synthetic gallates (sugar moieties esterified with galloyl groups) against CTA's ADP-rybosylation activity a small library of synthetic gallates. Some of compounds (12 for example) from their library exhibited strong inhibitory activity of CTAs ADP-ribosylation.

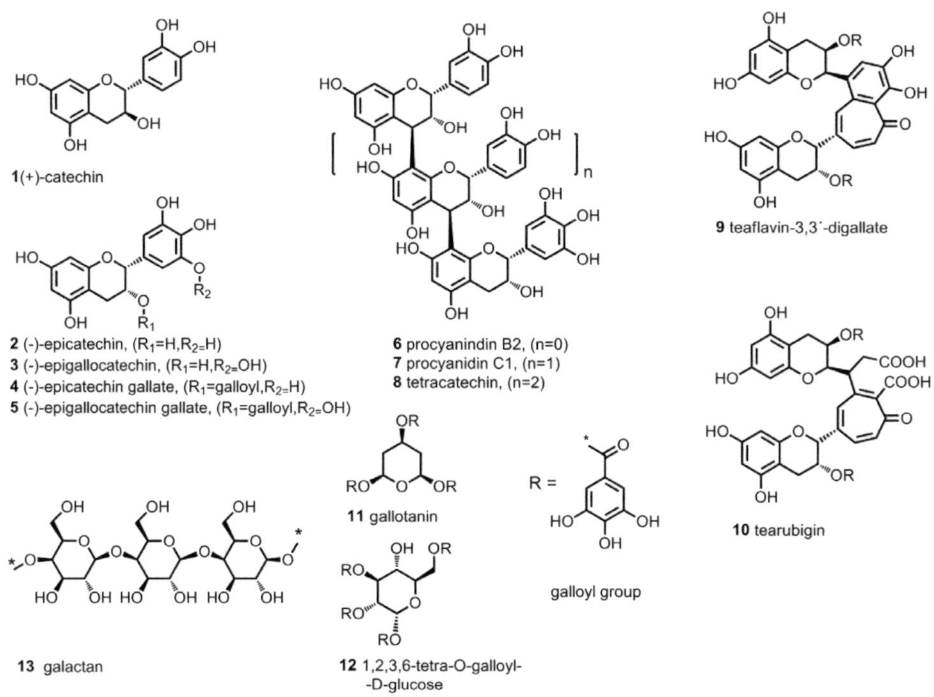

Fig. 4. Structures of natural products that could serve as CT inhibitors.

Politi *et al.* (2006) reported binding activity between a high molecular weight polysaccharide, galactan from garlic water extract and the B subunit of CT (CTB). The interaction was confirmed with Saturation Transfer Difference (STD) experiment, one of the NMR methods used to measure interaction between ligands and target receptor, and with fluorometric binding assays. This study indicates that one galactan polymer could bind with large number of CTB protein monomers. The ability of galactan to form high molecular weight aggregates with CTB and thus prevent adhesion to cell-surface could be the main reason for its inhibitory activity. A fragment of galactan 13 is shown in Fig. 4.

Podlipnik (2009) has collected polyphenol structures from different sources and described a structure-based model of inhibition of ADP-ribosyltransferase activity of Cholera toxin by polyphenol's. Compounds 1-12 (Fig 4) are members of the polyphenol´s library used for virtual screening against CTA_1 . For docking purposes a model based on a crystallographic structure of CTA_1:ARF_6-GTP complex (Hol, O'Neal et al. 2005) was prepared. From docking (Glide XP) results it is evident that mono catechines can penetrate deeply into the binding site of CTA (Fig. 5a). The inhibitory activity of polyphenols generally increases with their complexity, measured by number of hydroxyl groups attached to the scaffold. On the other hand, oligocatechins can not penetrate into the binding site in the whole extension, such compounds could additionally form numerous non-specific contacts with the protein surface, and hinder NAD^+ to access the binding site (Fig. 5c). Nice fits to CTA binding site have been also observed for theaflavin-3,3 digallate (Fig. 5d), 9 from black tea and Oi's synthetic gallate (Fig. 5b), 12, the results of molecular docking (Glide XP) indicate that these two compounds could act as strong inhibitors of CT´s ADP-ribosylation activity .

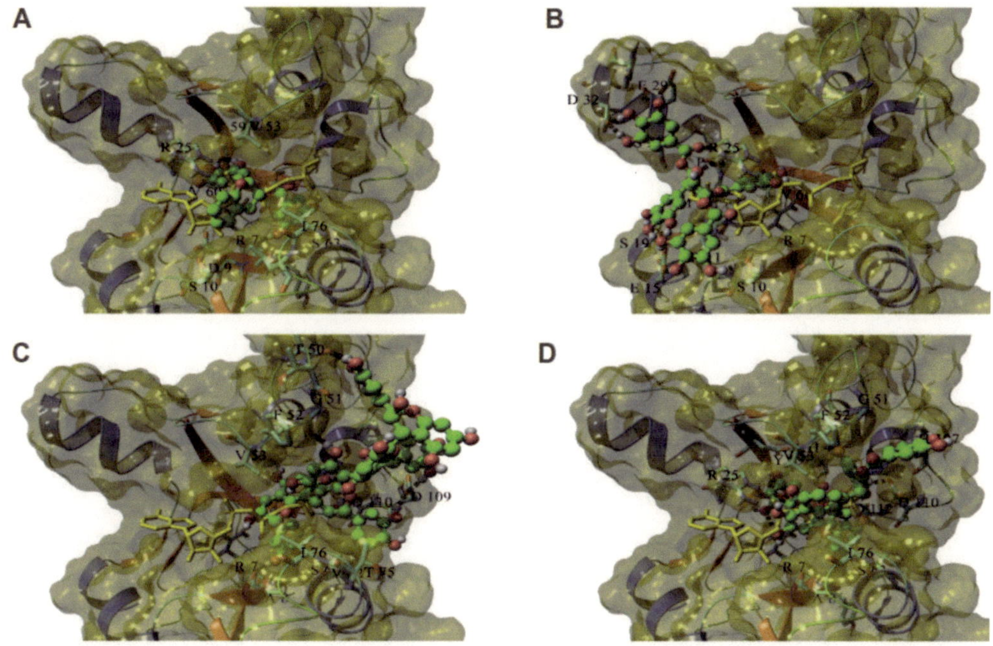

Fig. 5. Docking poses (GlideXP) for selected polyphenols. (A) epigallocatechin gallate; (B) 1,2,3,6-tetra-O-galloyl-D-glucose; (C) tetrameric catechin; (D) theaflavin-3,3-digalate. Yellow coloured NAD+ is appeared in each CTA:ligand complex as a reference.

Many other plants have been used for centuries around the world in traditional medicine as natural remedies for cholera and other diarrhoeal infections. Most of the current pharmacological studies are oriented to test antibacterial activity of some of these medicinal species from plant extracts against *V. Cholerae*. On the other hand, direct investigations of natural products as potential CT inhibitors are very rare, this field of research is still open and some additional founding of direct biological action of natural compounds to cholera toxin and other AB_5 toxins are more than welcome.

4. Rational design of GM1 mimics as Cholera toxin inhibitors

The synthesis of ganglioside GM1 itself is very complex (Sugimoto, Numata et al. 1986), therefore one of the strategies how to prevent adhesion of CTB to the cell surface involves design and synthesis of functional and structural mimics of oGM1 (Fig 6).

NMR and theoretical studies of the conformational behavior of GM1 and of other ganglioside head groups (e.g. GM2, GM3, and asialo GM1) have shown that the 3,4-

branching at Gal-II residue is the main reason for rigidity of oGM1 structure, so Gal-II residue appears to act as the scaffold that holds together the two terminal Gal-IV and Neu5Ac moieties at the proper orientation for optimal interaction with CT (Bernardi and Raimondi 1995; Bernardi, Arosio et al. 2002). Bernardi *et al.* have used the above structural hypothesis to develop and design ligands (14 for example) using conformationally restricted *cis*-1,2-cyclohexanediol, 15, as a replacement of Gal-II residue in oGM1 (Bernardi, Checchia et al. 1999; Bernardi, Arosio et al. 2001). The experimental results obtained by ELISA assays and fluorescence titration have shown that CT inhibition activities of Bernardi's mimics and oGM1 are more or less in the same range. The major problem in the synthesis of the "first generation" of the Bernardi's mimics is the stereoselective syalilation of *cis*-1,2-cyclohexanediol, this step represents the bottleneck of the synthesis. Therefore, a further simplification of oGM1 structure that has been based on the replacement of the sialic acid residue with simple α-hydroxyl acids, 16-20 was proposed by Bernardi's research group (Bernardi, Carrettoni et al. 2000).

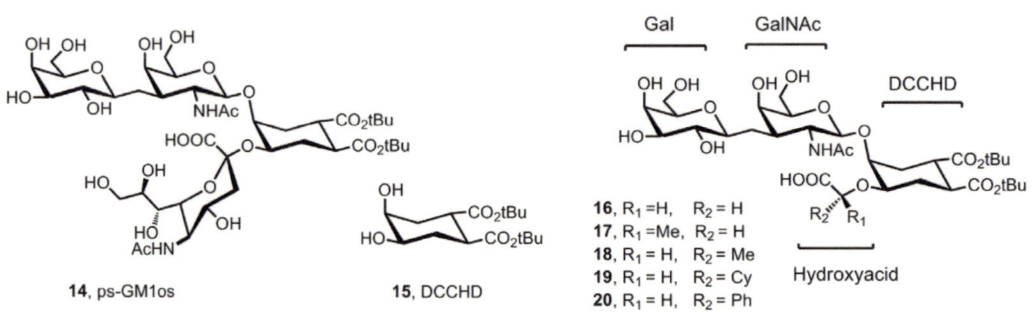

Fig. 6. Structures of Bernardi's GM1 mimics.

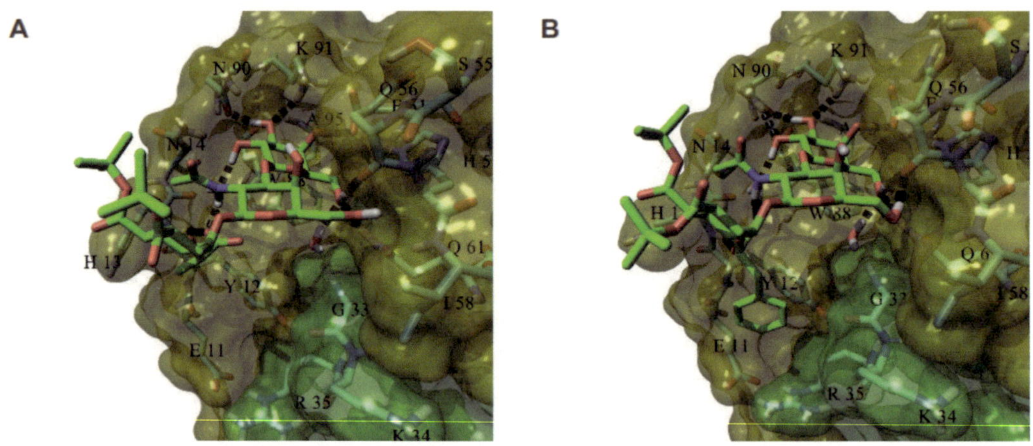

Fig. 7. Poses (Glide XP) of Bernardi's GM1 mimics: (A) 18 and (B) 20 to CTB .

The next widely used approach to design CTB inhibitors is to use the terminal galactose as an anchor to which various pharmacophores can be attached. Minke *et al.* (1999) have used fluorescence titrations and ELISA assays to screen a series of commercially available galactose derivates. The most active compound from this series was meta nitrophenyl α-D-galactoside (MNPG), 21. Its affinity for CTB (IC_{50} = 720 μM) is two orders of magnitude higher than it is found for galactose. (Minke, Roach et al. 1999) (Fan, Merritt et al. 2001) Further crystallographic studies have shown the displacement of a water molecule that is structurally bound to CTB by the meta nitro group of the MNPG's phenyl ring. The mentioned displacement leads to an increase in the entropy of the system and creates tight hydrogen bond interactions between the nitro group of MNPG and CTB could, which may be the reason for an increased CT inhibitory activity (Fan, Merritt et al. 2001). It has been also observed that m-carboyxphenyl α-D-galactoside (MCPG), 22, binds to the target with a different binding mode. Poses of MCPG and MNPG extracted from crystallographic structures are shown in Figs. 9a and 9b, respectively (Fan, Merritt et al. 2001).

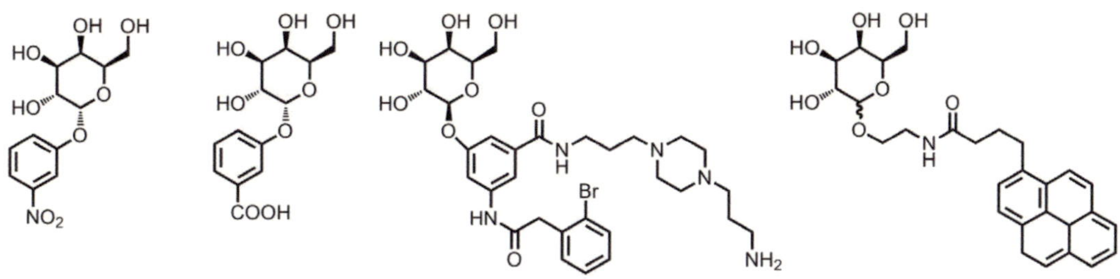

21, MNPG **22**, MCPG **23** **24**

Fig. 8. Some examples from MNPG (MCPG) library.

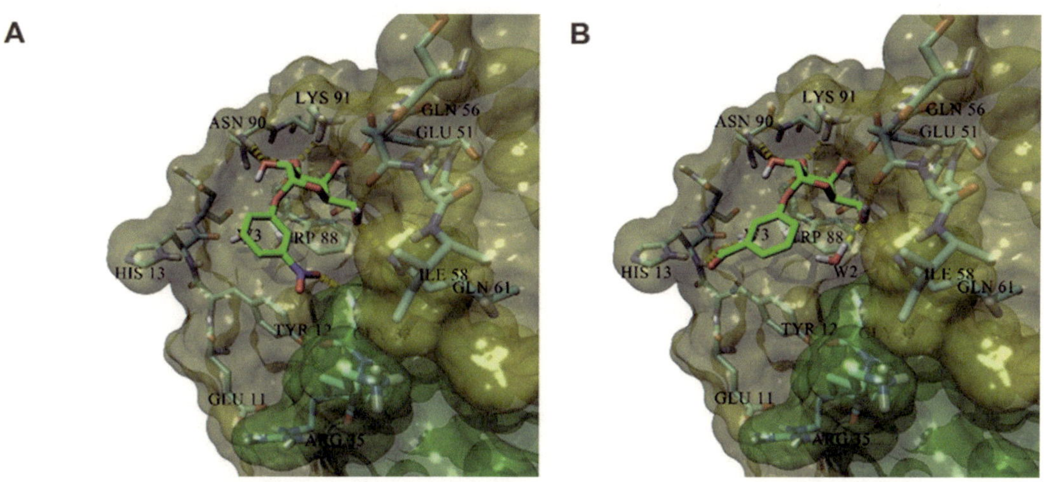

Fig. 9. Poses of (A) MNPG, 21 and (B) MCPG, 22 to CTB. Poses are extracted from crystallographic data.

Fan *et al.* designed a library of CTB antagonists where rigid hydrophobic rings were linked with different short and flexible aliphatic linkers to the meta position of phenyl ring of α-D-galactoside (Fan, Pickens et al. 2002). Some compounds from the mentioned libraries are shown in Fig. 9. This modification of MNPG allows to explore different regions of CTB binding site. Minke *et al.* (1999) explored a hydrophobic pocket in the bottom of the LT-II binding with series of galactosides that have large hydrophobic moieties, and found that compound 24 had the lowest IC_{50}=40 μM, which is more than three orders of magnitude lower from the IC_{50} of galactose . Docking (Glide XP) pose of 24, an α galactoside with large rigid hydrophobic moiety, to CT is shown in Fig. 12a.

Pieters *et al.* (2001; 2002) synthesized monovalent lactose-derived ligands for Cholera toxin, an example of such ligand is 25, where a thiourea moiety served as a spacer between lactose and aromatic system. A 72 fold enhancement of binding affinity of the compound 25 (K_d=248 μM) versus lactose (K_d=18 mM) to CTB determined by fluorescence titration was observed. The next step to improve Pieters' ligands was to increase the rigidity of a spacer between the lactose and a aryl group. The fluorescence study of 26 (Kd=23 μM) revealed one order of magnitude enhancement in the affinity of 25 for the CTB. Two examples from the library of Pieters' ligands based on lactose scaffold are shown in Fig. 10.

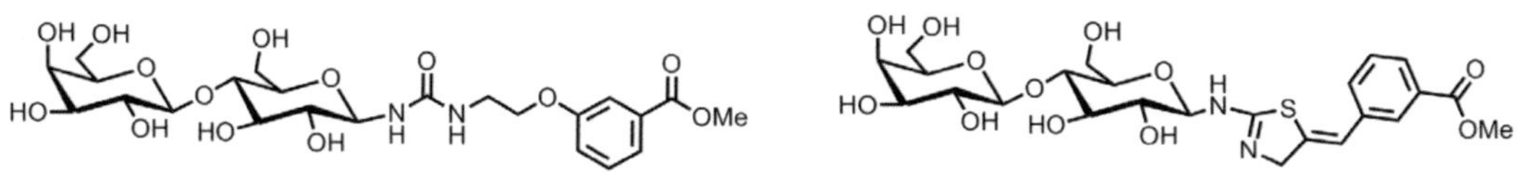

25 **26**

Fig. 10. Pieters' lactose derived ligands.

Mari *et al.* (2004; 2006) designed and synthesized a galactose-derived bi-cyclic scaffold, the rigid framework and possibility of functionalization at appended side-chain made these compounds interesting for further combinatorial development. NMR and conformational search analysis showed, however, that these compounds were more flexible than expected and did not fit the cholera toxin's binding site. An example, 27 from their library is shown in Fig. 11.

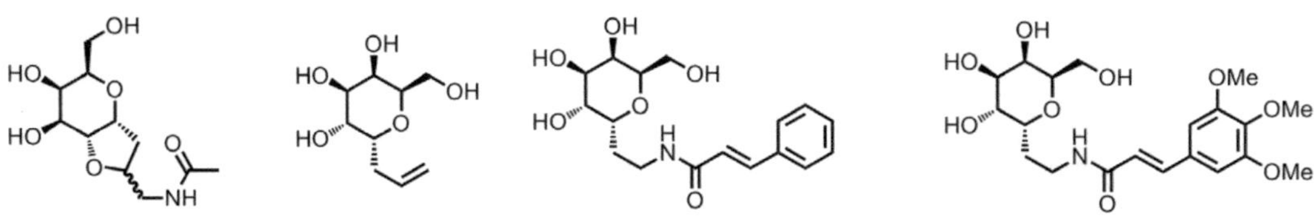

27 **28**, IC_{50}=3500 μM **29**, IC_{50}=3500 μM **30**, IC_{50}=125 μM

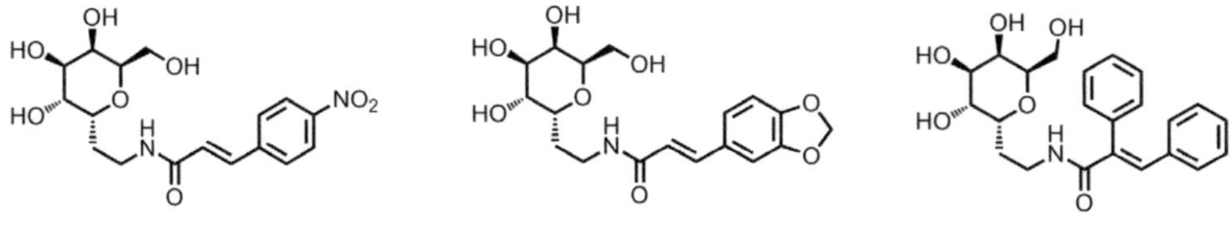

31, IC_{50}=233 μM **32**, IC_{50}=305 μM **33**, IC_{50}=595 μM

Fig. 11. Cholera toxin inhibitors: bi-cyclic inhibitor, 27 and cinnamic acid galactoconjugates 28-33.

Podlipnik *et al.* (2007) designed a small focused library of functionalized C-galactosides that could serve as non-hydolysable inhibitors of Cholera toxin. The fact that C-galactoside anchors (compound 28 from Fig. 11) can be synthesized in a few steps from galactose, thus avoiding the need for protecting groups, and their metabolical stability are the main reasons for the selection of the scaffold. The approach that has been adopted to identify CT inhibitors involves the following steps: the development and validation of a docking/scoring protocol based on a set of known pseudo-GM1 ligands; the design of a focused library of C-galactosides; the synthesis and affinity evaluation (by SPR) of selected elements of the library. The authors have tried to design relatively rigid ligands with α configuration on Galactose anomeric center that could fit CTB binding site. Cinnamic acids and their derivatives have been found as an ideal solution for conjugation functionalized C-galactosides (compounds 29-33 from Fig. 11). The best value of IC_{50} (125 µM) has been observed for compound 30. The pose of this compound within CTB binding site (Glide XP docking) is shown in Fig. 12b.

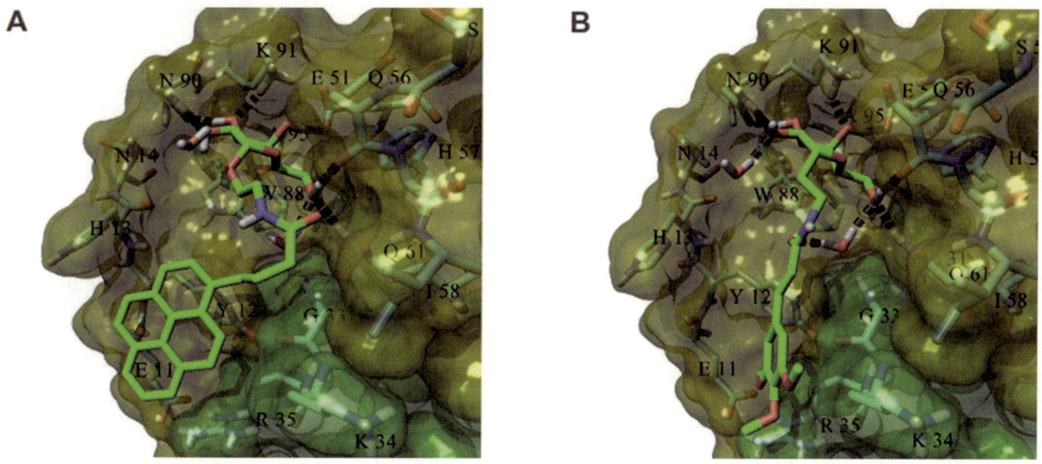

Fig. 12. Docking (Glide XP) poses of (A) Verlinde's ligand 24 and ligand 30 from cinnamic acid galactoconjugates library to CTB. Comparison of two galactoconjugates with α configuration on anomeric centre.

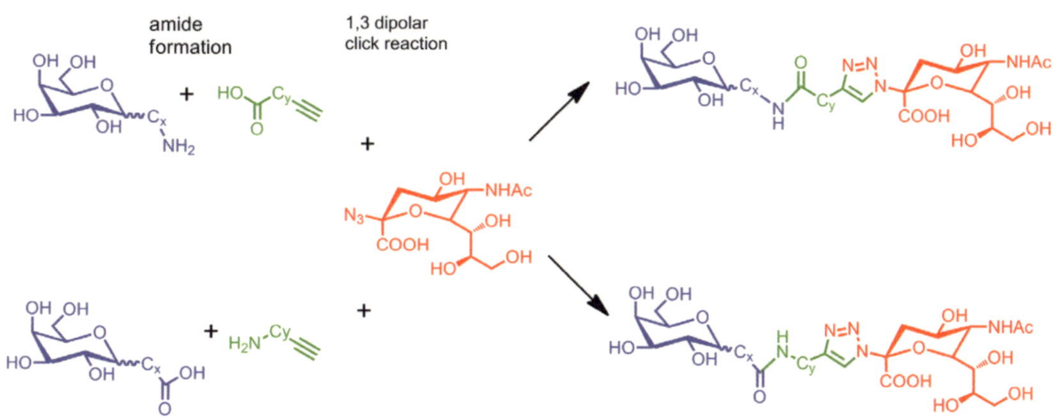

Fig. 13. General scheme for design of non-hydrolysabile Cheshev's bidentate CT inhibitors.

Cheshev *et al.* (2010) have used click chemistry to design a library of non-hydrolyzable bidentate CTB ligand, where two binding determinants, galactose and sialic acid, are connected to one other as they are in oGM1. All compounds from their library were synthesized from readily available precursors using high performance reactions, including click chemistry protocols, and avoiding glycosidic bonds. The general strategy of Cheshev's design is shown in Fig. 13. The affinity of bidentate ligands to CT measured by weak affinity chromatography could be enhanced up to one or two orders of magnitude relative to the individual pharmacological sugar residues. A further enhancement of CT inhibition could be accessed by conjugation of some of the compounds from the library with polyvalent aglycons. Two examples from Cheshev's library are shown in figure 14. Nice fit computed with Glide XP docking software of *R*-epimeric form of ligand 34 to CTB is shown in Fig. 14.

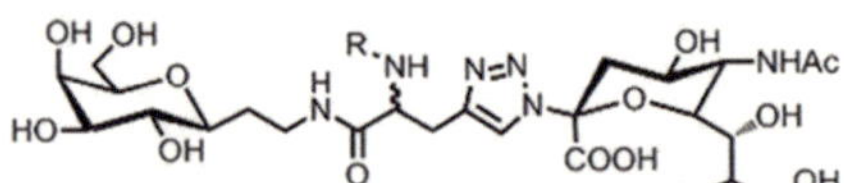

34, R = COPh
35, R = $COCH_2Ph$

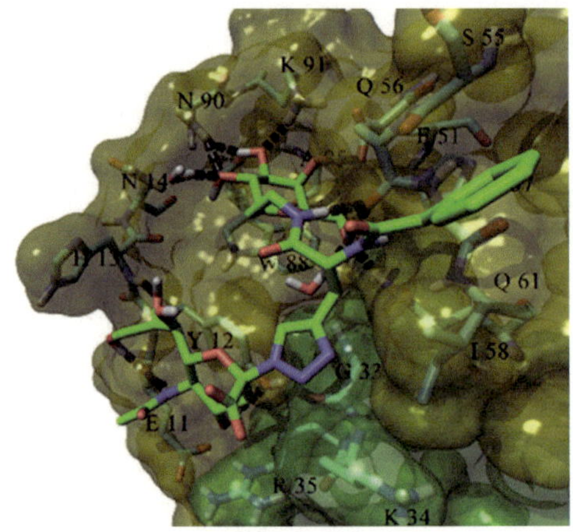

Fig. 14. Two examples from Cheshev´s design and docking (Glide XP) pose of R epimer of compound 35 to CTB.

In this section we shortly described a rational design of CTB antagonists derived from structural simplification of oGM1 - the natural receptor for CT. The presented structures are in the range of very close structurally related mimics of oGM1, such as psGM1, 14 and α-hydroxylacid derivatives, 16-20 with K_d that is close to value found for oGM1 itself, to very simple galactoconjugates MNPG, 21, cinnamic acid galactoconjugates, 29-33 for example. The affinity data for binding of simple galactoconjugates to CTB are still far from ideal, but by conjugation of these compounds with polyvalent aglycons the affinity could be enhanced by several orders of magnitude. The design of multivalent inhibitors will be described in next section of the review.

5. Design of multivalent inhibitors

A very effective way to enhance ligand's binding affinity toward its receptor target is to use the ligand in multivalent presentation. The Cholera toxin B-pentamer is an ideal target for studying multivalency and developing multivalent ligands against its action. Due to its high five-fold symmetry and the fact that it has five identical binding sites for GM1. A first attempt to improve oGM1 affinity using multivalency was reported by Schwarzmann *et al.* (1978), who designed and synthesized divalent oGM1 that has better affinity to CTB than oGM1 by itself. More recently, Schengrund *et al.* (1989) prepared highly active multivalent o-GM1 ligands by linking them to a polymer (poly-L-lisine) or to a dendrimer (octapropyleneimine) that serves as a core.

Fan *et al.* (2002) have designed a multivalent receptor-binding antagonists against CT and LT-II with particular focus on exploiting the 5-fold symmetry of the binding sites on the toxin B pentamer. A conceptual design of such symmetric pentavalent ligand where monovalent "fingers" that block the toxin receptor binding site are attached to symmetric core via modular linker units is shown in Fig. 15. Multivalent inhibitor 36 (Fig. 16) is shown as an example of symmetric pentavalent inhibitor with using MNPGs as monovalent fingers. The affinity of 36 for CTB was investigated using enzyme-linked addhesion assay, from which ED_{50}=0.9 μM was determined. This represents more than 250-fold enhancement of the activity found for MNPG, 21. Crystallographic studies of complex between 36 and CTB brought additional support for a 1:1 association model between the ligand and the toxin, the canonical water is displaced also in this case (Minke, Pickens et al. 2000; Hol, Zhang et al. 2002).

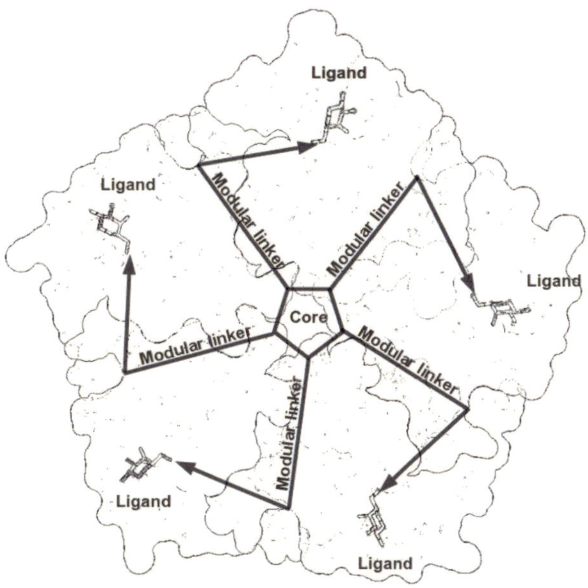

Fig. 15. General scheme of Fan's symmetric multivalent inhibitor design.

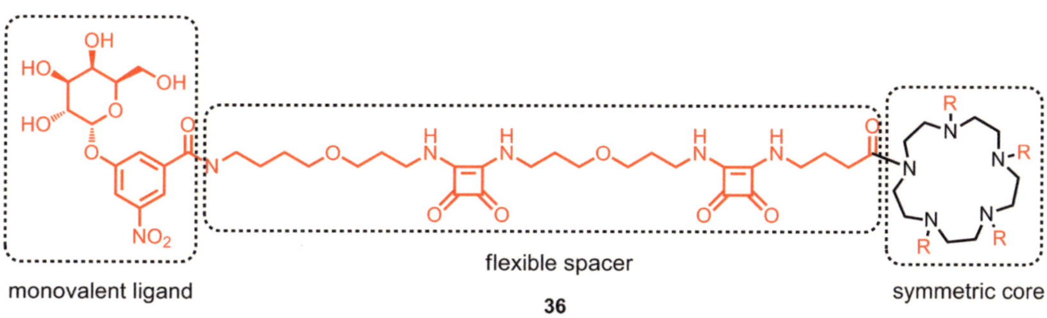

Fig. 16. An example of multivalent inhibitor with pent-fold symmetry designed by Fan.

Another strategy for the design of multivalent inhibitors involves the use of dendrimers. A typical example of such design was shown by Pieters and cooworkers (Pieters, Vrasidas, et al. 2001; Pieters, Vrasidas, et al. 2002), who derived denrimers from 3,5-di-(2-

aminoethoxy)benzoic acid repeating units with 2,4 and 8 end groups to which lactose isothiocyanate units, 25, were attached, providing thioureea-linked glycodendrimers 37 (Fig. 17). Analysis of fluorescence titration data showed that the affinity of these compounds for CT was increased by one order of magnitude relative to the monovalent ligands. It has been also shown that the branching of dendrimer provided only a modest increase in the potency of the ligand. The authors have also reported same indications that ligands are able to bind to multiple toxin molecules, rather than to single B pentamer.

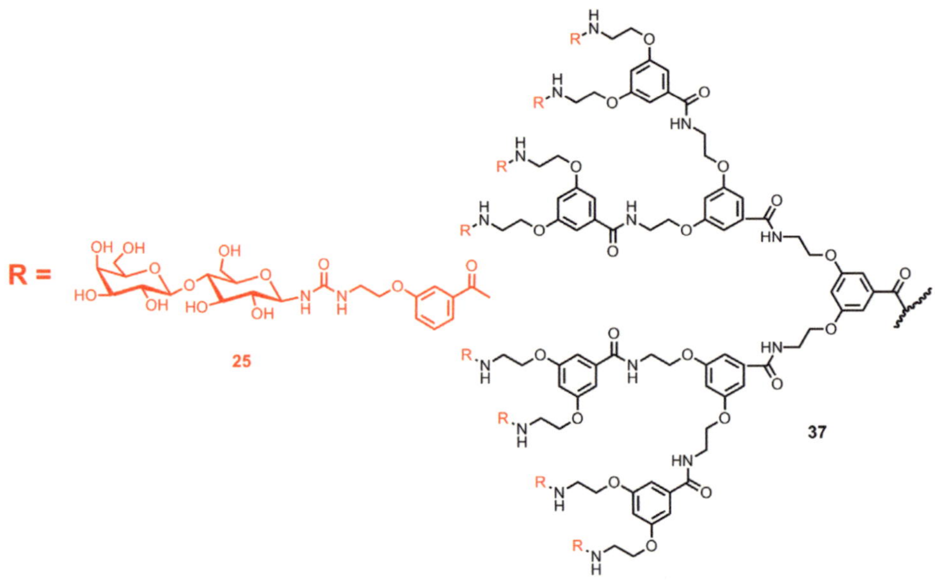

Fig. 17. A scheme of Pieters' multivalent inhibitor based on dendridic structure.

A further improvement of multivalent ligand's affinity for the toxin has been obtained attaching Bernardi's monovalent GM1 mimic 25 to Pieters' dendrimeric core (Arosio, Vrasidas et al. 2004). For further improvement, the polysaccharide scaffold was provided with elongated spacer arms. The analysis of surface plasmon resonance data revealed EC_{50}=0.5 μM for 38.

Another option of using Bernardi's GM1 mimics for multivalent inhibitor's design has been presented by Bernardi, Casnati and cooworkers (Bernardi, Arosio et al. 2005). They prepared a bivalent ligand 39 by hooking two units of GM1 mimic 18 to a functionalized calix-[4]-arene core. The size of affinity enhancement measured by fluorescence titration was found to be 3800-fold (1900-fold per sugar mimic). Recently, the huge affinity enhancement of 39 versus 18 to CT were confirmed in our laboratory with isothermal calorimetry titration (Prislan, et al. 2011).

The best known multivalent inhibitors up-to date have been reported by Pukin *et al.* (2007). In this study, GM1 containing compound was synthetized enzimatically starting from ω-azidoundecyl lactoside, that was then coupled onto Pieters' linker-extended dendrimers by cooper-catalysed azide-alkyne cycloaddition. Dendrimers bearing two, four and eight GM1 sugars were evaluated by ELISA, the IC_{50} values for these compounds were 2 nM, 0.2 nM and 50 pM, respectively.

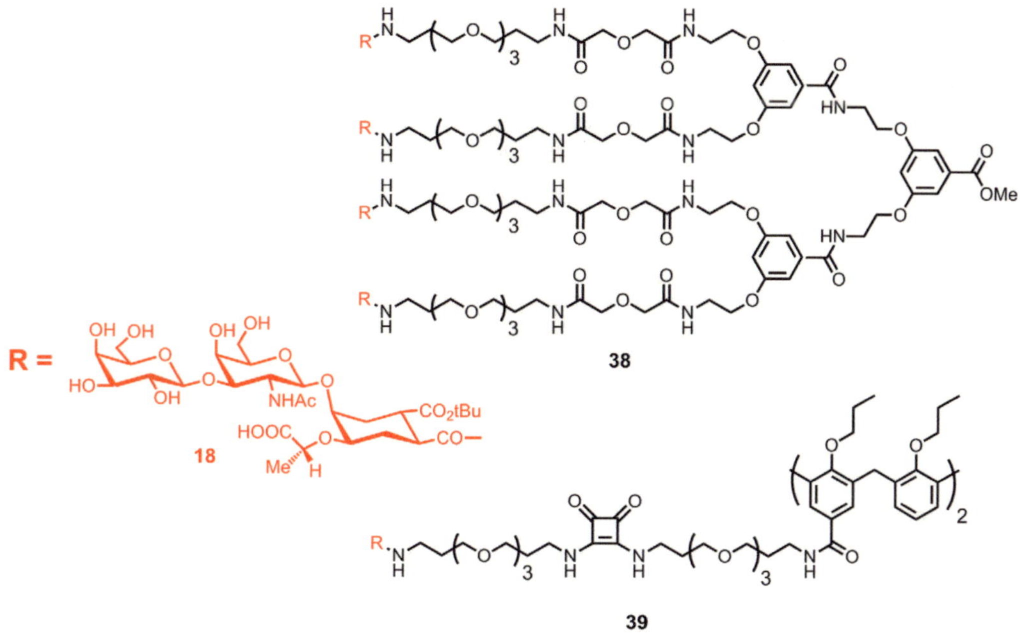

Fig. 18. A scheme of multivalent Bernardi-Pieters' inhibitor based on dendridic structure and Bernardi-Casnati's inhibitor based on Calix-[4]-arene core.

The most recent example of using multivalent strategy in the design of Cholera toxin inibitors presented in this chapter is based on the work of Tran and collaborators (Tran, Kitov et al. 2011). They are intensively working on designing a bidentate multivalent ligands. In their recent work they describe the synthesis and activities of a series of galactose conjugates on polyacryl amide and dextran. Nanomolar affinity of inhibitors against CT was obtained by conjugation of a second fragment (corresponding Neu5Ac's mimic), while galactose-only progenitors showed no detectable activity. The general idea of such inhibitor's design is shown in Fig. 19.

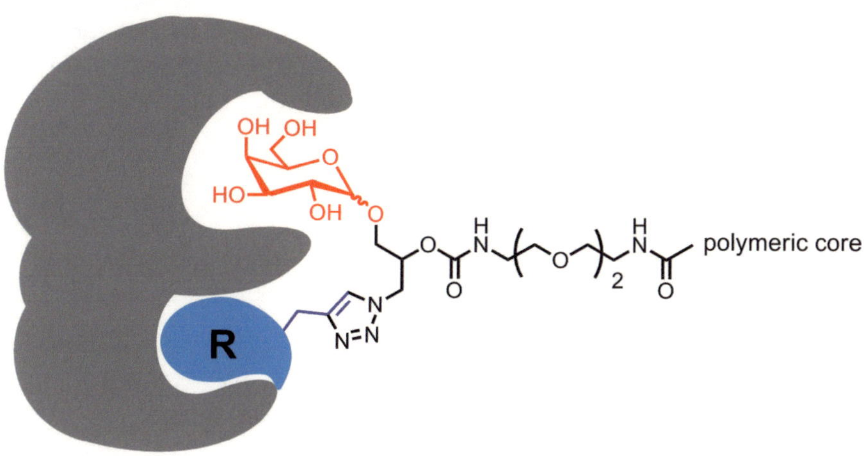

Fig. 19. Scheme for general design of multivalent Tran-Kitov's bidentate inhibitors.

A variety of multivalent inhibitors were described in this chapter. Basically, the multivalent inhibitors are designed using linkers to connect a galactose anchor to polymeric or dendrimeric cores or symmetric cores (5-fold symmetry). Recently, bidentate multivalent inhibitors were designed with conjugation of second fragment of that corresponds to Neu5Ac mimic. Generally, the above results showed that strategy of designing multivalent presentations of monovalent ligands can bring affinity closer to what is required for practical application against CT.

6. Novel binding site for blood group antigens in Cholera toxin: Potential target for the design of new Inhibitors?

At the end of the 1970s, two epidemiological studies established a dependency between the severity of Cholera infections and the blood group phenotype (Baura, Paguio 1977; Chaudhuri, De 1997). In these studies it was reported that people with blood group O were more prone to develop severe symptoms in comparison with people of blood group A, B or AB phenotype. Also, it was found that this dependency is strain specific, for example, in *V. cholerae* O1 "El Tor" (responsible of the seventh (current) pandemic) and *V. cholerae* O139 infections a connection with blood group phenotype of individuals was found (Glass et al. 1985, Swerdlow et al. 1994, Farruque et al. 1994, Tacket et al. 1995, Harris et al. 2005, Harris et al. 2008). On the other hand, for infection with classical *V. Cholerae* strains, no such association was observed.

The blood group phenotype of an individual is determinated by the presence or absence of antigenic substances on the surface of red blood cells. The ABO antigens are fucosylated oligosaccharide structures, carried on both glycolipids and glycoproteins. (Fig. 20) These antigens are not only on the surface of red blood cells, but are widely distributed throughout body fluids and tissues and are found also in the small intestine, the site of Cholera and ETEC infections. In this tissue, blood group antigens are presented on the intestinal epithelium cell surface (Finne 1989, Breimer 1984, Björk 1987), close to GM1 gangliosides. Structurally, ABO antigens are very similar, the H antigen (responsible of the O phenotype) is a tetrasaccharide characterized by a terminal fucose residue. The A and B antigens are pentasaccharides with a core similar to the H antigen, but each contain and additional saccharide residue- a terminal 2'-*N*-acetyl galactosamine (GalNAc) in the A antigen, or a terminal galactose for the blood group B antigen.

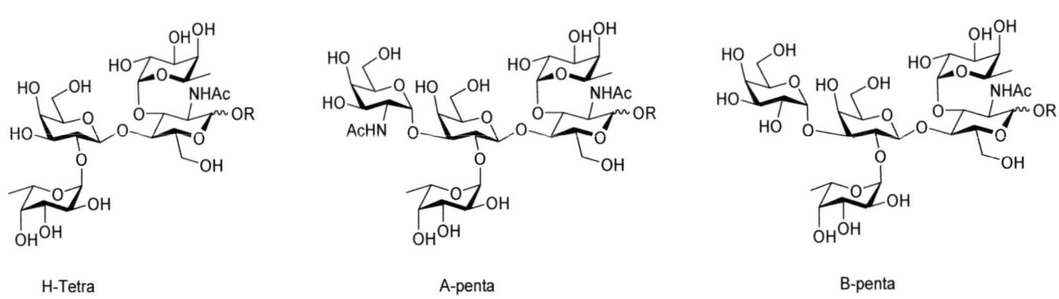

Fig. 20. Schematic representation of the Blood Group antigens H, A and B.

Following the discovery of the relation between blood group phenotype and cholera susceptibility, many studies have been conducted in order to investigate the ability of cholera toxin and of the highly homologous heat-labile enterotoxin (LT) from enterotoxigenic Escherichia coli (ETEC), to recognize blood group antigens of the ABO system (Bennun 1989, Monferran 1990, Barra 1992, Balanzino 1994, Balanzino 1999). It has been hypothesized that blood group antigens, with a preference for A and B epitopes, might disturb the action of the toxin by interfering with binding to GM1 ganglioside in the small intestine. However, the well-conserved GM1 binding site of CT is believed to be ganglioside-specific and cannot accommodate the fucosylated blood group antigens according to computer modelling. Consequently, the basis for the recognition of blood group antigens by Cholera Toxin at a molecular level is still unclear. In a recent investigation, Teneberg and co-workers have discovered a novel carbohydrate binding site studying a chimera between the B subunits of cholera toxin and the E. coli LT. This CTB/LTB chimera was shown to bind blood group A or B antigens on type 2 chains (Ångström 2000), and was subsequently characterized in complex with a blood group A analogue using protein crystallography by Krengel and co-workers (Holmner 2004). The structure of such complex is shown in Fig 21a. A follow-up study showed that native LTB, despite binding blood group antigens with lower affinity, also display the same mode of binding as the CTB/LTB chimera (Holmner 2007). In both cases, this binding site for blood group ligands is clearly distinct from the primary GM1 binding site. The blood group recognition site is located at the interface of two B-subunits, with one of the 2 subunits providing the majority of the contacts to the ligand. Based on the two crystal structures, it was possible to explain how the toxins discriminate between different ABH epitopes. The GalNAcα3 residue characteristic of blood group antigens binds with the toxin via several hydrogen bonds, including one involving its acetamido nitrogen (Fig 21b). The blood group B antigen is characterized by a terminal galactose residue and only differ from the A antigen at the 2-position, i.e. the acetamido group is replaced by a hydroxyl group. This hydroxyl group should preserve most of the interactions with the toxin and explains why the toxin does not discriminate notably between A and B epitopes. The fucose residue on the ABH antigens is also an important contributor to receptor recognition, however, blood group H determinants lack the entire terminal saccharide residue compared to blood group A and B determinant, and would therefore be expected to have significantly reduced binding affinities to cholera toxin. This assumption is substantiated by the finding that the loss of a single water-mediated hydrogen bond to the terminal GalNAcα3 residue results in a pronounced decrease in binding affinity (Holmner 2004), confirming the importance of the terminal GalNAc residue characteristic of blood group A antigens in molecular recognition. All these new contributions to understand the molecular basis of the interaction between blood group antigens and cholera toxin were reviewed in more detail by Krengel and co-workers (Holmner 2010).

In conclusion, the new information on the molecular recognition of blood-group antigens by Cholera Toxin should encourage medicinal chemist to development improved drug design strategies to prepare new pharmacological agents that inactivate cholera toxin. Inhibitors of the interaction of the cholera toxin with its primary receptor, the GM1 ganglioside, are especially attractive. Development of antagonists for the blood group binding site of cholera toxin could enable a more effective combined therapy together with GM1 antagonists and, furthermore, could be used as a tool to understand the variability of susceptibility to Cholera infection with the blood group phenotype of individuals.

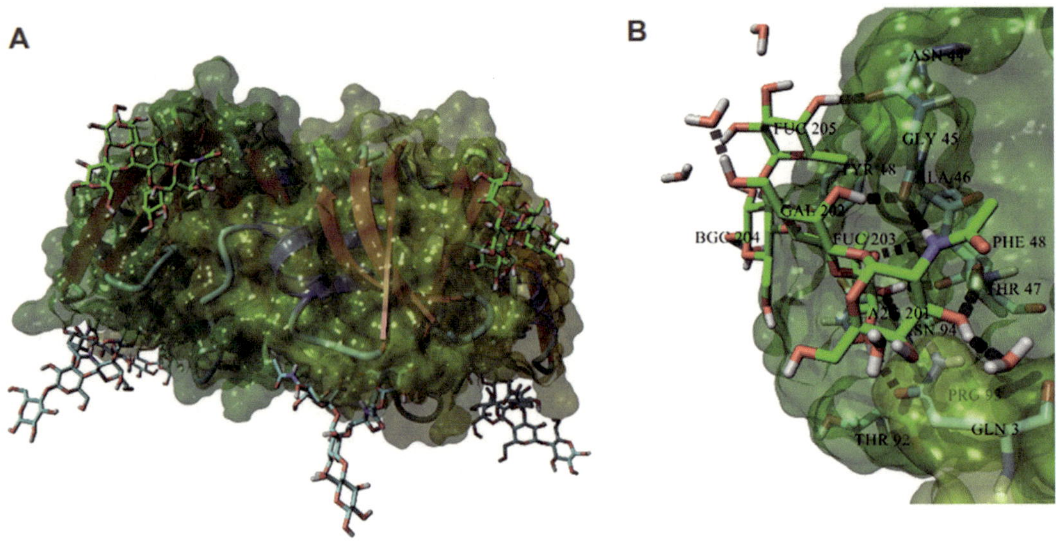

Fig. 21. (A) A crystallographic representation of CTB/LT chimera that shows the comparison between the binding site of blood group A pentasaccharide analog (green sticks) and GM1 ganglioside (sky-blue sticks) superimposed for comparison. (B) Interactions between blood group A and CTB/LT chimera - close view (Holmner 2010).

7. Methods and software

The methodology of structure based design of CT is described in several occasions (Podlipnik and Bernardi 2007; Zhang 2009). Structure based design starts with preparing a model of the protein receptor site. Models described in our review are based on receptor:ligand complex. In case of exploring of A-site ligands (Section 3) we have used a model based on crystallographic structure of CTA_1:ARF_6-GTP complex (PDB-ID: 2A5F)(Hol, O'Neal et al. 2005). A high resolution crystallographic structure (1.25 Å) of Cholera toxin B pentamer complexed with oGM1 (PDB-ID:3CHB) (Merritt, Kuhn et al. 1998) has been used as a template for generating a model in the case of exploring GM1 mimics (Section 4). The raw crystallographic structures were in both cases optimized with protein preparation wizard provided as part of the Schrodinger Suite 2011 (http://www.schrodinger.com). The interaction field grids that were used for docking were centered at the center of the ligand

(NAD^+ in case of CT's A-Site; oGM1 in case of B-Site). All ligands described in Sections 3 and 4 are prepared using Schrodinger's Ligprep. Glide XP (Murphy, Repasky et al. 2011) has been used for docking. The figures 1,2,5,7,9,12,14 and 21 representing poses were perpared with YASARA (http://www.yasara.com).

8. Conclusions

We reviewed different strategies to design an effective cure against cholera infections. The first strategy is based on exploring natural ligands as potential inhibitors of the ADP-ribosylation function of CT A subunit. The data collected from various sources indicate that catechin derivatives found in different natural sources could limit enzymatic activity of CT. Maybe this is one of the major reasons why during the centuries cholera pandemies have spared China and Japan, the catechin-consumig countries. The second approach is to design mimics in a mono- and/or multivalent presentation that could bind to the GM1 binding site in the B-pentamer, and thus prevent binding to GM1 receptors at the surface of epithelial cells, the first act necessary for Cholera toxin intoxication. The rational design of GM1 mimics is one of the most representative example of using structural information supported by molecular modelling methods in task to get an effective inhibitor. Nice examples of how multivalent presentation of single ligands can enhance affinity to CT by several orders of magnitude, and thus reach the levels of affinity required for practical applications against CT were presented. In addition we introduced a new strategy for developing CT inhibitors by targeting a newly identified binding site for blood group antigens in CT. This chapter describes examples of some successful application of knowledge that is connected with molecular structures and processes at the molecular level to design inhibitors toward Cholera toxin. The challenge to transfer the knowledge described in our review to achieve the practical, economic and scalable preparation of CT inhibitors remains still open.

9. Acknowledgments

Financial support (to Č.P.) from the Slovenian Research Agency (P1 0201) is greatly appreciated. J.J.R is supported by a Marie Curie Intra-European fellowship within the 7th EU Framework Programme (PIEF-2009-GA- 251763). The authors would like to thank Prof. Anna Bernardi (UNIMI) and Dr. Miha Lukšič (UNILJ) for helpful discussion and critical reading of manuscript.

10. References

Andrews, J. R. and S. Basu (2011). "Transmission dynamics and control of cholera in Haiti: an epidemic model." Lancet 377(9773): 1248-1255.

Ångström, J., Bäckström, M., et al.(2000) "Novel carbohydrate binding site recognizing blood group A and B determinants in a hybrid of cholera toxin and Escherichia coli heat-labile enterotoxin B-subunits." J. Biol. Chem. 275, 3231–3238.

Arosio, D., I. Vrasidas et al. (2004) "Synthesis and Cholera Toxin Binding Properties of Multivalent GM1 Mimics." Org. Biomol. Chem, 2, 2113-2124.

Balanzino, L. E., J. L. Barra, et al. (1994) "Differential interaction of Escherichia coli heat-labile toxin and cholera toxin with pig intestinal brush border glycoproteins depending on their ABH and related blood group antigenic determinants." Infect. Immun. 62, 1460–1464.

Balanzino, L. E., J. L. Barra, et al. (1999) Interaction of cholera toxin and Escherichia coli heatlabile enterotoxin with glycoconjugates from rabbit intestinal brush border membranes: relationship with ABH blood group determinants. Mol. Cell. Biochem. 194, 53–62.

Barra, J. L., C. G. Monferran, et al. (1992) Escherichia coli heat-labile enterotoxin preferentially interacts with blood group A-active glycolipids from pig intestinal mucosa and A- and B-active glycolipids from human red cells compared to H-active glycolipids. Mol. Cell. Biochem. 115, 63–70.

Bernardi, A., D. Arosio, et al. (2001). "Stereoselective synthesis of conformationally constrained cyclohexanediols: A set of molecular scaffolds for the synthesis of glycomimetics." Journal of Organic Chemistry 66(19): 6209-6216.

Bernardi, A., D. Arosio, et al. (2002). "Mimicking gangliosides by design: Mimics of GM1 headgroup." Neurochemical Research 27(7-8): 539-545.

Bernardi, A., D. Arosio, et al. (2005). "A synthetic divalent cholera toxin glycocalix[4]arene ligand having higher affinity than natural GM1 oligosaccharide." Journal of the American Chemical Society 127(11): 3660-3661.

Bernardi, A., L. Carrettoni, et al. (2000). "Second generation mimics of ganglioside GM1 as artificial receptors for cholera toxin: Replacement of the sialic acid moiety." Bioorganic & Medicinal Chemistry Letters 10(19): 2197-2200.

Bernardi, A., A. Checchia, et al. (1999). "Sugar mimics: An artificial receptor for cholera toxin." Journal of the American Chemical Society 121(10): 2032-2036.

Bernardi, A., Č. Podlipnik, J. Jiménez-Barbero (2006): "GM1 Glycomimetics and Bacterial Enterotoxins". pp- 73-91 in Protein-Carbohydrate Interactions in. Infectious Diseases C.A. Bewley Ed., RSC Publishing 2006.

Bernardi, A. and L. Raimondi (1995). "Conformational-Analysis of Gm1 Oligosaccharide in Water Solution with a New Set of Parameters for the Neu5ac Moiety." Journal of Organic Chemistry 60(11): 3370-3377.

Bennun, F. R., G. A. Roth, et al. (1989) Binding of cholera toxin topigintestinalmucosa glycosphingolipids: relationship with the ABO blood group system. Infect. Immun. 57, 969–974.

Björk, S., M. E. Breimer, et al. (1987). "Structures of blood group glycosphingolipids of human small intestine. A relation between the expression of fucolipids of epithelial cells and the AbO, Le and Se phenotype of the donor." J. Biol. Chem. 262, 6758–6765.

Breimer, M. E. (1984). Tissue specificity of glycosphingolipids as expressed in pancreas and small intestine of blood group A and B human individuals. Arch. Biochem. Biophys. 228, 71–85.

Cassel, D. and T. Pfeuffer (1978). "Mechanism of cholera toxin action: covalent modification of the guanyl nucleotide-binding protein of the adenylate cyclase system." Proc Natl Acad Sci U S A 75(6): 2669-2673.

Cheshev, P., A. Bernardi, et al. (2010). "Synthesis and Affinity Evaluation of a Small Library of Bidentate Cholera Toxin Ligands: Towards Nonhydrolyzable Ganglioside Mimics." Chemistry-a European Journal 16(6): 1951-1967.

Fan, E., E. A. Merritt, et al. (2001). "Exploration of the GM1 receptor-binding site of heat-labile enterotoxin and cholera toxin by phenyl-ring-containing galactose derivatives." Acta Crystallogr D Biol Crystallogr 57(Pt 2): 201-212.

Fan, E., E. A. Merrit, et al. (2002). "Characterization and Crystal Structure of a High-Affinity Pentavalent Receptor-Binding Inhibitor for Cholera Toxin and *E. coli* Heat-Labile Enterotoxin" Journal of the American Chemical Society 124(30): 8818-8824.

Fan, E. K., J. C. Pickens, et al. (2002). "Anchor-based design of improved cholera toxin and E-coli heat-labile enterotoxin receptor binding antagonists that display multiple binding modes." Chemistry & Biology 9(2): 215-224.

Faruque, A. S. ,G. Mahalanabis, et al. (1994) The relationship between ABO blood groups and susceptibility to diarrhea due to Vibrio cholerae 0139. Clin. Infect. Dis. 18, 827–828.

Finkelstein, R. A., P. Atthasampunna, et al. (1966). "Pathogenesis of experimental cholera: biologic ativities of purified procholeragen A." J Immunol 96(3): 440-449.

Finne, J., Breimer, et al. (1989). "Novel polyfucosylated N-linked glycopeptides with blood group A, H, X, and Y determinants from human small intestinal epithelial cells." J. Biol. Chem. 264, 5720–5735.

Glass, R. I., J. Holmgren, et al. (1985). "Predisposition for cholera of individuals with O blood group. Possible evolutionary significance." Am. J. Epidemiol. 121, 791–796.

Harris, J. B., A. I. Khan et al. (2005) "Blood group, immunity, and risk of infection with Vibrio cholerae in an area of endemicity." Infect. Immun. 73, 7422-7427.

Harris, J. B., R. C. LaRocque , et al. (2008) Susceptibility to Vibrio cholerae infection in a cohort of household contacts of patients with cholera in Bangladesh. PLoS Negl. Trop. Dis. 2, e221.

Hol, W. G. J., E. K. Fan, et al. (2004). "Structural biology and structure-based inhibitor design of cholera toxin and heat-labile enterotoxin." International Journal of Medical Microbiology 294(4): 217-223.

Hol, W. G. J., C. J. O'Neal, et al. (2005). "Structural basis for the activation of cholera toxin by human ARF6-GTP." Science 309(5737): 1093-1096.

Hol, W. G. J., Z. S. Zhang, et al. (2002). "Solution and crystallographic studies of branched multivalent ligands that inhibit the receptor-binding of cholera toxin." Journal of the American Chemical Society 124(44): 12991-12998.

Holmner, Å., M. Lebens , et al. (2004) Novel binding site identified in a hybrid between cholera toxin and heat-labile enterotoxin: 1.9 Å crystal structure reveals the details. Structure 12, 1655–1667.

Holmner, Å., G. Askarieh, et al. (2007) Blood group antigen recognition by Escherichia coli heat-labile enterotoxin. J. Mol. Biol. 371, 754–764.

Holmner, Å, A. Mackenzie, et al. (2010) Molecular basis of Cholera blood-groupdependence and implications for a world characterized by climate change. FEBS Let., 584, 2548-2555.

Hor, M., H. Rimpler, et al. (1995). "Inhibition of intestinal chloride secretion by proanthocyanidins from Guazuma ulmifolia." Planta Med 61(3): 208-212.

Koch, R. (1884). "An Address on Cholera and its Bacillus." Br Med J 2(1236): 453-459.

Mari, S., F. J. Canada, et al. (2006). "Synthesis and conformational analysis of galactose-derived bicyclic scaffolds." European Journal of Organic Chemistry(13): 2925-2933.

Mari, S., J. Jimenez-Barbero, et al. (2004). "Synthesis, conformational studies and mannosidase stability of a mimic of 1,2-mannobioside." European Journal of Organic Chemistry(24): 5119-5125.

Merritt, E. A., P. Kuhn, et al. (1998). "The 1.25 A resolution refinement of the cholera toxin B-pentamer: evidence of peptide backbone strain at the receptor-binding site." J Mol Biol 282(5): 1043-1059.

Merritt, E. A., S. Sarfaty, et al. (1994). "Crystal structure of cholera toxin B-pentamer bound to receptor GM1 pentasaccharide." Protein Sci 3(2): 166-175.

Minke, W. E., J. Pickens, et al. (2000). "Structure of m-carboxyphenyl-alpha-D-galactopyranoside complexed to heat-labile enterotoxin at 1.3 A resolution: surprising variations in ligand-binding modes." Acta Crystallogr D Biol Crystallogr 56(Pt 7): 795-804.

Minke, W. E., C. Roach, et al. (1999). "Structure-based exploration of the ganglioside GM1 binding sites of Escherichia coli heat-labile enterotoxin and cholera toxin for the discovery of receptor antagonists." Biochemistry 38(18): 5684-5692.

Minke, W. E., F. Hong, et al. (1999). "Using a galactose library for exploration of a novel hydrophobic pocket in the receptor binding site of the Escherichia coli heat-labile enterotoxin." Journal of Biological Chemistry 274(47): 33469-33473.

Monferran, C.G., G.A. Roth, et al.(1990) "Inhibition of cholera toxin binding to membrane receptors by pig gastric mucin-derived glycopeptides: differential effect depending on the ABO blood group antigenic determinants." Infect. Immun. 58, 3966–3972.

Murphy, R., M. Repasky, et al. (2011). "Evaluation of docking and scoring accuracy using a new version of Schrodinger's Glide XP and Induced Fit Docking (IFD) methodologies." Abstracts of Papers of the American Chemical Society 241.

Oi, H., D. Matsuura, et al. (2002). "Identification in traditional herbal medications and confirmation by synthesis of factors that inhibit cholera toxin-induced fluid accumulation." Proc Natl Acad Sci U S A 99(5): 3042-3046.

Pieters, R. J., I. Vrasidas, et al. (2001). "Synthesis of lactose dendrimers and multivalency effects in binding to the cholera toxin B subunit." European Journal of Organic Chemistry(24): 4685-4692.

Pieters, R. J., I. Vrasidas, et al. (2002). "Synthesis and cholera toxin binding properties of a lactose-2-aminothiazoline conjugate." Organic Letters 4(10): 1807-1808.

Podlipnik, Č. (2009). "Docking of Selected Natural Polyphenols to ARF Activated A1 Subunit of Cholera Toxin." Acta Chimica Slovenica 56(1): 156-165.

Podlipnik, Č. and A. Bernardi (2007). "Design of a focused virtual library to explore cholera toxin B-site." Acta Chimica Slovenica 54(3): 425-436.

Podlipnik, Č., F. Nicotra, et al. (2007). "First round of a focused library of cholera toxin inhibitors." Carbohydrate Research 342(12-13): 1651-1660.

Prislan, I. (2011). To be published.

Politi, M., J. Alvaro-Blanco, et al. (2006). "Screening of garlic water extract for binding activity with cholera toxin B pentamer by NMR spectroscopy - An old remedy giving a new surprise." European Journal of Organic Chemistry(9): 2067-2073.

Pukin, A. V., H. M. Branderhorst, et al. (2007). "Strong inhibition of cholera toxin by multivalent GM1 derivatives." Chembiochem 8(13): 1500-1503.

Ramamurthy, T., P. K. Bag, et al. (1993). "Virulence patterns of Vibrio cholerae non-O1 strains isolated from hospitalised patients with acute diarrhoea in Calcutta, India." J Med Microbiol 39(4): 310-317.

Ramamurthy, T., S. Garg, et al. (1993). "Emergence of novel strain of Vibrio cholerae with epidemic potential in southern and eastern India." Lancet 341(8846): 703-704.

Sack, D. A., R. B. Sack, et al. (2004). "Cholera." Lancet 363(9404): 223-233.

Saito, T., M. Miyake, et al. (2002). "Inhibition by apple polyphenols of ADP-ribosyltransferase activity of cholera toxin and toxin-induced fluid accumulation in mice." Microbiol Immunol 46(4): 249-255.

Schengrund, C. L., N. J. Ringler (1989). "Binding of Vibrio cholera toxin and the heat-labile enterotoxin of Escherichia coli to GM1, derivatives of GM1, and nonlipid oligosaccharide polyvalent ligands." J Biol Chem 264(22): 13233- 13237.

Schwarzmann, G., W. Mraz, et al. (1978). "Comparison of Interaction of Mono-Valent and Oligo-Valent Ligands with Cholera Toxin - Demonstration of Aggregate Formation at Low Ligand Concentrations." Hoppe-Seylers Zeitschrift Fur Physiologische Chemie 359(10): 1277-1286.

Spangler, B. D. (1992). "Structure and function of cholera toxin and the related Escherichia coli heat-labile enterotoxin." Microbiol Rev 56(4): 622-647.

Sugimoto, M., M. Numata, et al. (1986). "Synthetic Studies on Cell-Surface Glycans .50. Total Synthesis of Gangliosides Gm1 and Gm2." Carbohydrate Research 156: C1-C5.

Swerdlow, D.L., Mintz, et al.(1994) "Severe life-threatening cholera associated with blood group O in Peru: implications for the Latin American epidemic." J. Infect. Dis. 170, 468–472.

Tacket, C.O., G. Losonsky,et al. (1995) "Extension of the volunteer challenge model to study South American cholera in a population of volunteers predominantly with blood group antigen O. Trans. R. Soc. Trop. Med. Hyg. 89, 75–77.

Toda, M., S. Okubo, et al. (1992). "The Protective Activity of Tea Catechins against Experimental-Infection by Vibrio-Cholerae O1." Microbiology and Immunology 36(9): 999-1001.

Toda, M., S. Okubo, et al. (1991). "The protective activity of tea against infection by Vibrio cholerae O1." J Appl Bacteriol 70(2): 109-112.

Tran, H. A., P. I. Kitov, et al. (2011). "Multifunctional multivalency: a focused library of polymeric cholera toxin antagonists." Org Biomol Chem 9(10): 3658-3671.

Turnbull, W. B., B. L. Precious, et al. (2004). "Dissecting the cholera toxin-ganglioside GM1 interaction by isothermal titration calorimetry." J Am Chem Soc 126(4): 1047-1054.

Zhang, G. T. (2009). "Design and in silico screening of inhibitors of the cholera toxin." Expert Opinion on Drug Discovery 4(9): 923-938.

Zhang, R. G., D. L. Scott, et al. (1995). "The three-dimensional crystal structure of cholera toxin." J Mol Biol 251(4): 563-573.

Part 4

Treatment

10

Evidence Based Treatment of Cholera: A Review of Existing Literature

Marzia Lazzerini
Institute for Maternal and Child Health IRCCS Burlo Garofolo
Italy

1.Introduction

Cholera outbreaks are reported every year in more than 50 countries worldwide, both in emergency and non-emergency contexts. Every year there are an estimated 3–5 million cholera cases, and 100,000–120,000 deaths. Case fatality rates as high as 50% have been reported for untreated cholera, but can be reduced to 1% with rapid and comprehensive treatment. During cholera epidemics the number of cases can rapidly escalate to hundreds of patients in need for immediate therapy, and severe cases will survive only if effectively, timely and safely treated.

This chapter will review the evidence behind the treatment of cholera, providing an up to date description of what we know on cholera treatment from existing scientific literature. The review takes into consideration different aspects of cholera treatment, such as fluids, antibiotics, zinc, and anti-diarrhoeal agents. The types of evidence searched for this umbrella review includes guidelines, systematic reviews and, where needed, clinical trials. Systematic reviews were searched in the Cochrane Library and in MEDLINE (1966 to 2011). In areas of treatment for which no systematic review was retrieved, or when retrieved systematic reviews were over two years old, single studies were searched in the following databases of primary research: the Cochrane Central Register of Controlled Trials (CENTRAL), MEDLINE (1966 to 2011). Guidelines for cholera management were searched in the following databases: MEDLINE (1966 to 2011); World Health Organization (WHO); Center of Diseases and Control (CDC); National Institute for health and Clinical Excellence (NICE); National Guidelines Clearinghouse.

1.1 When to suspect cholera

Cholera should be suspected when a child older than 5 years or an adult develops severe dehydration from acute watery diarrhoea (usually with vomiting), or when any patient older than 2 years has acute watery diarrhoea when cholera is known to be occurring in the area. Younger children also develop cholera, but the illness may be difficult to distinguish from other causes of acute watery diarrhoea, especially rotavirus (WHO 2011).

Cholera differs from acute diarrhoea for other causes in three ways:

- it occurs in large epidemics that involve both children and adults;

- voluminous watery diarrhoea may occur, leading rapidly to severe dehydration with hypovolaemic shock;
- for cases with severe dehydration appropriate antibiotics may shorten the duration of the illness.

2. Assessment of the severity of dehydration

The very first step in the treatment of cholera, as well as of other diarrhoeal diseases, is the assessment of the severity of dehydration. The WHO criteria to assess the severity of dehydration are based on the evaluation of few simple signs and symptoms (Table 1).

Look at -Conditions [a] -Eyes [b] -Thirst	• Well, alert • Normal • Drinks normally, not thirsty	• Restless, irritable • Sunken • Thirsty, drinks eagerly	• Lethargic or unconscious • Sunken • Drinks poorly, or not able to drink
Fell -Skin pinch [c]	• Goes back quickly	• Goes back slowly	• Goes back very slowly
Decide	No Dehydration	Some dehydration	Severe dehydration

[a]Being lethargic and sleepy are *not* the same. A lethargic child is not simply asleep: the child's mental state is dull and the child cannot be fully awakened; the child may appear to be drifting into unconsciousness.
[b]In some infants and children, the eyes normally appear somewhat sunken. It is helpful to ask the mother if the child's eyes are normal or more sunken than usual.
[c]The skin pinch is less useful in infants or children with marasmus or kwashiorkor, or obese children. Other signs may be altered in children with severe malnutrition.

Table 1. WHO criteria for the assessment of dehydration in patients with diarrhoea

3. Treatment of dehydration

The treatment of patients with dehydration due to cholera follows the same guidelines given for patients with dehydration due to other diarrhoeal diseases, and is substantially consistent among different guidelines (WHO 2011, NICE 2009, WGO 2008, AAP 1996). Here are reported the WHO guidelines.

3.1 How to treat severe dehydration

Patients who develop the typical clinical picture of cholera with severe diarrhoea and rapid fluid loss risk to quickly develop hypovolemic shock, hypoglycemia, coma and seizures and are at risk of dying within a few hours of onset. These patients need to be treated with intravenous fluids, and need to be monitored very closely. The initial intravenous (IV) infusion should be given very rapidly to restore an adequate blood volume, as evidenced by normal blood pressure and a strong radial pulse. Typically, an adult weighing 50 kg and with severe dehydration would have an estimated fluid deficit of five litres. The first two litres should be given within 30 minutes, and the remainder in the following three hours.

With cholera, unusually large amounts of oral rehydration salts (ORS) solution may be required to replace large continuing losses of watery stool after dehydration is corrected. The amount of stool lost is greatest in the first 24 hours of illness, being largest in patients who present with severe dehydration. During this period, the *average* fluid requirement of such patients is 200 ml/kg of body weight, but some need 350 ml/kg or more. Patients whose stool losses fall in this range, or are higher, usually require intravenous maintenance therapy using Ringer's Lactate Solution with added potassium chloride. Additional potassium can also be provided by ORS solution as soon as the patient can drink.

After rehydration, patients should be reassessed for signs of dehydration at least every 1-2 hours, and more often if there is profuse ongoing diarrhoea. If signs of dehydration reappear, ORS solution should be given more rapidly. If patients become tired, vomit frequently or develop abdominal distension, ORS solution should be stopped and rehydration should be given IV with Ringer's Lactate Solution (50 ml/kg in three hours), with added potassium chloride. After this it is usually possible to resume treatment with ORS solution.

If possible, suspected cholera patients should be treated under observation until diarrhoea stops, or is infrequent and of small volume. This is especially important for patients who present with severe dehydration. Attention to intake and output is especially important for infants. Food should be restarted as soon as deficits are replaced to minimize the nutritional impact of the illness; refeeding does not affect purging rates or the duration of diarrhoea.

The WHO guidelines for treatment of severe dehydration (Table 2) are based on randomised controlled trials that have shown that severe dehydration due to diarrhoea can be effectively and safety corrected by a rapid infusion over few hours (NICE 2009). Intravenous treatment is recommended also in the rare event of ileus or carbohydrate malabsorption.

3.1.1 What to do if intravenous therapy is not immediately available

If IV therapy is not available at the facility, but can be given nearby (i.e. within 30 minutes), send the patient immediately for IV treatment. If the patient can drink, give the care-taker some ORS solution and show her/him how to give it to the patient during the journey.

If IV therapy is not available nearby, health workers who have been trained can give ORS solution by naso-gastric (NG) tube, at a rate of 20 ml/kg body weight per hour for six hours (total of 120 ml/kg body weight). If the abdomen becomes swollen, ORS solution should be given more slowly until it becomes less distended. If NG treatment is not possible but the patient can drink, ORS solution should be given by mouth at a rate of 20ml/kg body weight per hour for six hours (total of 120 ml/kg body weight). If the rate is too fast, the patient may vomit repeatedly. In this case, the ORS solution must be given more slowly until vomiting subsides. Patient receiving NG or oral therapy should be reassessed at least every hour. If the signs of dehydration do not improve after three hours, the patient must be taken immediately to the nearest facility where IV therapy is available. If neither NG nor oral therapy is possible, the patient should be taken immediately to the nearest facility where IV or NG therapy is available.

If rehydration progresses satisfactorily, the patient should be reassessed after six hours and a decision on further treatment should made as described above for patients receiving IV therapy.

<table>
<tr><th></th><th>Type of fluid</th><th>Quantity</th></tr>
<tr><td>No dehydration</td><td>ORS</td><td>Children<2 years: 50–100 ml, up to 500 mL / day
Children 2–9 years: 100–200 ml, up to 1000 mL / day
Patients >9 years: As much as wanted, to 2000 mL / day</td></tr>
<tr><td>Some dehydration</td><td>ORS</td><td>Infants<4 mos (<5 kg): 200–400 mL
Infants 4–11 mos (5–7.9 kg): 400–600 mL
Children 1–2 yrs (8–10.9 kg): 600–800 mL
Children 2–4 yrs (11–15.9 kg): 800–1200 mL
Children 5–14 yrs (16–29.9 kg): 1200–2200 mL
Patients >14 yrs (30 kg or more): 2200–4000 mL
Over 4 hours</td></tr>
<tr><td>Severe dehydration</td><td>Intravenous

Ringer Lactate or Normal saline and ORS</td><td>Age < 12 months: 30 mL/kg within 1 hour*, then 70 ml/kg over 5 hours
Age > 1 year: 30 mL/kg within 30 min*, then 70 ml/kg over 2 and ½ hours
*Repeat once if radial pulse is still very weak or not detectable</td></tr>
<tr><td colspan="3">Indications for monitoring the patient
• Reassess the patient every 1-2 hours and continue hydrating. If hydration is not improving, give the IV drip more rapidly. 200ml/kg or more may be needed during the first 24 hours of treatment.
• During IV rapid infusion the heart rate and the respiratory rate should decrease. If they increase, suspect a fluid overload.
• After 6 hours (infants) or 3 hours (older patients), perform a full reassessment. Switch from intravenous to ORS solution if hydration has improved and the patient can drink.</td></tr>
</table>

Table 2. WHO Fluid Replacement Recommendations

3.1.2 What types of fluids to avoid

Treating a patient with severe dehydration from infectious diarrhoea with hypotonic solutions such as 5% dextrose with 1/4 normal saline is unsafe. Severe dehydration usually occurs as a result of bacterial infection (such as cholera), which may lead to greater sodium losses in feces (60 to 110 mmol/L). A 1/4 normal saline solution contains sodium (Na) 38.5 mmol/L, and this does not balance the sodium losses. Intravenous infusion with 5% dextrose with 1/4 normal saline will thus lead to severe hyponatremia, convulsion, and loss of consciousness. (WGO 2008)

3.2 How to treat cholera with moderate or mild dehydration

Patients with cholera but no sign of severe dehydration can be treated with ORS (Table 2). Interestingly, historical events surrounding cholera epidemics have marked the transition to modern rehydration therapy. It was during a cholera epidemic at the time of the Bangladesh Liberation War in 1971 that ORS was proven to be an effective treatment for diarrhoea. As medical teams ran out of intravenous fluids to treat the spreading cholera epidemic, the staff was instructed to distribute ORS to the 350,000 people in refugee camps. Over 3,000 patients with cholera were treated. The death rate was only 3.6% as opposed to the typical 30% registered with intravenous fluid therapy (Bhattacharya et al. 1994). The physiological basis for ORS use lies in the knowledge that glucose can enhances sodium and water absorption through the sodium-glucose cotransport on intestinal mucosa, even during diarrhoea. Intestinal mucosa is not disrupted during cholera. Moreover, ORS can be given by family members instead of trained staff thus allowing for large populations to be treated even in emergency contexts (Sacks et al. 2004).

This ecological evidence was confirmed by a Cochrane systematic review of seventeen trials in children with gastroenteritis (Hartling et al.2006). The meta-analysis showed no clinically significant differences in outcomes between ORS and intravenous rehydration therapy. It's widely accepted that patients presenting with mild to moderate dehydration secondary to acute gastroenteritis, including cholera, should initially be treated with ORS. However, it must be remembered that mild cases of cholera, if not further investigated, can be misdiagnosed for other diarrhoeal diseases, while according to WHO estimates up to 80% of people with cholera present only mild diarrhoea. Patients with moderate or mild dehydration need to be followed up to ensure that they do not develop severe dehydration. The patients and their care-takers need to be instructed to come back and seek care should diarrhoea become more severe, or other danger signs appear (inability to drink, weakness and deterioration of the neurological state, blood in the faeces).

3.2.1 Rice based ORS

Polymer-based ORS contain whole rice (amylopectins), as in rice-based ORS or rice syrups (maltodextrins), or other sources of polymers such as wheat, sorghum, and maize (high amylase-resistant starch). In these polymer-based solutions, the glucose is slowly released after digestion and is absorbed in the small bowel, enhancing the reabsorption of water and electrolytes secreted into the bowel lumen during diarrhoea.

A 1998 Cochrane Review of rice-based ORS for the treatment of diarrhoea concluded that rice-based ORS significantly reduce the mean 24 hour stool output in adults and children with cholera or cholera-like diarrhoea, but results were inconclusive for infants and children with non-cholera diarrhoea (Fontaine et al. , 1998).

A recent Cochrane review evaluated all polymers (eg rice, wheat, maltodextrins, maize, sorghum, or corn)- based ORS for the treatment of diarrhoea (Gregorio et al., 2009).

- There were fewer unscheduled intravenous infusions in the polymer-based ORS group compared with glucose-based ORS (ORS < 310 and < 270 groups combined) (RR 0.75, 95% CI 0.59 to 0.95; 2235 participants, 19 trials)
- Adults positive for *Vibrio cholerae* had a shorter duration of diarrhoea with polymer-based ORS than with ORS < 270 (MD -7.11 hours, SD -11.91 to -2.32; 228 participants, 4 trials).
- Wheat-based ORS resulted in lower total stool output in the first 24 hours compared with ORS < 270 (MD-119.85 g/kg, SD -114.73 to -124.97; 129 participants, 2 trials).
- Adverse effects were similar for polymer-based ORS and glucose-based ORS.

WHO and the International Centre for Diarrhoeal Disease research (ICDDR) recommend using rice-based ORS in the treatment of cholera. Rice based-ORS may be available in packets containing pre-cooked rice powder. Alternatively, uncooked rice powder may be added to water, boiled for 5 minutes and allowed to cool before adding salts in the same concentration as in ORS (WHO 2004).

3.2.2 Low osmolarity ORS

For several decades, the most widely recommended formulation of ORS contained 90 mmol of sodium and had a total osmolarity of 311 mOsm/L. However, the amount of salts and glucose has always been a subject of debate, and other formulas have been experimented in the field (Table 3).

	Standard ORS	**Reduced Osmolarity ORS** (mEq or mmol/l)		
Glucose	111	111	75-90	75
Sodium	90	50	60-70	75
Chloride	80	40	60-70	65
Potassium	20	20	20	20
Citrate	10	30	10	10
Osmolarity	311	251	210-260	245

Table 3. Composition of standard and reduced osmolarity ORS solutions

Recently, reduced osmolarity ORS (osmolarity decreased to 245 mOsm/L or lower, reduced amount of sodium) have proved to be superior to high osmolarity ORS in treating acute diarrhoea (Hahn et al, 2001). Based on the greater efficacy of reduced osmolarity ORS solution, especially for children with acute, non-cholera diarrhoea, WHO and UNICEF now recommend that countries use and manufacture reduced osmolarity ORS in place of the previously recommended standard ORS solution (WHO 2004). However, since cholera is associated with significant electrolyte loss especially among children, there are concerns about potential adverse effects (i.e. hyponatraemia) of a reduced osmolarity solution in people with cholera. A Cochrane review set out to answer these questions (Murphy et al., 2004). The review included seven randomised controlled studies (RCTs) on adults and children with acute cholera (confirmed by stool microscopy or stool culture or presumed to be caused by *Vibrio cholerae).*

- Five trials (n=616) reported on need for unscheduled intravenous infusion and showed no difference between glucose-based reduced osmolarity and standard ORS (RR 0.86,95% confidence interval 0.66 to 1.12).
- Four trials (n=465) showed biochemical hyponatraemia was more common with glucose-based reduced osmolarity ORS (RR 1.67, 95% CI 1.09 to 2.57), but showed no difference in severe biochemical hyponatraemia between the groups (RR 1.58, 95% CI 0.62 to 4.04). No trials reported symptomatic hyponatraemia.

In conclusion, in a reasonably large sample of patients with cholera outcomes were similar if treated with reduced osmolarity ORS or standard ORS, apart from asymptomatic hyponatraemia, which was more common with reduced osmolarity ORS. The conclusion of the Cochrane authors is that while it may be easier to administer a single ORS formulation worldwide, the potential harms of, and limited evidence on improved efficacy, of reduced osmolarity ORS for patients with cholera should be kept in mind. No further studies have been published to date, and so far the conclusion of the Cochrane authors seems reasonable (Murphy et al., 2004).

4. Antimicrobial therapy

Several trials have proved the benefits of antibiotics in treating cholera. Antibiotics reduce the total volume of stool passed, reduce diarrhoea duration, and shorten the period of faecal excretion of *V. cholerae*, thereby reducing cholera transmission. WHO, ICCDR, CDC and several other agencies recommend that all cases of suspected cholera with severe dehydration should receive an oral antimicrobial known to be effective against strains of *Vibrio cholerae* in the area. WHO guidelines for antibiotic treatment of cholera are reported in Table 4.

Antibiotic(s) of choice	Alternative(s)
Doxycycline Adults: 300 mg once *or* **Tetracycline** Children: 12.5 mg/kg Adults: 500 mg 4 times a day x 3 days	**Erythromycin** Children: 12.5 mg/kg Adults: 250 mg 4 times a day x 3 days

All doses shown are for oral administration. If drugs are not available in liquid form for use in young children, it may be necessary to use tablets and estimate the doses reported in this table. The first dose should be given as soon as vomiting stops, which is usually 4-6 hours after starting rehydration therapy.

Table 4. WHO guideline of antimicrobial treatment of cholera

Tetracycline-resistant strains of *V. cholerae* O1 have appeared in many countries. Alternative antimicrobials for treating cholera in children are trimethoprim/sulfamethoxazole (TMP-SMX) (5 mg/kg TMP + 25 mg/kg SMX, b.i.d. [twice a day] for 3 days), furazolidone (1.25 mg/kg, q.i.d. [four times a day] for 3 days), norfloxacin (WGO 2008) and azitromicin (Saha et al., 2006, Nelson et al., 2010). The choice of antimicrobial should depend on the known resistance/sensitivity pattern of *V. cholerae* in the region. The information may be available from local health institutions. Otherwise, especially in the case of an epidemic, laboratory investigations are required. However, it should be noted that severe dehydration leads to death in cholera, and only rehydration will prevent death. Antibiotics, while useful, are not a lifesaving therapeutic measure, particularly for cholera (ICDDR).

It has been shown that 20-30% of patients' household contacts develop symptoms of cholera within 10-20 days (Wei et al., 2009). The prevention of transmission is based on hygienic measures (soap, sanitation, potable water). Chemoprophylaxis for the prevention of transmission is debated but not recommended at the moment (Framer et al., 2011). Some evidence from past epidemics in Tanzania and Ecuador suggest that chemoprophylaxis may lead to increased bacterial resistance, without compensatory gains in survival (Weber et al.,1994).

5. Zinc

Zinc deficiency, as well as other micronutrient deficiencies, is wide-spread in low and middle income countries and is thought to have importation health consequences, especially in children. Zinc influences the activity of over 300 enzymes, controlling different functions such as immunity, growth, and development of the nervous system (IZiNCG 2004). There are several different mechanism of action of zinc on acute diarrhoea (Berni Canani et al., 2010). Zinc has a direct effect on ion channels, acting as a potassium-channel blocker of adenosine 3-5-cyclic monophosphate-mediated chlorine secretion (Hoque et al., 2009, Hoque e tal., 2005). Zinc restores mucosal barrier integrity and enterocyte brush-border enzyme activity, and promotes the production of antibodies and circulating lymphocytes against intestinal pathogens, including cholera (Alberts et al., 2003):

A Cochrane review evaluated the efficacy and safety of zinc supplements in the treatment of diarrhoea in children (Lazzerini et al., 2008).

- In acute diarrhoea, zinc shortened the duration of diarrhoea (MD -9.60 h, 95% CI -18.25 to -0.96 h; 4242 children, 13 trials), with fewer children with diarrhoea by day three (RR 0.77, 95% CI 0.67 to 0.89; 1568 children, three trials), day five (RR 0.74, 95% CI 0.55 to 0.99; 1646 children, four trials), and day seven (RR 0.82, 95% CI 0.72 to 0.94; 5528 children, 10 trials). The benefit of zinc in children over six months was consistent in subgroup analysis.
- In children under six months, no benefit was demonstrated.
- No trial reported serious adverse events, but vomiting was more common in zinc-treated children with acute diarrhoea (RR 1.59, 95% 1.27 to 1.99; 5189 children, 10 trials).

One study evaluated the efficacy of zinc supplements selectively on cholera. The study enrolled only children and found a 12% reduction on the duration of diarrhoea compared to control patients and 11% less stool output (Roy et al., 2008).

Since 2004, zinc supplementation (10-20 mg for 10-14 days) is recommended by WHO, UNICEF and other agencies for all children with diarrhoea,, including cholera (WHO 2004). By continuing zinc supplementation for 10 to 14 days, the zinc lost during diarrhoea is fully replaced and the risk of the child having new episodes of diarrhoea in the following 2 to 3 months is reduced.

6. Racecadotril

Racecadotril is an antisecretory drug that inhibits enkephalinase. Enkephalins are endogenous opiate substances which act as neurotransmitters, especially along the digestive tract. By inhibiting enkephalinase, racecadotril reinforces the physiological activity of endogenous enkephalins, which is to elicit intestinal antisecretory activity without affecting intestinal transit time or motility.

To date, only one study has evaluated racecadotril in the treatment of cholera (Alam et al., 2003). The study is a double blind, randomised, placebo controlled clinical trial involving 110 adult male cholera patients who received either racecadotril or placebo in addition to standard cholera treatment. The major outcome measures (stool output, oral rehydration solution (ORS) intake, requirements for unscheduled intravenous fluid infusion, and duration of diarrhoea) were compared between the groups. The study demonstrated that racecadotril therapy, although safe, does not provide additional benefit in the treatment of severe cholera in adults.

7. Loperamide

No clinical study was retrieved on efficacy and safety of loperamide in cholera. WHO recommends that cholera antidiarrhoeal medicines, such as loperamide, should not be given (WHO 2011).

8. How to manage a cholera epidemic

ICCDR is a research centre with vast experience in cholera epidemics. Reported below are the ICCDR guidelines on how to manage a cholera epidemic (ICDDR 2004).

8.1 The risk associated with a cholera epidemic

Despite the advances made in treatments that can prevent deaths from cholera, a large number of patients still die each year, particularly during epidemics. Unlike any other diarrhoeal disease, the rate and volume of fluid loss in cholera can threaten life within hours of onset. Cholera deaths can only occur either due to lack of treatment or to inadequate treatment and can be easily averted by prompt and effective rehydration therapy. Deaths are always highest at the beginning of epidemics and are usually associated with areas that have communication difficulties. Access to treatment facilities is often the major problem for cholera patients requiring medical care, particularly in rural areas, where epidemics of the disease are common. It was demonstrated that temporary field treatment centres can be effective in averting deaths during cholera epidemics. The overall aim of makeshift treatment centre, therefore, is to provide quick access to treatment and thus to ensure prevention of deaths. The expected effectiveness of a makeshift treatment centre will depend on sound planning and on efficient running of the centre.

8.2 When is a temporary treatment centre needed?

There are no rigid rules to follow in deciding when to set up a makeshift treatment centre and what the ideal location for such a centre would be. However, experience suggests that a temporary treatment centre is usually needed when:

a. a large number of patients with acute watery diarrhoea accompanied with deaths are reported from an area from where transportation to the nearest health facilities is difficult;
b. an epidemic of acute watery diarrhoea involves a large area and is spreading;
c. natural disasters and diarrhoea outbreak occur simultaneously in many areas, such as in post-cyclone epidemics.

8.3 What would be the best location?

The specific objective of operating a makeshift treatment centre is to take the emergency health care services to the doorstep of patients who would otherwise be at risk of death during cholera epidemics. Given the limited resources available, providing door-to-door health care services in such emergencies is difficult. The optimum benefit of a temporary treatment centre can, therefore, be derived if the treatment centre is set up at a location, which is within easy reach of patients from the affected areas. In rural and remote areas, this is sometimes not an easy task.

Although health posts are ideal for the purpose, they may not be easy to access from the affected areas. Therefore, alternatives such as schools or any other available spaces that can facilitate access to the centre should be selected.

8.4 Who should be involved?

The success of a temporary treatment centre depends on the extent to which the treatment facilities are used. Efforts should be made to inform the local population of the physical presence of the treatment centre and its location. Community leaders, village practitioners, and union council members should be involved. The local community leaders and the union council officials are the key persons and should be consulted for providing space for the treatment centre, informing the population and organizing community members to run the treatment centre. The other important persons are the government employed Health Assistants and the village practitioners who are the providers of day-to-day health care at village level. Family members of the patients are to provide nursing care and food for the patient.

8.5 Resources needed for a temporary treatment centre

Once the local health care administrators have decided to set up a treatment centre, the next stage is to make plans for the mobilization of resources. While planning to set up a makeshift treatment centre it is important to keep in mind that the effectiveness of a makeshift treatment centre will depend on establishing the centre quickly and moving the logistics easily. One should plan for requirements that are basic and minimum. Due to difficulty of access, transportation of large quantity of supplies to the temporary treatment centre is difficult. Therefore, arrangements should be made to receive required supplies at regular intervals from the permanent source. The basis for estimating resources will depend on the expected patient-load for the treatment centre and the duration of the epidemic. To do this, one should consider these important points: a) at what stage of the local epidemic the treatment centre is to be set up; b) what the magnitude of the epidemic is, in terms of area and population affected. This can be assessed by analyzing the information available locally. In a cholera endemic area such as Bangladesh, seasonal outbreaks usually last 6-8 weeks. However, in newly- infected areas, in refugee camps or in the case of disaster-induced epidemics the period may be longer. The basic and important resources needed are:

a. personnel,
b. rehydration fluids,
c. antibiotics, and
d. a few other essential items such as butterfly needles, etc.

8.5.1 Personnel, drugs, and supplies needed for a temporary treatment centre

Experience has shown that during diarrhoea epidemics in rural areas, 10-20 persons per 1000 population may complain of diarrhoea and most of them may have cholera infection.

Many patients with less severe diarrhoea tend to remain at home. Usually 10% to 20% of the patients who seek treatment at the health facilities during epidemics may have severe dehydration. Between 150 and 200 patients may seek treatment in a temporary treatment centre that covers up to two unions (approx. pop. 40,000). Nearly half of the diarrhoea cases seeking treatment don't show signs of dehydration. Between 25% and 30% of the cases, however, may show signs of some dehydration and can be, to a large extent, treated with ORS. Approximately, 15% to 20% of the cases may need treatment for severe dehydration. They will be needing initial rehydration therapy with IV fluids. Resource requirements were estimated on the basis of a temporary treatment centre expecting to handle at least 100 diarrhoea patients during an epidemic.

8.6 Assessment of the magnitude and spread of epidemic

Assessment of the magnitude of epidemic, particularly with relation to the number of persons affected and the geographic distribution of the epidemic is important for planning and for operating the temporary treatment centre. A temporary treatment centre will be less useful if patients fail to use it and when the epidemic moves away from the catchment area. It has been seen that many cholera patients remain at home during epidemics because of the difficulty to access the health facilities or due to milder forms of disease, which escape attention. Many of these patients are inadequately treated or not treated at all. Organizing a local surveillance system to identify cholera patients and to monitor the course of the epidemic is, therefore, essential.

Objectives of the epidemic surveillance:

- Identify cholera patients
- Provide quick treatment
- Assess the magnitude of the epidemic
- Assess the adequacy of available stock of essential supplies
- Identify the pathogen involved and its drug sensitivity patterns
- Set up control measures and monitor progress.

Type of information needed:

- Who are affected and where they are
- Which are the organisms causing the epidemic
- What is the drug sensitivity patterns of the organisms

Source of information:

- Local public health establishments
- Permanent treatment facilities
- Local field health staff
- Private health care providers
- Available records of laboratory investigations
- Community leaders

Box 1. Epidemic surveillance of cholera

8.6.1 Identify cholera cases

One common problem with cholera surveillance is the case definition. The clinical manifestations of cholera cases vary widely. Nevertheless, the use of a standard case definition can facilitate detection of suspect cases. The following definition will assist the field workers to identify cases:

- A patient who is above 2 years of age, suffering from acute watery diarrhoea with rice watery stool, with or without vomiting and with signs of dehydration, should be suspected as a case of cholera during a cholera outbreak.

However, it is still difficult to predict an epidemic and to detect it early in its course because epidemics usually start abruptly, and affect many people within days. Furthermore, the inadequacy of laboratory diagnostic facilities and information systems contributes to delaying both detection and response. Useful indicators for suspecting an outbreak of cholera are: 1) incidence of adult death due to watery diarrhoeal illness of short duration, or 2) increase in hospitalization rates due to acute watery diarrhoea with or without vomiting, particularly in individuals over 2 years of age.

8.6.2 Collecting illness information

Information on age, gender, location of the patient, onset of diarrhoea, dehydration status, diagnosis, and treatment administered, should be collected and recorded on a simple form. Information relating to other cases and deaths in the family or in the neighbourhood should also be collected. The mapping of the location of cases is important for the identification of the affected areas and of the source of infection and to monitor the course and spread of the epidemic.

8.6.3 Laboratory identification of organisms causing an outbreak

The identification of *Vibrio cholerae* and their drug sensitivity patterns can only be established by laboratory methods. Laboratory analysis of specimens from suspected cases are, therefore, essential for establishing the cause of an outbreak. However, laboratory tests are expensive. During a suspected cholera epidemic, isolation of *V. cholerae* from a sample of patients' specimens can contribute to establishing the cause of the epidemic. A sample of specimens (Rectal swabs) collected in Carry-Blair medium should be sent to the nearest reference laboratory for culture and to determine antibiotic sensitivity patterns. Furthermore, results of antibiotic sensitivity and resistance patterns from different regions of the country will be useful for the formulation of standard drug protocols. Before collecting rectal swabs one should make sure that the patient did not receive any antibiotics.

8.7 Control and prevention of local spread of an epidemic

8.7.1 Disposal of wastes and disinfecting contaminated material

It is virtually impossible to provide patients with regular hospital beds in a temporary treatment centre. Contamination of cholera patient surroundings is therefore unavoidable.

Bedding, including mats, can be disinfected by thorough drying in the sun. After drying, all soiled and contaminated materials should be washed with detergents. A pit-hole in the ground for draining the water used for washing can minimize chances of further contamination. Bleaching powder should be used to disinfect the pit. The pit can also be used to dispose of cholera stool. The floor of the treatment centre can be disinfected by washing, swabbing or sprinkling with bleaching powder solution. Attendants should be advised to wash their hands and clothes thoroughly with detergents.

8.7.2 Water

Drinking safe water is a basic requirement. Tubewell water for drinking and for domestic use, if available, should be encouraged. Boiling of water makes it safer. Stored water can also be easily contaminated. Use of narrow-necked itchers for water storage greatly reduces the risk of contamination. Use of bleaching powder solution can disinfect contaminated water. The risk of infection can be further reduced by washing hands with soap and water after defecation and before handling or eating food. Ponds receiving drainage from latrines should not be used to wash utensils or for bathing. Washing stool-contaminated clothes and bedding of diarrhoea patients can contaminate the surface water (ponds) used for domestic purpose. Drying these materials in the sun before washing can reduce the risk of contamination. Potentially contaminated water can be disinfected with 6 mL of bleaching powder solution per 10 L of water (33 g of bleaching powder dissolved in one litre of water makes the stock solution). Treated water should be left to sit for at least 30 minutes before use.

8.7.3 Food

Many raw foods, such as fish and vegetables, are contaminated with cholera bacteria. Raw food should not be eaten. All foods should be well-cooked and kept covered. Left-overs should be thoroughly re-heated and stale food should be discarded. Food should be eaten as soon as it is cooked or while still hot.

8.7.4 Washing hands

Washing hands with water and soap after defecation, before preparing, serving and eating food will reduce the chances of getting infected with the cholera bacteria.

8.7.5 Health education

Simple health education messages include: eat freshly cooked food; reheat leftovers and eat while still hot; drink tubewell water or boiled water; wash utensils in clean water and dry them in the sun; wash hands before handling or eating food and after defecation.

9. Conclusions

The effective management of cholera is based on few simple rules and procedures, summarized in Box 2.

1. Assess the severity of dehydration.

2. Replace fluids:
- severe dehydration: IV infusion, replace 10% of the body weight within 3–6 hr.
- moderate or mild dehydration: standard ORS, rice-based ORS if possible.

3. Monitor the patient:
- repeate the evaluation of the severity of dehydration
- monitor stool output (use cholera cot if possible).

4. Maintain hydration:
- replace continuing fluid losses until diarrhoea stops.

5. Give an oral antibiotic to dehydrated patients as soon as vomiting stops.
- based on the local known resistance/sensitivity pattern

6. Provide food as soon as patient is able to eat (within a few hours).

7. Recognize complications such as hyponatriemia.

8. Give to children zinc supplementation
- dose 10-20 mg for 10-14 days

9. In case of cholera epidemic:
- Aggressive case finding and efficient transport.
- Set up treatment centres for remote areas.
- Start epidemic surveillance.
- Strengthen control and prevention measures.

Box 2. Synthesis of recommendations for the management of cholera

10. References

Alam NH, Ashraf H, Khan WA, Karim MM & Fuchs GJ (2003) Efficacy and tolerability of racecadotril in the treatment of cholera in adults: a double blind, randomised, controlled clinical trial. *Gut.* 2003;52:1419-23.

Albert MJ, Qadri F, Wahed MA, Ahmed T, Rahman AS, Ahmed F, Bhuiyan NA, Zaman K, Baqui AH, Clemens JD & Black RE . (2003). Supplementation with zinc, but not vitamin A, improves seroconversion to vibriocidal antibody in children given an oral cholera vaccine. *J Infect Dis.* 2003 Mar 15;187:909-13.

American Academy of Pediatrics, Provisional Committee on Quality Improvement, Subcommittee on Acute Gastroenteritis. (1996). Practice parameter: the management of acute gastroenteritis in young children. *Pediatrics.* 1996 ;97:424-35.

Bhattacharya SK. History of development of oral rehydration therapy. Indian J Public Health. 1994;38:39-43.

Berni Canani R, Buccigrossi V& Passariello A. (2011). Mechanisms of action of zinc in acute diarrhea. *Current Opinion Gastroenterology* 2011;1: 8–12.

Farmer P, Almazor CP, Bahnsen ET, Barry D, Bazile J. (2011) . Meeting 's Challenge to Haiti and the World: A Joint Statement on Cholera Prevention and Care. *PLoS Negl Trop Dis* 2011; 5(5): e1145.

Fontaine O, Gore SM & Pierce NF.1998). Rice-based oral rehydration solution for treating diarrhoea. *Cochrane Database of Systematic Reviews* 1998, Issue 4. [DOI: 10.1002/ 14651858.CD001264.pub2]

Gregorio GV, Gonzales MLM, Dans LF & Martinez EG. (2009). Polymer-based oral rehydration solution for treating acute watery diarrhoea. *Cochrane Database of Systematic Reviews* 2009, Issue 2. Art. No.: CD006519. DOI: 10.1002/14651858.

Hahn S, Kim Y, Garner P. Reduced osmolarity oral rehydration solution for treating dehydration caused by acute diarrhoea in children. *Cochrane Database of Systematic Reviews* 2002, Issue 1.

Hartling L, Bellemare S, Wiebe N, Russell KF, Klassen TP & Craig WR. (2006) . Oral versus intravenous rehydration for treating dehydration due to gastroenteritis in children. *Cochrane Database of Systematic Reviews* 2006, Issue 3. Art. No.: CD004390. DOI:10.1002/14651858.

Hoque KM, Rajendran VM & Binder HJ. (2005). Zinc inhibits cAMPstimulated Cl secretion via basolateral K-channel blockade in rat ileum. *American Journal of Physiology, Gastrointestinal and Liver Physiology* 2005;288:956–63.

Hoque KM, Sarker R, Guggino SE & Tse CM. (2009). A New Insight intoPathophysiological Mechanisms of Zinc in Diarrhea. *Annals of the New York Academy of Sciences* 2009;1165:279-84.

International Zinc Nutrition Consultative Group (IZiNCG), Hotz C, Brown KH, editors. (2004). Assessment of the risk of zinc deficiency in population and options for its control [Technical Document]. *Food and Nutrition Bulletin* 2004;25 (1 Suppl 2):94–204.

Lazzerini M, Ronfani L (2008). Oral zinc for treating diarrhoea in children. *Cochrane Database Syst Rev.* 2008;3:CD005436.

Murphy CK, Hahn S &Volmink J.(2004).Reduced osmolarity oral rehydration solution for treating cholera. *Cochrane Database of Systematic Reviews* 2004, Issue 4. Art. No.: CD003754. DOI: 10.1002/14651858.

Nelson E, Nelson D, Salam M & Sack D. (2010). Antibiotics for both moderate and severe cholera. *N Engl J Med* 2010;364: 5–7.

National Institute for Health and Clinical Excellence (NICE). Diarrhoea and vomiting caused by gastroenteritis: diagnosis, assessment and management in children younger than 5 years. (Clinical guideline 84.) London: NICE, 2009.

Roy SK, Hossain MJ, Khatun W, Chakraborty B, Chowdhury S, Begum A,Mah-e-Muneer S, Shafique S, Khanam M & Chowdhury R. (2008). Zinc supplementation in children with cholera in Bangladesh: randomised controlled trial. *BMJ.* 2008 2;336:266-8.

Saha D, Karim MM, Khan WA, Ahmed S & Salam MA. (2006). Single-dose azithromycin for the treatment of cholera in adults.*N Engl J Med* 2006;354: 2452–2462.

Sack DA, Sack RB, Nair GB, Siddique AK. Cholera. *Lancet.* 2004 Jan 17;363:223-33.

Siddique AK, Asib Nasim SM. (2001). Guidelines for operating makeshift treatment centres in cholera epidemics, international centre for diarrhoeal disease research (ICDDR). Mohakhali, Dhaka-1212, Bangladesh, 2001.

Weber JT, Mintz ED, Canizares R, Semiglia A & Gomez I. (1994). Epidemic cholera in Ecuador: multidrug-resistance and transmission by water and seafood. *Epidemiol Infect* 1994;112: 1–11.

Weil AA, Khan AI, Chowdhury F, Larocque RC & Faruque AS. (2009). Clinical outcomes in household contacts of patients with cholera in Bangladesh. *Clin Infect Dis* 2009;49: 1473–1479.

WHO. The Treatment of diarrhoea: a manual for physicians and other senior health workers. - 4th rev. Geneva, 2004.

WHO. Cholera. Basic Facts availabl e at http://www.searo.who.int/EN/Section10/Section391.htm

World Gastroenterology Organisation. (2008). WGO practice guideline: acute diarrhea. Munich, Germany: World Gastroenterology Organisation; 2008 Mar. 28 p.